MW00999876

Covenant of Care

Covenant of Care

NEWARK BETH ISRAEL AND
THE JEWISH HOSPITAL
IN AMERICA

ALAN M. KRAUT
DEBORAH A. KRAUT

Rutgers University Press
New Brunswick, New Jersey, and London

Library of Congress Cataloging-in-Publication Data

Kraut, Alan M.
  Covenant of care: Newark Beth Israel and the Jewish hospital in America / Alan M.
  Kraut and Deborah A. Kraut.
    p. ; cm.
  Includes bibliographical references and index.
    ISBN-13: 978-0-8135-3910-2 (hardcover: alk. paper)
    ISBN-10: 0-8135-3910-2 (hardcover: alk. paper)
  1. Newark Beth Israel Medical Center—History. 2. Jewish hospitals—New Jersey—
History. I. Kraut, Deborah A. II. Title.
  [DNLM: 1. Newark Beth Israel Medical Center. 2. Hospitals, Religious—history—
New Jersey. 3. History, 19th Century—New Jersey. 4. History, 20th Century—New
Jersey. 5. Hospitals, Voluntary—history—New Jersey. 6. Judaism—New Jersey.
  WX 28 AN4 N532K 2006]
  RA982.N492N495 2006
  362.110974932—dc22

                                                                      2006005655

A British Cataloging-in-Publication record for this book is available from the British
Library.

Manufactured in the United States of America

To all those who gave their hearts to the Beth

CONTENTS

Covenant of Care

Introduction

*T*he history of Newark Beth Israel Hospital and Medical Center chronicles the transformation of a twenty-eight-bed converted house in the midst of a teeming immigrant neighborhood to a modern regional medical center serving the city of Newark and the state of New Jersey. This history offers a prism though which to comprehend the broader experiences of voluntary hospitals created under Jewish auspices.

Early in the twentieth century, hospital administrators of a progressive bent argued that the modern hospital had the potential to be an engine of social change, as well as a place to heal and care for the sick. The 1913 inaugural issue of the journal *Modern Hospital* proclaimed in its editorial that each "hospital of the future" was to be a "social service," a "new human melting pot, wherein the weak and the poor and the unfortunate are blended in the warm fires of a common brotherhood with the rich, the strong, and the self-reliant; and the process must bring forth a new humanity, a new moral code, a new religion." The editorial resonated with the values that gave rise to Jewish hospitals, especially the core values expressed in the Hebrew word *tzedakah*. Although often taken to mean "charity," *tzedakah* quite literally means "justice," and to bring justice to those in need is part of the even larger mission that Jews undertake, *tikkun olam*, "repairing the world." How similar that notion of justice was to *Modern Hospital's* vision that the "social service of today is no charity, but a meager and halting attempt to mete out a common justice, to right the wrongs which are the accumulated transgressions of all the ages." Inherently modern in their mission, then, Jewish hospitals still needed to transform themselves into modern medical institutions of distinction. The history of Newark Beth Israel Hospital epitomizes that struggle as it unfolded across the twentieth century.[1]

This volume offers the history of Newark Beth Israel Hospital ("the Beth") as a prism through which to comprehend the broader experiences of voluntary hospitals created under Jewish auspices as they navigated the variable currents of U.S. medical culture. It traces the Beth's odyssey from immigrant institution to modern hospital, as its physicians, surgeons, nurses, and lay board members sought how best to offer culturally sensitive cure and care to their patients and community while ensuring their institution's survival. While the experience of Newark Beth Israel and other Jewish hospitals is not unique among that of voluntary hospitals generally, its example illuminates the significant contribution such institutions have made to health care in this country. The fate of such institutions may also offer a cautionary note to those who regard our modern health care system as the ultimate achievement rather than merely a new and uncertain course taken by the U.S. medical mainstream.

A Brief History of the Jewish Hospital

Jewish hospitals in the United States exist at the intersection of immigration history, Jewish history, and the history of the voluntary hospital, a critical chapter in the larger history of U.S. medicine but one little studied by scholars.

Jewish hospitals have a venerable history arising from the twin traditions of community self-help and resistance to anti-Semitism. Evidence suggests that as early as the eleventh century, synagogues in cities such as Cologne had one room, a *hekdesh*, reserved for the care of sick itinerants. By the eighteenth century, little had changed in most communities other than to relocate the *hekdesh* outside the town, often near a cemetery. Rarely were there more than two rooms, with a few beds in each room. If most who came could not be cured, at least they could die with dignity in the care of coreligionists. More elaborate facilities, *Krankenhausen*, or "houses for the sick," were erected in larger Western European cities. A 250-bed hospital opened in Breslau in 1726; two decades later, London's Sephardic community opened another; and by the end of the century, Berlin and Vienna opened still others. Elsewhere, Jewish facilities were not built until the nineteenth century. The first Jewish hospital in Paris opened its doors in 1836, followed by Amsterdam in 1840, and Hamburg in 1841. In Jerusalem, the Mayer de Rothschild Hospital was established in the Old City in 1854. Jewish hospitals appeared in Eastern Europe, as well. By the first third of the twentieth century, forty-eight hospitals in Poland identified themselves as Jewish, including a one-thousand-bed facility in Warsaw.[2]

Until the early twentieth century, hospitals were not places where the application of scientific medicine by highly trained physicians and surgeons restored most patients to health. Instead, they were charitable institutions where those who had no families to care for them at home went to receive the care of strangers. The almshouse, largely regarded as a warehouse for society's poor and dependent, had taken on some of the duties of a hospital by the late eighteenth century in many U.S. communities. But the increasing number of indigent sick in cities, especially seaports, resulted in a growing number of institutions devoted exclusively to their care, while orphans, poor, and the mentally ill were shuttled into other institutions specific to their needs.[3] Still, in an era when physicians commanded a limited arsenal of therapeutics and surgical options, hospitals offered custodial care more often than cure. The religious groups and community interests who administered hospitals carefully distinguished between insiders and outsiders, those welcome in such institutions and those unwelcome.[4]

In mid-nineteenth-century America, Roman Catholics and Jews (then called Hebrews) were often regarded as outsiders, their souls valued far more than their bodies. As immigration brought an increasing number of Roman Catholics and Jews among the 4.5 million newcomers who arrived between 1840 and 1860, clergy from some religious traditions saw the vulnerabilities of sickness and death as opportunities to effect religious conversions. Hospitals became fields of religious combat, as evangelically inclined Protestant clergy sought converts among sick and dying Roman Catholics and Jews.[5] Apart from the fear of deathbed conversion, for the religiously observant Jewish patient, kosher food, the regular ministrations of a rabbi, and access to religious services required care in an institution under Jewish auspices.

In the United States, early Jewish communities cared for their own from death to life. The first community effort of Jewish settlers in a city was to form a burial society to purchase land for a Jewish cemetery. There, Jews could be buried with others of their faith. Hebrew Benevolent Societies composed of merchants and businessmen soon undertook additional responsibilities, including the founding of orphanages and provision of institutions for invalids, as in Newark, whose Hebrew Benevolent Society established an orphanage in 1861. The first U.S. Jewish hospitals emerged in response to urban epidemics of cholera or yellow fever in the mid–nineteenth century.[6] The 1849 cholera epidemic in Cincinnati, a commercial city populated by German Jewish merchants and craftspeople, spurred the founding of Jewish Hospital a year later. Jewish Hospital was intended by its founders to serve the approximately four thousand Jews who lived in the city, as well as impoverished and homeless peddlers who moved from place to place throughout the Midwest and clung to their Jewish identities.[7] New York City, ravaged by waves of cholera, in 1852 chartered the Jews' Hospital (renamed Mount Sinai during the Civil War). After three years of fund-raising, much of it personally guided by businessman Samson Simson, the hospital opened its doors in 1855 "for the purpose of affording surgical and medical aid, comfort and protection in sickness to deserving and needy Israelites for all purposes appertaining to hospitals and dispensaries, a benevolent, charitable, and scientific hospital."[8]

In 1868, another businessman, Judah Touro, in yellow fever–infested New Orleans, spearheaded the founding of a Jewish hospital that took his name. After an epidemic of typhoid fever, the German Jews who had come to San Francisco as peddlers and shopkeepers during the Gold Rush founded the Mount Zion Hospital Association. In Chicago, the rebuilding of the city after the great fire of 1871 included the construction of Michael Reese Hospital, named for the Bavarian-born businessman whose family inherited the fortune he had amassed in San Francisco. Reese's family donated his legacy to build a Jewish hospital in Chicago and his relatives sustained the legacy by continuing to support its expansion.

In the late 1890s a second surge of Jewish hospitals responded to a new wave of immigrants from Eastern Europe. During the years 1880 to 1921, more than 2.25 million Jews arrived. These newcomers, most of whom were poor, needed a charitable institution where their identities and religious beliefs would be respected and allowed expression. The presence of so many Jewish immigrants, including large numbers of poor and Orthodox Jews from Eastern Europe, sparked a new wave of anti-Semitism. Their philanthropic coreligionists sought to spare the newcomers the deprecating gaze of non-Jewish physicians such as Richard C. Cabot, a distinguished Boston physician, who admitted in his memoir:

> As I sit in my chair behind the desk, Abraham Cohen, of Salem Street, approaches, and sits down to tell me the tale of his sufferings; the chances are ten to one that I shall look out of my eyes and see, *not* Abraham Cohen, but a *Jew*; not the sharp clear outlines of this unique sufferer, but the vague misty composite photograph of all the hundreds of Jews who in the past ten years have shuffled up to me with bent back and deprecating eyes, and taken their seats upon this stool to tell their story. I see a Jew,—a nervous, complaining,

whimpering Jew,—with his beard upon his chest and the inevitable dirty black frockcoat flapping about his knees. I do not see *this* man at all. I merge him in the hazy background of the average Jew.[9]

As if such disparaging looks were not enough, non-Jewish physicians' cultural insensitivity could shape their diagnoses. Physicians who were not conversant in Yiddish or informed as to the customs and problems of Eastern European Jewish immigrants sometimes diagnosed neurasthenic symptoms presented by these patients as a uniquely Jewish ailment that they dubbed "Hebraic Debility."[10] Those so diagnosed were said to be highly nervous and having difficulty adjusting to life in the United States. Jewish physicians had the necessary cultural sensitivity to avoid such diagnoses, but anti-Semitic barriers kept them off the staffs of many U.S. hospitals. The need to train Jewish physicians and give them access to hospital privileges, then, was yet another strong argument in favor of establishing Jewish hospitals.

New discoveries and new technologies transformed the hospital's role. In the Progressive era at the dawn of the twentieth century, Americans increasingly saw the hospital as an institution that epitomized modernity. There, physicians and surgeons grounded in an understanding of germ theory and infectious disease marshaled human and technological resources to cure the ill and heal the injured. The number of Jewish hospitals increased fivefold in this period.

In New York, the borough of Manhattan's Mount Sinai was joined by hospitals named Beth Israel, Beth David, Sydenham, Jewish Memorial (formerly Philanthropin), and further north, in the Bronx, by Lebanon, Montefiore, and the Bronx Hospital and Dispensary. Brooklyn sprouted its own Jewish Hospital, as well as United Israel Zion, Beth Moses (formerly Bokur Cholim), and Beth-El (formerly Menorah Hospital). Each borough also established a Jewish maternity hospital.

Hospitals named Sinai were founded in Los Angeles, Hartford, Chicago, Cleveland, Philadelphia, and Milwaukee. The name "Jewish Hospital" was used in Louisville and St. Louis (a second Jewish Memorial Hospital in Kansas City was renamed Menorah Hospital). There was a Boston and a Newark Beth Israel. Other hospitals took names of renowned Jews, such as Sir Moses Montefiore in Pittsburgh and Isaac Wise in Omaha. San Francisco established the only Mount Zion hospital, and Providence, Rhode Island, the only hospital named Miriam.

The hospitals founded during the great influx of immigrants shared their formative years with the drive for the formation of the American

Hospital Association; the reformation of the American medical schools in response to the Carnegie Report; the standardization of the education and training of U.S. medical school students promulgated by the American Medical Association Council on Medical Education, requiring them to serve internships in hospitals; and establishment of a hospital accreditation system by the American College of Surgeons (ACS). Many hospitals and dispensaries had short existences, unable to achieve ACS accreditation or to sustain their community's support. Thus, there were many other hospitals whose names briefly appeared in the *American Jewish Yearbook*, such as the Mount Sinai hospitals in Delaware and Virginia. The Jewish maternity hospitals located in New York and in other cities, such as Newark and Philadelphia, were amalgamated into general Jewish hospitals at the onset of the Depression. (See Appendix, Table 1.)

By 1940, on the cusp of World War II, there were only thirty-six Jewish general hospitals that were accredited by the ACS, providing a full range of services and training interns. Other Jewish hospitals specializing in the treatment of tuberculosis, arthritis, and chronic joint diseases, still flourished, raising the total number of general and specialized hospitals to approximately fifty.

In the post–World War II period, there was a third surge of Jewish hospitals as a product of the suburbanization of Jewish communities and the ability to utilize matching grant support from the Hospital Survey and Construction Act of 1946. These new hospitals included the Denver Maurice Rose Medical Center, the New York Long Island Jewish Hospital, the Miami and the Minneapolis Mount Sinai hospitals, and Chicago's Weiss Hospital. A few other hospitals were able to relocate to new suburbs during this period, exemplified by Sinai Hospital in Baltimore. The Jewish hospitals that were unable to relocate remained in their aging industrial cities, caring for new waves of migrants. Late twentieth-century government regulations and cost-containment programs forced mergers or buyouts of Jewish hospitals into large health-care conglomerates. They were absorbed into other networks or became their own health care networks, such as Barnes Jewish Health Care, Jewish Hospital Health Care, and the Sinai–New York University system. (See Appendix, Table 2.)

Newark's Jewish Community

The history of Newark Beth Israel Hospital is inseparable from the history of the Newark Jewish community. There had long been Jews in

New Jersey, but until the nineteenth century too few to need a hospital. Not long after the first Jews entered the Dutch colony of New Amsterdam in 1654, a group of English Puritans from the Connecticut towns of Branford, Guilford, Milford, and New Haven, under the leadership of Robert Treat, settled on the opposite side of the Hudson in 1666. The town that would become Newark got its name from Newark-on-Trent in England.[11] How many of Newark's colonial residents were Jewish is unclear, but there were some, although most Sephardim in the mid-Atlantic colonies resided in either New York or Philadelphia, where there were substantial Sephardic Jewish communities. Sephardic names, including Hendricks, Gomez, and Nathan, appear in the records of post-Revolutionary New Jersey communities such as Belleville, where Harmon Hendricks founded a copper mill in 1813.[12]

By the first third of the nineteenth century, Ashkenazic Jews were arriving in New Jersey as part of the larger German migration to the United States. Many were tradespeople, including tanner Louis Trier, whose son Abraham, born in 1845, was the first Jewish child to receive a Newark birth certificate; by 1855, the Jewish community of Newark consisted of two hundred individuals. In 1848, there was sufficient piety in the small community to support the founding of the city's first Jewish congregation, B'nai Jeshrun. Polish Jews founded a small synagogue that would evolve into B'nai Abraham, one of the city's most important congregations. And in 1860 an intracongregational dispute at B'nai Jeshrun resulted in the formation of a third major congregation, Oheb Shalom. Originally all three followed the Orthodox ritual, but B'nai Jeshrun eventually became Reform, the other two Conservative.[13]

Some of the Jewish women in the community took the lead in offering assistance to Jews too poor and too sick to help themselves. In 1852, they formed the Frauenverein Naechstenliebe (Friendly Sisters).[14] Accounts of their meetings suggest a fierce independence that did not appreciate or silently suffer the advice or interference of husbands in the women's organizational affairs. After one clash of men and women at a meeting, "breathing defiance to the trembling males, the outraged women decided that never, never, never thereafter shall men be invited to meetings of the organization."[15]

The charitable needs of the Newark Jewish community multiplied with the great Eastern European migration, which lasted from the 1880s until it was curbed by restrictive legislation in the 1920s. Of the approximately 2.25 million Jews who emigrated to the United States between 1880 and 1924, some 45,000 settled in Newark. Jobs for skilled, semi-skilled, and unskilled labor in Newark's burgeoning industrial economy were the magnet. More than two thousand factories and a plethora of trolleys and trains not only made Newark a bustling and productive city but also required workers and maintenance. And, as in all Jewish communities, there were ample opportunities for entrepreneurship founded on the ritual needs and cultural preferences of Eastern European Jews, who tended to be more Orthodox than their German Jewish coreligionists, many of whom had embraced Reform Judaism. Along streets such as Prince Street, which ran through the heart of the Eastern European Jewish enclave just a few blocks from the Passaic River, pushcarts and small stores abounded. Here observant Jews could find everything from kosher beef to Sabbath candlesticks. Here, too, were the secular necessities of life—milk, bread, fruits, and vegetables, as well as garments, some hung outside shops to lure customers in. One observer of Prince Street in its heyday dubbed it "Baghdad on the Passaic" because of its aggressive salespeople, willing to bargain over everything they sold.[16]

For some, memories of those days evince sweet nostalgia. One Newarker whose family lived behind their shoe store at the corner of Ferry and Congress Streets recalled that most of the neighbors, Jewish and non-Jewish, earned a living from hard work: the Italians swung their pickaxes or repaired shoes; the Germans sweated in their breweries; the Poles worked in foundries; the Irish built the factories and bridges or worked for the city, and the Jews owned the establishments that formed his personal geography, "the Rivoli Theater, that dim beatific manufactory of dreams. Reuben's Sweet Shoppe next door where we sipped our sodas. . . . Further up, the Ironbound Theater, where the Westerns galloped across the screen. Weintraub's Women's Wear, Jaffe's Grocery Store, Shulman's Hardware."[17]

But for the poor, especially the immigrant poor, the very neighborhoods they would recall so fondly festered with danger. The factories' whirring machines could mangle or sever human limbs. Trolley cars could crush the body of a child who dashed into the street after a ball. In the dark, dank, crowded tenements lurked pathogens that attacked bodies weakened by poverty. There was a critical need for care for the sick and comfort for their families. There was a need for a Jewish hospital.

Throughout the remainder of the twentieth century the history of Newark Beth Israel Hospital was intimately intertwined with the history of the city in which it was located and the Jewish community that founded it. A bustling industrial city, its factories and shops fueled with foreign-born labor, Newark experienced waves of infectious disease, often in epidemic bursts such as the polio epidemic of 1916 and the influenza pandemic of 1918, creating the demand for clean water, adequate sanitation, safe housing, and the other public health measures to remedy urban ills. It survived economic crises such as the Great Depression of the 1930s and postwar recessions. The exodus to suburbia experienced by many American cities recast Newark's population as well. As the immigrants and their children moved to the city's periphery, their places were taken by African American migrants from the South seeking economic opportunity and in flight from Jim Crow. By the 1960s, patterns of poverty and prejudice exploded in racial tensions. Controversy over the land and location of the University Medical and Dental School of New Jersey exploded in citywide protests by African American residents who were at risk of being displaced by the school. Riots left Newark synonymous in the media and minds of many Americans with urban blight. As many hospitals and other health-care institutions exited the city or succumbed to the economic pressures of late twentieth-century medicine, others were born or recast. Newark Beth Israel Hospital completed a multiphase construction program already under way that kept state-of-the-art medical care in a Newark community where it was needed. If the Jewish community dwindled, its premier medical institution in Newark assumed a fresh luster.

By the last decade of the twentieth century, the Beth felt the same economic pressures as other voluntary nonprofit hospitals. The high cost of medical technology, the tangle of government regulations, and the competition with large, strong medical conglomerates made further institutional growth problematic. In 1996, Newark Beth Israel Medical Center was sold to the Saint Barnabas Healthcare System.

A condition of sale was that the original name and Star of David remain on the premises and visible to remind all those who entered of the institution's rich heritage. The Beth's service to the people of Newark was a gift of the city's Jewish community. In its early years and in moments of financial exigency, well-known Jewish philanthropists such as Felix Fuld and department store magnate Louis Bamberger sustained the hospital with their generosity and support, but so did less famous Newark Jews who contributed their dimes and dollars directly and through Jewish charitable organizations. Local Jewish businessmen such as tannery owner Abraham Lichtman, furrier Adolph Hollander, builder Alan Sagner, and engineer Lester Z. Lieberman took valuable time from their affairs to lead the Beth in the board room. Community women such as Augusta Parsonnet and Ruth Schindel served the Beth with their organizational skills. In the wards and operating rooms Jewish physicians, often not welcome at other medical institutions because of anti-Semitism, contributed their careers to forging a top-flight medical staff for the hospital. Drs. Max Danzis, Victor and Eugene Parsonnet, Samuel Diener, Abraham Bernstein, Rita Finkler, and so many others relieved the suffering of Newarkers who came to the Beth whatever their religion or ethnicity.

A gift from the Jewish community that has kept on giving, the Newark Beth Israel Medical Center continues to serve the city of Newark, including those most recently arrived in the United States, even as it did a century ago.

Newark Beth Israel Hospital's history encompasses institutional change that spanned the twentieth century. As did all other voluntary hospitals, the Beth evolved from a charitable institution to a business enterprise that reflected the industrial organization of U.S. medicine and finally to inclusion in a much larger medical services corporation. The Beth's story is also the story of its staff, and patients; as a federal government administrator once observed, "a building does not exist until people use it. It then becomes an entity."[18]

The Arrangement of *Covenant of Care*

Chapter 1 describes the tumultuous founding of the Newark Beth Israel Hospital, which was first called to public attention by the 1900 *Newark Evening News* lead: "There's Trouble in the Betch Israel Hospital Association." The rift between the female-led Daughters of Israel Hospital Association and the male-led Hebrew Dispensary Association was resolved by their merger and the founding of a hospital under Jewish auspices. The first Newark Beth Israel would be a nonsectarian hospital, treating all who entered, although its beds would fill with the city's growing Jewish immigrant community. The opening of the first hospital, a converted nineteenth-century mansion, and the second hospital, built on the same site, were both celebrated by Newark's German and Russian Jewry with "Prince Street" parades.

Chapter 2 describes the formative years of the hospital, bringing to life its memorable founding physicians, set in the context of Newark, an industrial city, and the epidemics the city experienced—smallpox, the 1916 outbreak of polio, and the 1918 influenza pandemic.

Chapter 3 describes the successful campaign to relocate the hospital to the Weequahic community; its efforts to regain ACS accreditation and transform itself into a modern hospital; and the creation of Miss Beth Israel, who garnered the affection of the Jewish community and asked the Newark community, "Is your heart with the hospital?"

Chapters 4 and 5, chronologically parallel, span the era from the 1928 triumph of the Beth as "Modern Hospital of the Month" through the Great Depression to the end of World War II. Chapter 4 describes the hospital's near bankruptcy and recovery, the impact of the Depression on its patients, and the operation of the hospital during wartime. Chapter 5 offers the perspective of the Beth's Jewish physicians and hospital staff during in the same time period, when its research program and its laboratories made tremendous advances. The role of the Jewish hospital is presented in the context of the anti-Semitism experienced by medical students and physicians.

Chapters 6 and 7 are also chronologically parallel, covering the twenty years from the end of World War II through 1969. Chapter 6 describes the transformation of Newark, the Weequahic community, the geographic distribution of the Jewish community, the professional and unskilled hospital workforce, and the way in which patients paid for their hospitalizations. The expanded role of federal funding also transformed Newark and its Jewish hospital, the tumultuous urban violence ultimately exerting a complete transformation of Newark and other cities. Chapter 7 chronicles the continued development of the hospital's research program as reflected in its own medical journal, the impact of the struggle to bring a medical school to Newark, and the work carried on by the departments through the first days of Medicare and through the years when urban violence made the city's name synonymous with urban despair.

Chapter 8 traces the tensions of developing a regional medical center in the era of regional planning and cost containment, while continuing to serve the local community.

Chapter 9 examines the decisions made by the Beth's leadership for the future of the Jewish hospital in the context of the changes affecting all other Jewish hospitals.

An epilogue provides perspective on the century of Jewish hospitals, their assets and their weaknesses, as seen through the eyes of one of the great Jewish hospital administrators, Dr. S. S. Goldwater, and through the contemporary efforts of the Healthcare Foundation of New Jersey, established with the funds from the Beth's sale.

The Contemporary Resonance of the Beth's Story

The history of the Jewish hospital in America is more than another chapter in the U.S. Jewish experience or even in the broader history of the U.S. hospital. It has contemporary resonance, for the United States is again in the midst of a great wave of immigration, largely from Southeast Asia and parts of Africa and Latin America. Once again newcomers need culturally sensitive and economically accessible medical care. While the U.S. social and cultural landscape is generally more open to those from other cultures than was the case at the turn of the twentieth century, issues remain for the hospital staff in the medical, professional, nursing, ancillary, and supportive services of hospitals. As long as the United States remains a nation of nations, there will be a need to look to the past to guide contemporary behavior.

While some newcomers from abroad have resources for medical care, others do not. While some accept the Western allopathic medical tradition, others do not. And while some are quick to adapt to new ways of maintaining their bodies' health, others are not. The story of Jewish medical institutions suggests that today's concerns among medical professionals have antecedents worth consulting.

CHAPTER 1

"Trouble in the Betch Israel Hospital Association"

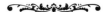

*I*n Newark, New Jersey, as in other U.S. cities of the early twentieth century, the evening newspaper was the key source of metropolitan news. The *Newark Evening News* appeared on Newark's streets late each afternoon, filled with racy headlines that newsboys could shout to passersby. The 1900 *News* was fourteen pages long: the front page for headlines and breaking news, followed by national and international news and separate pages devoted to obituaries, business, department-store advertisements, comics, and sports. Page 3 was the first of several devoted to reports of important events that had occurred the previous night.

In 1900, the *News* was distributing its papers on the streets of a thriving industrial mecca that had enjoyed nearly fifty years of growth of breweries and tanneries, powered by the rushing water of its Passaic River. Its industries were spreading west of the shoreline with thousands of thread manufacturers, varnish factories, jewelry makers, and silverware producers for companies such as Tiffany.[1] And Newark was a city of inventors, epitomized by resident inventor Thomas Edison. The *News* ran a weekly column that listed the patents registered by local citizens, from improvements in smelting to the invention of celluloid.

Rail lines connected Newark to other U.S. industrial cities. Trains stopped at the city's rail depots before heading farther east, crossing the Passaic, a narrow strip of Jersey land, and the Hudson River to greater New York, a new city created in 1898 by the merger of the boroughs of Brooklyn, Queens, Manhattan, the Bronx, and Richmond.

Every day many thousands of skilled and unskilled workers labored in the factories that stretched along Newark's shoreline and lined its streets.

And daily the press reported the illnesses and accidents that were the byproducts of this industrial life—stories of workers with limbs mangled by machinery, others who fell into vats of toxic chemicals, and still others who were killed going or coming from their jobs by fast-moving streetcars.[2]

As the nineteenth century progressed, the laborers whose skulls and legs were crushed under wheels, whose lungs were seared by smoke, and whose bodies dissolved in bubbling vats were increasingly foreign-born and poor. The press of population by the mid–nineteenth century—many Irish and German arrivals—rendered Newark an unhealthy place to live and raise a family.[3] Then, beginning in the 1880s and extending through the early twentieth century, nearly 23.5 million immigrants entered the country. In 1890, 55,571 documented persons of foreign birth lived in Newark; another 15,782 had joined them by 1901. The proportion of foreign-born in Newark's population, many from southern and eastern Europe fluctuated between 29 and 34 percent. Many of the newcomers lived and earned their living on Prince Street, which ran south from Springfield Avenue to West Kinney Street, and where one found "rows of houses that had been converted to apartment flats with small stores on the ground level, filled with poultry butcher stores, bookstores, delicatessens, and cafes that are scenes of great activity at night, filled with members of an ambitious, energetic class."[4] It was this very ambition that exposed the foreign-born to illness and injury.

In 1900, the victims of industrial and traffic accidents were being admitted to Newark's four charitable hospitals, which Newarkers increasingly regarded as places where they might have a better chance of recovery than if they were transported to their homes. By the time founding a Jewish hospital in Newark was under debate, existing hospitals were expanding. Saint Barnabas Hospital (Episcopal), founded in 1867 by the Sisterhood of Saint Margaret, moved from its original location to the Lamassena mansion on High Street and erected a new wing in July 1900, displacing a grove of oak trees.[5]

In September 1900, the new Saint James Hospital (Catholic), founded by the Sisters of Saint Francis, opened in the down-neck section near the river. Its top floor was devoted to surgery, boasting the most modern operating rooms in Newark. In an era without electrical lighting, large windows and massive skylights were designed to illuminate the room with natural light in which surgeons would labor to save lives and limbs.[6]

Saint Michael's Hospital (Catholic), founded in 1867 by the Franciscan Sisters of the Poor, was located on High Street, and was known for its surgeons' skill in treating victims of industrial and traffic accidents. German

Hospital, founded in 1870 by German immigrants, with its own excellent nursing school, was engaged in a fund-raising campaign featuring concerts to support expansion of its facilities.[7]

As the names of these voluntary charitable hospitals suggest, faith and ethnicity were driving impulses of their founders. The members of Christian congregations would receive nursing care in a culturally sensitive environment that offered spiritual comfort. Here physicians and nursing nuns understood the connection between the needs of mind and of body, and the words of comfort would be in the patients' own languages. By opening its doors to those of other faiths and national origins, each charitable hospital hoped to demonstrate its benevolence and willingness to contribute to its neighbors' well-being. This generosity might also defuse any desire in the community to stigmatize a group as "other" and marginalize its members. Moreover, for some Christian groups, well-treated patients were potential converts.

But for those who were not members of these communities and were not comfortable with the ministrations of nuns, the presence of ministers or priests, and crosses on the walls, there was the City Hospital, Newark's municipal hospital, which admitted African Americans and impoverished Newarkers, including the Hebrew poor. In 1900, a grand jury convened to investigate conditions at City Hospital pronounced them appalling, reporting, for example: "In the bathroom, the bottoms of the porcelain tubs were covered by a thick scum, the accumulation of several weeks." One juror, touring the building, was reported to have traced several words in the scum with a pencil. An inspection by a city councilman revealed that the operating room was inadequately ventilated and the electrical wiring frayed.[8] The medical care was careless and deplorable. According to one press report, a severely burned man and his son brought to City Hospital in a police ambulance left at 4:00 A.M., untreated, to walk home to the ruins of their scorched home.[9]

The Daughters of Israel

For Newarkers, the report of the founding of the Newark Beth Israel Hospital began on page 3 of the October 22, 1900, *News* with the headline, "At Odds over a Hospital" and a memorable first line hawked by newsboys: "There is trouble in the Betch [sic] Israel Hospital Association."

A subhead promised colorful characters and continuing controversy: "Hebrew Women Cannot Agree with the Men and Desert the Betch Israel Hospital Association." The colorful characters were Eastern European Jews who had been arriving in the United States through Ellis Island in increasing numbers, many taking the short ferry ride to the Passaic River landing and settling into the crowded tenement area just west of old High Street, known as "the Hill." A new hospital stirred interest. Jewish or not, turn-of-the-century Newarkers needed more health-care services than its city's existing hospitals, dispensaries, and physicians could provide.

The twin impulses of philanthropy and self-help that are intrinsic to Jewish consciousness had already inspired Jewish Newarkers to create a Hebrew Ladies Immediate Relief Society, a Hebrew Burial Society, a Hebrew Benevolent Society, a Hebrew Sewing Circle, and a Hebrew Orphan Association.[10] In 1899, at the opening of the new Orphan Asylum building, Mayor James Seymour had noted that "this institution is one of the numberless proofs that the Jews as a race look out for themselves."[11] In early 1900, two new associations had formed to address the increasing numbers of injuries and illnesses of the Hebrew immigrants: the Hebrew Hospital and Dispensary Association and the Beth Israel Hospital Association.

The two associations agreed to create a unified strategy to meet the needs of the immigrants, but their merger plans were not successful. They could not agree on whether to treat immigrants in an ambulatory setting, through a dispensary, or in an inpatient facility, that is, a new hospital.

Two meetings were held on Sunday afternoon, October 21, 1900, one in the home of Max Harris and the other in the home of Mrs. Reuben Barnhard. Newarkers learned from the *News* that within the Jewish community, "the women have become divided against the men because they want a Hebrew hospital immediately, whereby the men declare themselves for a dispensary or temporary quarters for the treatment of patients—arguing that the funds in hand and those of possible availability are not adequate to build a hospital."[12]

The *News* favored the women's position—a new hospital would more fully meet the increasing demand for treatment of injuries and illnesses suffered by the immigrants of the Hill than would a storefront dispensary. But there were issues involved in the establishment of a charitable hospital that were unique to the Jewish population. Unlike hospitals under Christian auspices that derived financial support from the church coffers of a particular institution and the hierarchy of an order of nuns, a Jewish hospital would require the support of a patchwork of Reform and Orthodox synagogues founded by congregants who differed markedly in their ethnic origins and religious practices. The financial support for a Jewish hospital would be derived from hospital fees paid by private patients, stipends for the treatment of those Newarkers eligible for the city's workmen's compensation program, contributions by the Jewish lodges, the legacies of individuals, and coins placed in the charity boxes on the countertops of stores on the Hill.

The Daughters of Israel, composed of the women and a few young idealistic Jewish physicians, believed that the campaign for a hospital would unite the congregations and associations, as well as the Jewish labor lodges, in one common cause. Those who attended the meetings felt that "the spirit that pervaded [them] ran high, there was an attitude of intensity and fervor, akin to a religious crusade."[13] The members of the Newark Hebrew Dispensary Association, including many of the more established Jewish physicians, believed that the storefront dispensary would be sufficient to meet community needs, and that the community was not financially ready to support the operation of a hospital.

The second installment of the Jewish hospital saga appeared in the October 26, 1900, *News* under the headline "Hebrew Societies Still at Odds." The two societies, clashing "so emphatically that each determined to work independent of each other," incorporated separately. On October 25, 1900, the Jewish community had two new incorporated organizations: the Daughters of Israel Hospital Association and the Hebrew Dispensary Association.

The Hebrew Dispensary Association pressed forward, purchasing an old building on Prince and Charleton Streets, and in less than two months sent fifteen thousand invitations to physicians, attorneys, and other professionals, as well as city and county officials, to the December 16, 1900, dedication of a new dispensary. A dozen pharmacists were contracted to fill the prescriptions written by dispensary physicians, and plans were made for an on-site pharmacy. Doctors would be available to see patients from 11:00 A.M. to 6:00 P.M. Women sympathetic to the dispensary plan formed a women's auxiliary to assist with fund-raising and in other material ways.[14]

The *News* paid scant attention to the opening of the dispensary. On January 8, 1901, scarcely a month after the dispensary began operation, the Daughters of Israel held an evening meeting at Columbia Hall to announce to eight hundred people that the Jewish women had purchased the old Pennington mansion on the corner of Kinney and High Streets.[15] "Passing of a Famous Old Homestead," a *News* article published November 10, 1899, hinted at the mansion's faded glory: "Everything in it was old and told of a bygone period; the small panes in the windows and the clumsy lock on the door; the marquetry of the mahogany." When William Pennington, New Jersey's Whig governor from 1834 to 1843, built the house in 1840, the view from its windows was "unbroken by black columns of smoke from rows of factories along the Passaic riverbank known as 'Down Neck.' " In the early nineteenth century, New York Harbor shone clear in the distance and groves of oak trees rustled with cooling sea breezes.

Newark's wealthy families had built their mansions on the first rise of land west and above the colonial settlement that became High Street. The Penningtons included William S. Pennington, secretary of the legation at Paris during the Lincoln administration. The Newark family once entertained Napoleon's brother in their parlor, which featured a harpsichord once owned by Martha Washington. After the Civil War, the heirs of Newark's first families moved west to the Oranges and south to the land above Weequahic Lake. Mansions once owned by brewers were converted to meeting spaces such as Krueger Hall and Columbia Hall. In November 1899, William Pennington, son of Edward R. Pennington and grandson of the builder, sold the house, no longer elegant, the November 10 *News* article reported, as "change and decay went on until the homestead was in a state of dilapidated repair."

At the turn of the twentieth century, the Pennington mansion was in the midst of a Jewish immigrant enclave, a neighborhood created by the pattern of urban transition known as ethnic succession. It was sufficiently spacious to be converted into a hospital.[16]

With the support of those at the January meeting, the Daughters of Israel pressed ahead. The price of the Pennington homestead was $14,000, and the women had raised $750 toward a $4,000 down payment. Nettie Katchen, the Daughters of Israel recording secretary, recalled that when she learned of the purchase plan, "from that day on, my interest in the movement became a part of my daily life," as she went door-to-door collecting dimes and quarters.[17]

Their fund-raising activities had mixed success. In February 1901, they held a successful Purim Ball, imitating the annual fund-raising ball of the Newark Hebrew Benevolent and Orphan Asylum Association. The hall was festooned with flags and a "grand march" was played by Gluckman's Orchestra as forty children of members of the Daughters of Israel filed into the hall in time to the music.[18] In April, the Daughters sent letters to all the Hebrew societies and relief associations requesting their financial help and inviting them to attend a meeting at the Anshe Russia Synagogue. Thirty-two organizations each sent two representatives to the synagogue meeting and each demanded a place on the Daughters of Israel board, prompting thirteen of the original board members to resign in protest.[19] And their fund-raising picnic on a Saturday in June was canceled when another member resigned, denouncing the event as inappropriate for a

Jewish hospital whose members would be observing the Sabbath on Saturdays.[20]

United in Peace and Purpose

Quietly, without press coverage, a Peace Committee was formed, and representatives of both associations again began negotiating a merger. Physicians took the lead in creating the new alliance. On July 18, 1901, the medical staff of the Hebrew Hospital and Dispensary Association and the physicians who had joined the Daughters of Israel Hospital Association met in the assembly rooms of the dispensary to "work in harmony for the welfare of the hospital movement."[21]

The physicians from both associations met to establish a single medical staff. Scarcely two weeks later, a tragic event contributed to the urgency with which Jewish Newarkers regarded the hospital debate. On August 5, 1901, the *News* printed a photograph of beautiful eighteen-year-old Esther Newman above her obituary. One of the first female graduates of the New Jersey School of Pharmacy, Newman had been appointed chief pharmacist for the Hebrew Dispensary. In July, she resigned from her position at the Jewish-owned Schwarz pharmacy and began a brief vacation in a boardinghouse near Lyon's Farm, in the rural farmland above Lake Weequahic, two miles south of the Hill neighborhood. But she quickly fell ill and returned to the city. The Hebrew Dispensary physicians rushed her to Saint James Hospital, whose physicians diagnosed her with advanced appendicitis and issued a terminal prognosis. The Jewish physicians persuaded them to perform an emergency surgery. The young woman survived the surgery and briefly rallied but died two days later, with her father and brother at her bedside.

Although the poignant *News* story did not imply that treatment in a Jewish hospital would have saved her life, Newman's death amid strangers kept the issue in the spotlight for Newark's Jewish community. On September 8, 1901, a month after the funeral, the *News* reported under the headline "Hebrew Societies May Now Unite" that the physicians of the Hebrew Dispensary staff had met with the women of Daughters of Israel and negotiated an agreement to abandon their organizations' names and unite under the banner of the Beth Israel Hospital Society.

Conversion of the Pennington home into the Jewish hospital would take nearly a year. In the meantime, the Jewish hospital again became a public issue. In early 1902, Dr. Victor Parsonnet, an earnest young immigrant physician, was quoted in the *News* as stating that the mission of the new Jewish hospital would be to admit and treat individuals who were "sick."[22] The word "sick" spurred indignation and outrage in the city, as Newarkers assumed that the Hebrew physicians were going to build a hospital to treat patients sick with infectious communicable diseases right in their midst.

Their mistaken thinking grew from the two distinct categories of hospitals in 1902: general hospitals for the treatment of accidents and for illnesses thought to be noncommunicable, and special isolation hospitals for those diagnosed with communicable infections—diphtheria, scarlet fever, measles, mumps, and smallpox. A patient diagnosed with a communicable infection was "sick" and was either quarantined at home or transferred to an isolation hospital at a distance from any community, an alternative to legally enforced home quarantine. The year that the Daughters of Israel acquired the Pennington mansion, the Newark Board of Health had appropriated funding for the construction of a special isolation hospital in the northern outskirts of the city, near Belleville.

The isolation hospitals were never far enough away for a community's fearful residents. Newark had experienced a smallpox outbreak in 1901; that same year, an Italian mob in Orange, New Jersey, burned an isolation structure for smallpox victims being built near their community, as the *News* reported on March 10, in an article titled "Pest House Burned." In Newark, property owners along High Street began to raise objections to the opening of the new hospital and turned to the state legislature in Trenton.

On February 10, 1902, Assemblyman J. Henry Bacheller from Essex County introduced in the New Jersey State Assembly Bill Number 102, "An Act to regulate the erection of hospitals for sick and diseased persons." The bill, which was referred to the Committee on Public Health, made it unlawful to build a hospital "within any city, town, township, borough or other municipal corporation of this state, without first obtaining the consent theretofore of the governing body of such city, town, township, borough or other municipal corporation within the territorial limits of which it is proposed to locate or maintain any such structure."[23]

The members of Newark's Jewish community working to create Beth Israel Hospital thought the purpose of Bill 102 was to prevent Jews from having their own hospital. The dispute turned ugly. Angry members of the Beth Israel Hospital Association played upon the racial prejudices of their new neighbors by putting the word out on the street that if the hospital was blocked, they would establish a "combination of tenement for colored people, livery stable and meat market" on the site. Faced with this alternative, the residents urged the bill's promoters to permit the proposal to die "an easy death in a committee-room pigeon hole." Newark city treasurer Albert T. Guenther went to Trenton and dissuaded Bacheller from pursuing the divisive legislation.[24] While it is unclear that the intent of the bill was anti-Semitic, the episode suggests how raw social tensions were in the increasingly multi-ethnic Newark community, readily spilling over into discussions of what was best for the public's health and well-being.

On Sunday, August 31, 1902, the Beth Israel Hospital opened its doors with a celebratory procession through the streets of the Hill in what came to be known as a "Prince Street parade." Six marching bands and more than three thousand men, women, and children followed a zigzag route from Springfield Avenue to Prince Street and South Orange, to Broom, to Spruce, to High Street, and finally to the hospital building.[25] At the corner of High and West Kinney Streets, the paraders watched a member of the Beth Israel Hospital Association present hospital officials with ceremonial keys. The old mansion had been converted to a twenty-eight-bed hospital staffed with eight nurses. The hospital board had issued a nonsectarian policy for patient admissions. No patient would be turned away because of religion, ethnicity, or race. The dream of the tenacious Daughters of Israel had become a reality.[26]

One among the Many

When Newark's Beth Israel Hospital opened its doors in 1902, it joined the many Jewish hospitals founded at the beginning of the twentieth century to accommodate the needs of Eastern European Jews who were arriving in the United States in ever larger numbers. A handful of Jewish hospitals had been established by the wave of German Jewish immigrants in the mid–nineteenth century. During the forty-year period from 1880 to 1920, the number of Jewish hospitals in the United States increased fivefold, concentrated in the cities being transformed by immigrants. Newark's congested immigrant neighborhoods and hazardous industrial environment epitomized the urban elements that created the demand for dispensaries and hospitals. These crowded neighborhoods included the factories and shops where the newcomers labored by day, returning at night to overcrowded housing with inadequate ventilation and sanitation. Diseases and industrial accidents were perennial menaces. While charitable hospitals served these communities, such institutions were often under sectarian auspices and excluded Jews, or offered them environments culturally insensitive to Jewish ritual needs and sensibilities. The opportunity to found a Jewish hospital in such a community was often enhanced by the availability for purchase of a large vacant house or mansion once owned by a family of wealth and reputation.[27] Such structures were frequently abandoned in a process of ethnic succession as the native-born fled to avoid sharing space with newcomers from abroad. Leadership in the founding of Jewish hospitals often emerged from two groups. One group was Jewish physicians who shared with their non-Jewish colleagues a belief that hospitals, not homes, were the best places for increasingly sophisticated therapeutics and surgical solutions to illness and injury, but who were excluded from many such institutions by prevailing patterns of anti-Semitic prejudice. Another group was made up of community-minded Jewish women who individually and in their voluntary societies channeled their attention and energies toward meeting the healthcare needs of coreligionists and non-Jews, as well.

The role of women in the establishment of Jewish hospitals was consistent with the enthusiasm of many for Progressive reform. Beginning in the 1890s and continuing throughout the Progressive era, women in the United States took an ever-increasing role in shaping social welfare policy: two brick-and-mortar establishments that exemplified this trend were Chicago's Hull-House, created by Jane Addams, and New York City's Henry Street Settlement House, founded by Lillian Wald.[28] Some suffragists, such as Carrie Chapman Catt, believed that the way to secure the vote for women was to demonstrate by their work that women were able to make the world better.[29] Often the portal to activism was a religious institution.[30] Mary Lowe Dickinson, the president of the National Council of Women and the general secretary of the Christian benevolent organization the International Order of the King's Daughters and Sons, observed that women could not vote but they could engage in civic and charitable duties, including improving health and sanitation, declaring that "two thirds of the women of the world battle with dirt with their hands upon a broom handle. The knowledge of what ought to be done, which every intelligent woman can acquire, can be wielded much more effectively than can the broom stick."[31]

Middle-class women who had discretionary time and resources often led the way in shouldering the burden of social reform. These women became skilled fund-raisers and organizers and frequently focused their attention on matters of sanitation and public health. One tactic employed was to raise funds to support the appointment of women to positions that demonstrated their qualifications, such as paying the salaries of women to be health inspectors. In 1901, the Board of Health of South Orange, New Jersey, appointed Elizabeth M. Devine to be a health inspector: "Her salary was fixed at the nominal sum of $1 per year; . . . several women's clubs will pay the salary to the inspector."[32] Newspapers reported the work of the women's associations, printing lists of every female participant, and reprinted the speeches and articles of women leaders. In April 1901, as the Newark Daughters of Israel advocated for a Jewish hospital, the *News* printed Dickinson's statements, which included her exhortation for women's groups to engage in religious, educational, and philanthropic endeavors, which included the opening of many faith-based hospitals.[33]

In communities needing a Jewish hospital, Jewish women's associations took advantage of the opportunities for purchase of large houses such as Newark's Pennington mansion. In Pittsburgh, the Hebrew Ladies Hospital Aid Society was able to purchase the old Blackmore estate. The Young Ladies Hebrew Association of Cleveland opened a twenty-nine bed Mount Sinai Hospital in a converted mansion. And in Los Angeles, the Kaspare Cohn Hospital, operating in a nineteenth-century mansion, became the Cedars of Lebanon in 1902.[34] Milwaukee's Sinai Hospital may have been unique among these hospitals as it opened in a converted YMCA building. The converting of a house in the first decade of the twentieth century was accomplished quickly: the women's associations cleaned the large houses and filled the many rooms with beds and chairs, and the physicians purchased the equipment and surgical instruments to perform their work. Linens were made by sewing circles, and food was supplied largely by donations.[35]

In addition to general hospitals, Jewish associations founded institutions for the specialized care of Jewish tuberculosis (TB) patients. An awareness that the disease was sometimes characterized as the "Jewish disease" or the "tailor's disease" triggered the nationwide effort of Jewish organizations to establish sanitaria such as National Jewish Hospital and the Jewish Consumptive Relief Society, both located in Denver.[36] Similarly, in 1914, the national B'nai Brith organization established the Leo N. Levi Hospital in Hot Springs, Arkansas, specifically for the treatment of arthritis.[37] In Newark, the founding of the Essex Mountain Sanatorium for TB in 1907 was achieved by two non-Jewish women, who lobbied the Board of Health and, ultimately, every assemblyman in Trenton, New Jersey.[38]

Jewish physicians often encouraged Jewish women's organizations to found hospitals. The second wave of Jewish hospitals was driven, in part, by the needs of Jewish physicians. In the last decade of the nineteenth century, U.S. hospitals maintained closed medical staffs. Physicians who wished to admit their patients had to pass muster with the hospital's board of governors, the body responsible for administering the institution.[39] In the early twentieth century, paying patients sought the advanced medical and surgical care hospitals offered. Because Jewish physicians were often denied staff privileges at voluntary charitable hospitals operating under religious auspices, they began to open dispensaries, the precursors of outpatient clinics, in order to practice medicine. These dispensaries often expanded to include a small annex with beds; thus, many became clinics for the poor and small proprietary hospitals for one or several physicians. In 1897, a San Francisco physician offered his proprietary hospital and dispensary to the Mount Zion Hospital Association to be used rent free until the association was able to purchase its own structure in 1899, then merged with the nearby Temple Emanu-El Sisterhood Polyclinic in 1905.[40]

Not all leaders in Jewish communities supported establishing a Jewish hospital. In Pittsburgh, Rabbi J. Leonard Levy initially denounced the plan for a Jewish hospital, declaring that there was ample room for Jews in the city's nonsectarian hospitals. However, when Passavant and Mercy Hospitals denied admission to Jewish patients sent to them by the Hebrew Ladies Hospital Aid Society, Rabbi Levy relented. Pittsburgh's German and Russian Jewish communities united to raise $60,000 to open Montefiore Hospital, a sixty-five-bed nonsectarian hospital, in 1908.[41] In Detroit, similar objections, made by physicians, delayed the opening of Sinai Hospital until 1949.[42]

Questions of religious perspective and ritual practice often stalled efforts to open a Jewish hospital. Should the hospital be sectarian, admitting only Jews, or nonsectarian and open to all? Should the hospital offer kosher food? Where should the hospital be located in relation to the Jewish community?

Such was the story in St. Louis. Like those in Cincinnati and New Orleans, St. Louis's Jewish community made the initial decision to build a hospital in 1853. But not until 1891 did the St. Louis Jewish Hospital Association incorporate to "afford medical and surgical aid, comfort and relief to deserving and needy Israelites and to such of other denominations." Even with a lot purchased, nearly nine years passed before the Missouri secretary of state officially endorsed a revised constitution for the hospital, which pledged to "afford medical and surgical aid and nursing to sick or disabled persons of any creed or nationality," while "the religious services of the hospital shall be conducted in conformity with the doctrines and forms of the Jewish religion." The hospital, though nondenominational in its admissions policy, had a decided religious complexion. And still fund-raising floundered, until Elias Michael, a merchant and civic activist, donated $10,000. Finally, in 1902, the Jews of St. Louis opened their hospital, five months before Newark Beth Israel began treating patients.[43]

In Providence, Rhode Island, Miriam Lodge No. 1 raised $1,000 over fifteen years to purchase four adjoining brownstone buildings that were already functioning as a maternity hospital. It would still take nearly four years to convert the buildings to a general hospital.[44]

In Cleveland, the newly established Federation of Jewish Charities took over the funding of Mount Sinai Hospital. However, less than a decade later, religious differences menaced the hospital's existence when members of the Orthodox community refused treatment at the hospital because it lacked a kosher kitchen. Religious Jews demanded a second facility, and the federation had to negotiate an agreement so that Mount Sinai would satisfy everyone.[45]

In Brooklyn, New York, the Jewish Hospital was delayed nearly nine years because businessmen funding the project insisted that the community raise in advance all the funds needed for construction. Each year the community raised more funds, but escalating projected construction costs kept things at a standstill. Finally, in 1909, the hospital was built at twice the original estimated cost.[46]

The First Beth Israel Hospital

In 1902, Saint Michael's Hospital was affectionately called "the great house on the Hill" by Newarkers. The first Newark Beth Israel hospital, in the Pennington house, quickly earned the nickname of "the little house on the Hill." Its bed number decreased from twenty-eight to twenty-five within the first two weeks, when the ground floor was converted to a seven-bed adult-male ward and the upstairs became the domain of a ten-bed adult-female ward. Private rooms were allocated for paying patients. Anecdotes describe Dr. Victor Parsonnet carrying his patients downstairs in his arms after surgery, which suggests that the operating room was also on the top floor.

The Daughters of Israel continued to raise money for the hospital and to link the hospital with the larger social and economic concerns of Newark Jewry. Many of the Daughters served on the new hospital's board of directors, while others formed the Sewing Circle to create and mend the thousands of bandages, garments, and linens needed.[47]

Daily operation of Beth Israel was the responsibility of Caroline Feitzinger, the nursing superintendent. The title was a misnomer: Feitzinger, a trained nurse, served as hospital manager, chief operating-room nurse, and founder and chief instructor of the new nursing school. She began each workday by personally scrubbing the steps from the first to the second floor of the converted home. Feitzinger was a formidable presence.[48]

To guarantee its patients adequate care, Beth Israel needed a nurses' training school. No organization existed within the formal denominations of Judaism equivalent to those in Christian communities, where a charitable faith-based hospital founded by an order of sisters was part of the church organization structure, the intraorganizational structure of the order, and its mission. Thus, the head of an order, whose capabilities and commitment had enabled her to rise as a leader, might also serve as the superintendent of a hospital. The sisters who lived in a building adjacent to the hospital would perform both nursing duties and the daily tasks of their religious order. Because Jewish denominations offered only the numerous sisterhoods and women's associations that functioned in an auxiliary capacity in synagogue congregations, Jewish hospitals needed to create in-house diploma schools that recruited women, Jewish and non-Jewish, to study and to receive on-the-job nurses' training.

In 1904, Beth Israel's medical staff granted Feitzinger authority to issue diplomas to student nurses.[49] Feitzinger developed a three-year curriculum for the Beth Israel Training School of Nursing, similar to other nurse diploma schools of that time, including a series of twenty lectures for students delivered by the medical staff.

The curriculum would remain essentially unchanged for the next quarter century. For the first six months, nursing students, wearing blue uniforms with white aprons, attended daily classes. Upon successful completion of the course work, they would don white uniforms and caps designed specifically for the hospital; the candlelight capping ceremony included reciting the nurses' oath composed by Florence Nightingale. The student nurses then embarked upon another two and one-half years of part-time courses and intensive clinical experience in the hospital, progressing from the simpler tasks of changing bed linen and serving meals to the care of acutely ill patients. Their caps reflected their year of study: plain caps in the first year, caps with a blue stripe in the second, and caps with a black stripe for graduates. During these three years, students and their supervisors were an integral part of the Beth Israel Hospital community, sleeping on the premises and eating all meals there. In May 1906, the entire medical staff attended the first commencement of three graduating nurses.[50]

The First Annual Report of the
Newark Beth Israel Hospital

In 1906, the Newark Beth Israel Hospital Association published its first annual report, a summary of its first four years, with separate reports from its chief of medical staff, president, and nursing superintendent. Superintendent Feitzinger's report declared that "the success of this Hospital has been phenomenal; few institutions of its kind can boast of similar success, within comparatively so short a period of existence." She wrote with great pride that 50 of the 450 operations performed were appendectomies, and not a single fatality had occurred. The hospital medical staff and nurses had engaged in "strict adherence to the proper aseptic and antiseptic measures and observance of correct surgical technique."[51] The hospital surgical staff was among the increasing number in the United States who approached appendicitis as an infection to be treated with surgery as the first, not the last, resort. The Beth Israel surgeons performed appendectomies with sufficient frequency to ensure the skills and experience required for such high rates of success.[52]

The annual report presented inpatient statistics for the hospital census that indicated that in less than four years, each of its twenty-one beds had been filled thirty-four times.[53] From September 6, 1902, to January 1, 1906, 854 patients were treated in the hospital (402 males and 452 females), and "no distinction was made in receiving patients; all classes regardless of nationality or creed obtained the same care and attention in the Hospital, as well as in the Dispensary." The hospital had attended to its mission to provide care to all those in need: 573 admissions, more than 67 percent, were charity patients. The 281 paying patients were charged eight to ten dollars per week, which covered "bed and board," as well as ancillary services such as laboratory tests. A physician with hospital privileges admitted each patient, who was also charged separately for that physician's fees. The dispensary had continued to provide services to the Hill community, treating 13,806 patients during the same period.

The 1906 treasurer's report described the hospital as solvent, with a bank balance of $8,493.15 after expenditures. The Sewing Circle, while churning out linens, had raised $2,500 from the years of whist parties and a grand ball that netted $830.[54] The Beth Israel Hospital Women's Auxiliary, meanwhile, gathered donations of $4,444.89 and supervised the items donated as charitable contributions to the hospital, a routine practice in the nineteenth and early twentieth centuries. What kinds of items might a hospital receive? In the annual report, donations of linen went on for three pages of the list, in small font, followed by pages of items that included boxes of seltzer, bottles of whiskey, containers of fruit syrup, eggs, soup greens, baskets of potatoes and rolls, a fifteen-pound lamb, sewing machines, pillowcases, towels, bedsheets, yards of unbleached muslin for bandages, laundry soap, crutches, rocking chairs, coffeepots, medicine cups, two gas stoves—and hundreds of pounds of matzos for use during the eight days of Passover. There were annual donations from eighty-seven Jewish societies and lodges, whose names proclaimed the origins of their members (e.g., Este Lemberger Frauen, Kiever K.U.V.), their work in Newark (e.g., the United Hebrew Butchers Association, the Baker's Union, Local 167, the Independent Carpenters Verein), or their aspirations as Americans (e.g., Martha Washington Lodge, Success Lodge).[55] The savings to the hospital were considerable; for example, from these donations, volunteers were able to completely stock with cooking utensils the main kitchen and the diet kitchens on every ward.[56]

The presidency of the Newark Beth Israel Board of Directors passed during its first three years from Mrs. Reuben Barnhard to Dr. Armin Fischer, a prominent German Jewish physician, who wrote his annual report in German, confident that those for whom it was intended could read it.[57] By 1904, Dr. Victor Parsonnet directed the hospital, and in 1905, the president of the board was neither a member of the Daughters of Israel nor a physician but a businessman, Louis Lewis, who was succeeded by Joseph Okin, a real estate developer on the Hill.

The order of succession suggests perceived practical realities and a hierarchy of institutional needs: Drs. Fischer and Parsonnet reflected the need to establish a positive medical image for the new hospital, followed by Lewis and Okin, because the medical institution needed the guidance and support of the Jewish business community. Potential donors who might contribute funds during their lifetimes or designate the hospital in their wills would be concerned that their legacies would be managed well.

Transnationalism

Immigration scholars who speak of "transnationalism" refer to the ongoing relationship of migrants to people and events in their home countries, a connection that often endures for several generations.[58] Most of the Jews in

Newark had been in the United States for well under twenty-five years. The sounds and flavors of Eastern Europe could be heard in the Yiddish and Russian spoken in the streets on the Hill and tasted in the steaming breads and rolls sold over the counters of local bakeries.

Strolling near the Pennington house that had become the Newark Beth Israel Hospital, one writer was startled to see cupping glasses in the barbershop windows, instruments of an "ancient medical process . . . now practically obsolete except to a country so far behind the progressive spirit of the age as Russia." He described the flavor of the neighborhood:

> If one who had lived in a Russian city should happen to be dropped into a certain section of Newark called the "hill" he would likely think that he was still in the regions ruled over by the great white czar. The people seem to have brought over with them the salient characteristics of their native land and a goodly portion of the Russian costume. Men who have been here for many years still wear the boots they had on when they arrived in steerage. . . . On Prince Street, the signs over most of the shops are in Hebrew characters and every one does business on the sidewalks from early spring until the cold weather drives them indoors.[59]

Transnational sentiments that caused newcomers to remain intellectually and emotionally involved in the places of their birth, where friends and relatives still struggled to live, were heightened by news of outbursts of violence by Russians against their Jewish neighbors, pogroms, met with government indifference under Czar Alexander III.

The bloody Kishinev massacre of 1903, in which forty-nine people were killed and more than five hundred injured, made front-page news across the United States.[60] The May 20, 1903, *News* published a letter from the janitor of a synagogue in Russia who had witnessed the atrocities and wrote that "Basha, a mother was beaten to death and her daughter thrown out a window. Moses Atlansa was tied up, taken to the top of the Zetomistick Hotel and hurled to the ground. David Tanzus' daughter was found with her body cut to pieces." On April 3, 1904, the *News* reprinted the anti-Jewish proclamation published in a Russian newspaper urging right-minded Russians to kill Jews in retribution for Jews supposedly using the blood of Christian children in the making of Passover matzo. To its credit, the *News* refuted the accusation with an eight-column description of how Newark's Jews celebrated Passover.[61] However, the Jewish community in Russia needed more than sympathy from their brothers and sisters in the Americas.

In Newark and elsewhere, dollars needed by local institutions were diverted into relief funds for communities abroad. In 1905, the renowned New York Jewish philanthropist Jacob Schiff requested that Newark initiate its own campaign for relief efforts. Two recent arrivals stepped forward to lead the effort: Felix Fuld had come to Newark to work for Louis Bamberger, who had opened a department store; Solomon Foster, a reedy, clean-shaven, twenty-eight-year-old, was the new assistant rabbi at Temple B'nai Jeshrun. Fuld organized a massive meeting at the temple and was so successful that by the end of November, his Relief Fund of Sufferers from Russian Outrages had raised pledges of nearly $12,000.[62]

This generous giving, however, drained potential financial support and attention from local Jewish institutions, including Newark Beth Israel Hospital. But, in January 1905, there was a thirteen-week waiting list for admission. When the board met that month to discuss adding a wing onto the Pennington mansion to accommodate fifty additional beds, Parsonnet convinced board members to replace the old structure with a new building that would better accommodate both surgery and patient care.[63] The decision would require the physicians to continue to operate the Charleton Street dispensary for both outpatients and limited inpatient services while the new facility was being built.

When the fund-raising campaign began, Louis M. Frank, the third partner in the Bamberger Department Store, was among the early major contributors.[64] Rabbi Foster joined the campaign, at every opportunity promoting the hospital as an expression of the altruism of Newark Jews: "While Beth Israel makes no distinction of creed, it would enable the Jews to receive treatment in an institution supported primarily by persons of their faith." The goal was to meet this perennial need with a "commodious building modern in its appointments in every respect."[65]

By January 1906, the building budget had tripled to $80,000. Morris Rachlin, who had built many of the houses in the Clinton Hill area, chaired the Building Committee. Nathan Meyers, who had recently designed the Anshe Russia Synagogue, designed a modified H-shaped building, a central section for administration connecting the two wings. Each of its six wards would have twelve beds, toilets, baths, and a diet kitchen, in addition to the main kitchen. The first floor would be devoted to medical cases, the second floor to surgical cases, and the third floor to rooms for private or "paying" patients. The fourth floor would include nurses' quarters and sleeping suites for the nurse superintendent and house physician. Newarkers were assured that the building would "be constructed according to the very latest scientific and sanitary rules . . . and every effort will be made to have the hospital the equal of the best of its kind."[66]

On October 27, 1906, a grandstand was erected above the foundation of the second Beth Israel hospital building. A brief cornerstone laying ceremony began with a flourish by the fife-and-drum corps boys from the Hebrew Orphan Asylum, who had marched through the neighborhood from Gross's Café, which had provided a special lunch for them. Nettie Katchen placed in the cornerstone for the foundation of the new hospital building a copper box filled with news clippings that described the role of Newark's Jewish women in the hospital's founding, a history of the hospital, committee reports, a Mason union card, a Jewish calendar, and some U.S. coins.[67]

Shortly after the ceremony, newly elected president Joseph Okin reported that he hoped the new building would open by June 1907, but his hope proved illusory; on September 11, all Newark learned from the *News*: "Beth Israel Is Sorely in Need—Work on New Jewish Hospital Building Stopped for Lack of Money." With the building just two weeks from completion, the contractors had pulled all workers off the project pending the availability of the remaining funds. Monies that had been secured before construction were exhausted; unless a sum sufficient to satisfy the demands of the contractors could be secured, they would foreclose on the property. A letter asking for assistance had been circulated to the city's clergy of every denomination.

In October, tensions flared between Okin and some of the women on the hospital board. When recognized to deliver a report during a meeting open to the public, Augusta Parsonnet, wife of Dr. Victor Parsonnet, turned her back to Okin and did not acknowledge him in her opening greeting. An insulted Okin declared that he would not hold office while the doctors of the hospital were able to sit on the planning boards and committees and their wives were eligible to serve as board members.[68] Newspaper reports of Augusta Parsonnet's public rebuff of the board president created such a stir that some suggested the next meeting be held in an auditorium so more people could attend. The press report of the following Sunday's meeting noted that although Okin's resignation was accepted by a hand vote of nearly two hundred attendees, he was severely criticized for resigning before the end of his term in December, "especially in view of the obstacles now confronting the association."[69]

The matter was hardly closed. Several days later, another group of nearly two hundred assembled in a hall at Prince and Morton Streets and voted for Okin to continue as the Beth's president. Augusta Parsonnet told *News* reporters that the meeting was only for Okin's friends and that her husband had to force his way to the platform when he attempted to say something. Surprisingly, Okin was supported by Rabbi Foster, who said that unless the bickering ceased, his congregation would withdraw its support from the hospital.[70] Foster echoed Okin's view that the physicians and their wives should not be members of the board of directors but should defer to Okin and the other businessmen in the group because of their financial expertise.

The *News* editors, who reserved a column on their first page for a report of the next meeting, were not disappointed. The headline on October 15, 1907, read: "Continue fight over Hospital—Fuel Added to Beth Israel Rumpus by Conditional Offer of Assistance." On the previous night, the paper reported, the Columbia Hall had an overflow crowd and many stood outside in the cool autumn air. The tense meeting began with an announcement by Vice President Henry Gross that he had received Augusta Parsonnet's letter of resignation from the board. The crowd was stunned as every woman on the hospital board stood to offer her own resignation. As all decorum was discarded, heated words were hurled across the auditorium. One rabbi who rose to speak to the group in Yiddish was admonished by members of the crowd to "keep to the point." When Mrs. Rostow said that she wished to comment on some of the points Okin had made in his letter of resignation, Okin sprang to his feet and said "he would allow no one to throw dirt upon him."

Finally, Rabbi Foster stepped to the podium and attempted to halt an impending brawl by observing that this particular hospital was so ill that in fact surgery might be advisable. As the crowd quieted, he offered a proposal "generous to the extreme," announcing the names of fifteen community businessmen who were willing to collectively guarantee the mortgage on the new building's property. The rabbi added the conditions for such an arrangement, specifically that the hospital board would be limited in membership and exclude physicians and women. Foster took pains to defend the latter condition on the grounds that he did not think women were as capable as men of attending to the financial affairs of an institution.

According to the *News* reporter, a silence fell in Columbia Hall, which the rabbi thought signaled approval; he did not realize that Mrs. David Laskowitz, a hospital board member, sitting behind him on the platform, had risen from her seat. She came forward to the podium and, in carefully chosen Yiddish sentences, explained that if the hospital association agreed to accept the sum from the fifteen businessmen as guarantors under their proposed conditions, the Beth would de facto be theirs. Fearing that the Newark Beth Israel Hospital Association would become a trust of the kind that aroused Progressive fears because of the stranglehold such arrangements often exerted on the marketplace, Laskowitz asked: "When we need this money must we sell our hospital to what I call a trust? If we do this, these men will put out those who have been the most zealous workers to the cause." Growing increasingly passionate in her rhetoric, she turned to Rabbi Foster: "When we wanted this money at the very start they did not come to our aid." Her words hung in the air for a moment until a young man, Peter Nehemkis, strode to the stage. With a flourish, he drew two dollars from his pocket and placed them on the podium. A queue of men and women followed him to the podium, voting their rejection of the rabbi's proposal with their dollar bills and coins.

The spontaneous outpouring of small donations, though moving, failed to resolve the hospital's financial woes. Quiet negotiations proceeded behind the scenes, led by Dr. Clarence Rostow, until finally the *News* could report on October 23: "Beth Israel Hospital Trouble Is All Over—Warring Factions in Management Forgive and Forget—Mr. Okin Retracts Rostow Charges." According to the article, "peace once more reigns among the managers of the Beth Israel Hospital." Okin agreed to remain as president and subsequently, made a public apology at Gross Hall for his comments on the "undesirability of having the wives of the active attending physicians on the board of managers." Rostow told the reporter covering the story that everyone concerned had agreed to work in harmony for the hospital's best interests; soon donations from the business community resumed, and sufficient sums were raised to pay the construction contractor. As the work proceeded, the building committee "saw the light of day" and reconsidered items earlier judged "extras" and deleted from the building contracts; they let additional contracts to construct an elevator and a laundry, and to install kitchen equipment, electric service, gas ranges, window shades, lighting fixtures, and fire hoses.[71]

The Second Beth Israel Hospital

The dedication ceremony on Wednesday, January 30, 1908, in honor of the new facility suggests an elaborate attempt to mend all fences within the community and heal all rifts created by the controversy over the construction of the new hospital. The ceremony began at 3:00 P.M. on the front steps of the completed building with addresses by the community's rabbis. Rabbi Foster proclaimed the hospital "its own best interpreter" and described it and its nonsectarian admissions policies in terms designed to transcend the past year's turmoil and bitterness. The edifice was a "sermon in stone, a deep emotion crystallized into bricks and beams, a lofty purpose shaped into doors and windows, floors and ceilings, earnest effort transformed into a building." Addressing the entire Newark community, he observed: "While this hospital shall be mainly supported by Jews it will open its doors just as wide as they can swing to receive the non-Jew who may desire to enter and his religious sentiments shall be carefully safeguarded." Perhaps hoping to catch the attention of the German Jews in Newark, Foster made a point of observing that the hospital was testimony to the positive contribution of the Russian Jews now residing on the Hill:

> The Beth Israel Hospital is to me an indication of what the Russian Jews will accomplish in this land of freedom and enlightenment. Hounded and persecuted in Russia beyond the power of words to describe . . . they come to the United States, eager to breathe the air of freedom, anxious to repay the country for this blessing that she offers . . . [and] with the opportunities of learning and advances they enjoy, they will indicate more fruitfully than is appreciated the depth of their patriotism.[72]

Then the symbolic keys to the building were passed from architect Nathan Myers to William S. Rich, the chair of the Beth Israel building committee, who in turn handed them to Henry Gross, the new president of the board. The mayor of Newark, Jacob Haussling, offered brief remarks, and the ceremony ended with the playing of the *Star-Spangled Banner*. That evening, the dedication ceremonies resumed at the B'nai Abraham Synagogue on High Street, with its distinctive Moorish dome visible for miles around. After musical selections by a local band and remarks by Reverend Edmund A. Wahl, the director of Saint Barnabas Hospital, New Jersey governor Franklin Fort delivered a speech, his presence demonstrating to Newark and the state the hospital's importance. After generalizing about advancements in science and improvements in sanitary conditions nationwide, Fort spoke of the role that states were playing in improving the health and hygiene of their citizens. Even so, Fort observed: "Disease is bound to come. Man is prone to disease as sparks fly upward. Everyone must come to it and so when we are looking to the erection of public buildings, we must not forget the urgency of efficient hospitals. The increase of intelligence among the human race has resulted in bringing out these institutions for the care of the sick." The governor concluded with a prophesy about the future of health care: Because of its essential nature, he believed "that ultimately these institutions should be taken over by the state and the time will come when that will be done, the general uplifting of the people as well as the care of the sick will be borne by the state."[73]

For nearly a week, the hospital held open house so that the community could marvel at the modern wards, operating room, sterilizing rooms, dietary kitchens, and space for clinics. Then, to conclude the dedication festivities, the Jewish community held a Prince Street parade. On Sunday, February 2, 1908 the joyous procession stepped out, led by Glickman's Marching Band. All the businesses and homes on High Street were draped in red, white, and blue bunting and flew U.S. flags. A crowd in excess of seven thousand braved winter winds to follow the 1902 zig-zag route through the streets of the Hill, ending finally at West Kinney Street in front of the new hospital steps. Behind the band came the parade marshals, long-time board member Adolph Hollander and Isaac Shoenthal, the mayor of Orange. Fourteen open carriages carried dignitaries and honored guests. The first held Mayor Haussling, hospital president Gross, and Building Committee chair Rich. In the second were Katchen, Barnhard, and other women founders. The third carriage carried the rabbis, and behind them came the medical staff and board members. Four more parade divisions followed, each with its own band and grand marshal, followed by thousands of men wearing the sashes of their Jewish lodges, unions, and associations.[74]

Newark Beth Israel Hospital was recognized by Newark's Jews and non-Jews alike as a permanent institution that could in the years to come make an important contribution to the health and well-being of the entire community. However, none who were present during the hospital's rocky beginning could fail to wonder whether the Beth would grow and evolve with the rest of Newark or fall prey to the financial difficulties and internecine wrangling that had almost obliterated the hospital during its first decade of existence.

Of all those who spoke during the days of celebration, perhaps none mixed pride with caution better than Rabbi Julius Silberfeld:

> Take care, my friends, that this monument of mercy should stand on a solid foundation. See to it that even when the inspiration of this day shall have faded away you shall keep up your enthusiasm and your love for this institution, support it with the same heroic self-sacrifice and devotion that you have displayed until now. And thus will Newark Beth Israel Hospital stand as a perpetual memorial to the honor and glory of the Jews and Judaism.[75]

CHAPTER 2

The Formative Years

*L*ucifers, locofocos, flambeaus, torches, fusees—early twentieth-century nicknames of the little wooden stick with the dab of sulfur at one end. With one swift striking movement against a hard surface, the tip could glow incandescent for a second and ignite the kindling in stoves, the oil in lamps, the wicks of candles—and the corners of pinafores. Matches were in every room of a tenement apartment or house. Children learned to strike matches early in life and carried the sticks in their pockets. They would gather debris in a pile, strike a match, and run around the bonfire singing songs, louder, faster, and closer to the crackling flames. The sparks of the bonfire would fly up and outward, carried by the fire breeze, and gently land on the children's flimsy clothing.

On an August evening, just as her parents were observing the closing hours of the Jewish holiday of Tisha Ba'av, the sad commemoration of the fall of the Second Temple to the Romans, six-year-old Annie Krotowitz went into a narrow alley behind her tenement flat on the Hill and built a bonfire. A policeman who saw the smoke and heard the screams scooped up the charred, moaning child and ran three blocks north on High Street to Saint Barnabas Hospital, placing her into the arms of the physicians and nurses who were the most experienced with burns. They first tried to save her and then sadly labored to ease the pain of her last minutes of life.[1]

Newarkers lived with the danger of fire in their workplaces, as well as their homes. And for a great many of the city's immigrant poor the workplace was a factory. Between 1900 and 1910 an estimated 3,500 small factories were bustling in Newark. In 1907, at a Newark symposium on future development, the annual value of production was estimated at $14 million in leather, $10 million in jewelry, $4 million in chemicals, $7 million in machinery, and

$20–$30 million in paints and colors and varnishes.[2] Each factory, had open vats of flammable chemicals—for tanning and dyeing leather, for altering the texture and color of textiles, and for electroplating of metals, and for concocting paints—all capable of igniting into fireballs that imploded factory buildings.

On Saturday morning, November 26, 1910, a small fire ignited bolts of fabrics producing fiery embers that showered in arcs across the hot workrooms, landing on the heads and backs of women hunched over their sewing machines; in minutes the four-story Wolf Muslin Company factory at 216 High Street burst into flames. The extra editions of the *News* ran banner headlines and front-page stories that described the horror of women and girls running to the top of the building, their clothes and hair ablaze and then: "The dead girls jumped into eternity. They had been seized with fear that forced them to plunge wildly from the third and fourth floors to the ground below."[3] Only four months later, women and men garment workers would jump to their deaths from the top floors to escape the flames engulfing the Triangle Shirtwaist factory in a high-rise building in New York City. In Newark, many of the women survived their thirty-foot jumps and lay writhing in agony from their broken bones and burns, their bodies embedded in the concrete sidewalk.[4]

As the firemen directed fire hoses at the flames, the policemen checked the bodies on the sidewalk and sent those still alive to the city's public hospital or to one of Newark's charitable hospitals. The women whose injuries were minor were sent to Saint Barnabas Hospital. Eight women who had fallen or jumped were sent to Saint Michael's Hospital and seven survived. The thirty-one most severely injured were transported to City Hospital, which had developed the best emergency services through sheer volume and variety of clinical cases. The entire City Hospital staff assembled to meet the ambulances. Twenty-three victims were still alive when they were wheeled through the door, and five more died within thirty minutes. The remaining victims were not expected to live, but the efforts of the City Hospital staff would enable them to see or hear their relatives for a few minutes before they died. Their forewoman, Caroline Haag, who had suffered smoke inhalation after she had returned repeatedly to the building to lead the surviving women to safety, died in Saint Barnabas Hospital three days later.[5]

In 1909, five charitable hospitals had been designated as official Newark hospitals as a result of a *cy pres* adjudication providing a large legacy to "The Newark Hospitals."[6] Two of these official hospitals, Saint Michael's and Saint Barnabas, were receiving patients and two others, Saint James and German, were too far from the fire to receive patients. But as the acrid smell of smoke spread south on High Street and men ran north, including Morris Gottlieb, who found only the charred remains of his three daughters, no ambulances arrived at the fifth official Newark hospital on the corner of High Street and West Kinney.[7]

The physicians and nurses of the Newark Beth Israel Hospital, at 631 High Street, could only watch the mayhem in the distance. They stood on the front steps of a four-story solid brick structure with operating rooms on the top floor, complete with skylight, an elevator, fully-equipped kitchen and laundry, and state-of-the-art heating, plumbing, electrical wiring, and telephone systems. The Jewish hospital treated more than 700 inpatients each year and more than 10,000 in its outpatient clinics, many of which were tents pitched in the yard near its front door.[8] But, the Jewish hospital remained in the eyes of Newark's police and firemen "the little house on the Hill," in the shadow of Saint Michael's Hospital, "the great hospital on the Hill."

The Founding Medical Staff

In contrast to the image portrayed in *News* articles, the history of the Newark Beth Israel Hospital from 1901 to 1919, as described in the handwritten ledger of the medical staff and the minutes of its committee meetings, was not one of a struggle of women against men, but of the efforts of a group of young Jewish physicians and nurses to establish a progressive medical institution.

The Official Ledger of the Medical Staff begins with a declaration that the medical staffs of both the Hebrew Hospital and Dispensary Association and the Daughters of Israel Hospital Association are "officially joined to work in Harmony for the Welfare of the Hospital Movement." The ledger then lists fourteen physicians who agreed to hold meetings in the assembly room of the Charleton Street Hebrew Dispensary in order to forge the organization of the medical staff.[9] The result of their meetings held throughout the blistering summer of 1901, punctuated by Miss Esther Newman's tragic death, was the establishment of five divisions, each of which would offer a clinic in the dispensary building: surgical, medical, gynecological, pediatric, and dermatological.

Thus, by September 6, 1901, as the *News* reported that the two associations were about to merge, their medical staffs were already meeting regularly to discuss medical advances elsewhere and their own clinical cases. The physicians themselves raised funds to buy equipment and instruments for the Beth's first operating room.[10] By the time the hospital officially opened on August 31, 1902, each member of the medical staff was required to contribute $275 as an initial staff membership fee.

The opening of the "Pennington" hospital had closed the rift dividing the Daughters of Israel and the Hebrew Dispensary, although there were divisions that remained among the physicians from both organizations. Shortly after the hospital opened, a controversy erupted when several older physicians with established private practices tried to write bylaws that would automatically make all paying patients (those able to pay five dollars per week) private patients, who would be admitted and treated only by themselves. Such a change would make the Beth Israel a proprietary, or privately owned, hospital and was voted down as "injudicious" and inconsistent, with its mission.[11] The minutes also record that a three-bed ward converted to an operating room was kept locked after surgery to secure surgical instruments and to prevent any unauthorized surgeries.[12]

The construction of the second hospital necessitated a reorganization of the staff. In June 1907, the executive committee created the positions of house physician, house surgeon, and interns, increased the nurse staff positions to four trained nurses and six student nurses, and hired two orderlies. The medical staff also announced a 1907 examination for internships, aimed at graduating students from Cornell Medical College, Bellevue Medical College, the College of Physicians and Surgeons, and Long Island Medical College.[13] The decision to create intern positions and to develop standards for their qualifications was innovative, and preceded the American Medical Association (AMA) Council on Medical Education 1914 recommendation to add a hospital internship as a requirement for the last year of medical college training; medical interns in the early twentieth century were thus a rarity in the hospitals' labor force.[14] The qualifications required by applicants included proficiency in German, so that an intern could benefit from the research emerging from German laboratories and published in German medical journals.[15]

Junior staff duties were classified as: house surgeon, house physician, and intern. The house surgeon had charge of all inpatients who were not attended by a private physician with hospital privileges and was expected to assist at every surgery procedure. The house physician had charge of all medical cases, took patient histories, made initial physical exams of incoming patients, and administered anesthesia during surgeries. The interns or surgical assistants reported to the senior physicians and were responsible for taking the histories of surgical patients upon their admission and also were responsible for completing specimen analysis and related pathology laboratory work.[16] All interns were required to live on the hospital premises so that they were available around the clock to the attending physicians and their patients.[17]

Max Danzis and Victor Parsonnet

A hospital derives its identity in part from its human face, the physicians and nurses who provide cure and care. Dr. Edward Ill's prowess as a physician gave luster to Saint Michael's reputation, and the German Hospital's reputation for care was in no small measure derived from the nurses who walked in the footsteps of Clara Maas, who had sacrificed her life volunteering to be exposed to mosquitoes in order to determine whether yellow-fever virus was an insect-vector disease.[18] City Hospital operated the largest emergency room and the Newark Board of Health bacteriological laboratory, whose "germ hunters" received and cultured swabs from physicians throughout the city, critical for the containment of outbreaks of infections such as diphtheria. The name of Newark Beth Israel Hospital, in its formative years, was associated with two physicians: Drs. Max Danzis and Victor Parsonnet.

A native of Russia, Danzis arrived alone in the United States at the age of sixteen. Typical of many poor Russian immigrants, he held a series of jobs, from newspaper delivery boy to truck driver to hatter, until in 1899 he graduated from Bellevue Medical College. An immigrant physician, Danzis did not endear himself to the Newark Board of Health, whose members may well have judged this foreign-accented, bearded young medical man as not up to their standards.

The Newark Board of Health, with its separate division of contagious and infectious diseases, wielded considerable power in Newark, and had championed programs for vaccination, and for closing pumps and water wells that were sources of cholera. The board was legally empowered to enforce quarantines. When a physician diagnosed a person with a contagious disease, the board was informed and the front door of the home placarded. The physician was expected to continue to make house calls until he determined that the patient and family members were no longer contagious, at which point the house would be fumigated to purge it of remaining contagion. For their efforts, physicians received a stipend for the initial house call.[19] After Danzis had cleared two homes that had been quarantined for scarlet fever, a fumigation inspector reported to the Board of Health that both families were still sick. The young physician was summoned to a board meeting, where Dr. Herman C. H. Herold, the board president, publicly scolded him and a second physician, Marcus Seidman. Herold fumed: "I am a practicing physician and I never report a case of contagion for disinfection until the last vestige of contagion has entirely disappeared. You are probably one of those physicians who are the cause of so much scarlet fever in our city."[20]

Another board physician implied that the two Jewish physicians knew they would be paid by the city for only one house call and had simply estimated when the period of contagion would be over rather than make a second house call that would not be reimbursed. Certainly other physicians had been called before the board for disciplining. However, the board physicians' pointed stereotyping of immigrant Jews sensitized Danzis to anti-Semitic slights.

Victor Parsonnet also was a native Russian, born in 1871 in Balta. He emigrated to the United States in 1889, changing his family name, Petzetzelski, to that of a friend who had died during a wave of czarist persecution. Parsonnet pursued a law degree at Boston University, transferred to Tufts Medical College, and continued his studies at the Long Island Medical College, graduating in 1898. Standing 5 feet 8 inches, he was "built like an ox with broad shoulders" and was always immaculately dressed, with a freshly starched white collar and disposable white tie.[21] Parsonnet was considered an excellent physician with a memorable public-speaking style, his delivery studied, scholarly, and convincing. In the face of opposition, he spoke with vehemence and vivid imagery. Politically, Parsonnet was a committed socialist and named his eldest son Eugene V. after his political friend and idol, Socialist leader Eugene V. Debs. Parsonnet did not let his personal leanings interfere with the mission of the Beth Israel Hospital. In 1907, two members of the Women's Circle, a socialist organization, attended a Beth Israel Hospital fund-raising costume ball wearing on their costumes an advertisement to attend the New Year's Eve Socialist Ball; Parsonnet, chair of the ball's floor committee, thought this unseemly and ejected them forcibly.[22]

Parsonnet was the first physician in New Jersey to be prosecuted by law, sued by a patient who charged him with committing assault and battery during surgery. He had diagnosed a ruptured left hernia and recommended surgery, but as he began the operation, he located a much more serious hernia rupture on the patient's right side, and so he repaired the right rupture, leaving the left hernia to be dealt with after the patient had recovered from the first surgery. The patient's suit stated that he had not authorized the right hernia repair, and Parsonnet was fined $1,000. The case was appealed to the New Jersey Supreme Court, which overturned the lower court and ruled that a surgeon who has been authorized by a patient to perform an operation becomes an agent of the patient, empowered to act for his best interest during the period of unconsciousness. This ruling created an important precedent for surgeons.[23]

Parsonnet and Danzis were familiar members of the Hill community; they practiced in their homes on High Street, walked to the hospital, and made house calls to the tenements where their immigrant patients lived. Parsonnet began his working day at 8:00 A.M., when he saw private patients on a first-come, first-served basis. His son Eugene recalled that on his way to school, he would scoot down the front steps past a line of ten or fifteen men and women holding numbered appointment tickets in their hands, waiting for his father. After Parsonnet had seen all those patients, he walked across High Street to the hospital. On days when there was no school, Eugene Parsonnet remembered, at a certain point his father would stop walking, whirl around, and glance back at the house to see if his rambunctious son was perched on the roof, one of the youngster's favorite spots for scanning the neighborhood. If Eugene was there, all of High Street would hear the doctor bellow, "Sonny, get off the roof or you'll break your neck!" In the evening, Parsonnet walked home for a brief rest and then climbed into his beloved Pierce Arrow to be driven by his chauffeur, Joe, to make house calls. Back home, he conducted late evening meetings on hospital business in the parlor.[24]

On Saturdays, especially in the summers, the Parsonnet and Danzis families piled into the Pierce Arrow, the women wearing goggles and dusters, the doctors taking turns hand-cranking the engine, and set out for the Coney Island amusement park in Brooklyn, New York. Eugene recalled:

> We invariably reached Coney Island in time for lunch. Our mothers would chaperone us kids, and Pa [Max Danzis] and Dad would walk along the boardwalk and perhaps bowl a game or two. I shall never forget watching them bowl . . . and I recall the pinboys jumping out of the way of the flying pins. The families assembled at a seafood restaurant and, having our innards well stoked, we made our return trip, which took two and a half hours.

During these outings and gatherings, Eugene Parsonnet and Rose Danzis became sweethearts; eventually, they married.[25]

Parsonnet, who quickly became the hospital chief of staff, continually earned the enmity of Dr. Clarence Rostow, who resented being supervised by a much younger doctor. At one staff meeting, Rostow complained that his younger colleague had redone the surgical dressings for his patients. Parsonnet, who never held back in these situations, said that Rostow was right, but that he dressed these cases only after he had determined that they had been incorrectly dressed in the first place.[26]

Rostow's colorful clashes continued through the formative years of
the hospital; the minutes record a memorable scene when he burst into an
operating room to berate another surgeon, screaming: "Are you operating
on this patient? If I knew you would operate on him I never would have sent
him in!"[27]

In addition to performing inpatient surgeries, Danzis supervised the
operation of the outpatient clinics that had replaced the Charleton Street
dispensary and provided critical free services to the Hill neighborhood. But
the clinics suffered from personnel and administrative problems. The gynecology clinic could not receive patients at noon because the hospital pharmacist and nurse left together for lunch. A physician refused to see clinic
patients when patient gowns and towels were not available. A directive had
to be issued to physicians reminding them that they must stay for a full hour
when they drew a clinic assignment, because so many were showing up late
and leaving early. When one chronically late physician arrived and began to
remove his coat, the senior physician on duty told him not to bother and
fired him in front of the waiting patients.[28]

By 1911, the hospital's senior medical or visiting staff, in addition to
Rostow, Parsonnet, and Danzis, included Drs. Maurice Asher, Max Feldman,
Solomon Greenbaum, Bernard Greenfield, George Rogers, and Emanuel
Schwarz. Six noted physicians from other hospitals served as consultants,
including Edward Ill. The medical staff was organized by seniority, as it was
at most hospitals of the era.[29] Twelve physicians had been added to perform
duties as first assistants or junior medical staff; they were in turn assisted by
six interns. There were separate departments of medicine; surgery; diseases
of women; diseases of children; pathology; eye, ear, nose, and throat; and
dental surgery.[30] At each evening meeting, the medical staff mediated such
situations as the invariable clash of an intern with Rostow, the continuing
aggravation over finding a suitable nurse superintendent willing to remain in
the difficult position, and the quality of the nursing staff.[31]

Nurse Superintendents and the Nursing Staff

Caroline Feitzinger had served as the founding nurse superintendent
from 1902 to 1908; then she resigned, informing *News* reporters that after
clashes with the hospital executive committee, her position became "undesirable."[32] Carolyn Schmoker, her assistant and head nurse, simultaneously
announced her resignation to return to her position as assistant principal of
the City Hospital Training School for Nurses. Lavinia Ward, the next superintendent, remained only from May to December 1908 before she, too,

returned to City Hospital, accepting the position of instructor at City's nurses' training school.[33]

Ward's resignation was prompted in part by an error that came to light only in the wake of a tragedy. Ward had hired Rosa Rosensohn, an immigrant from Vienna, who claimed to have had extensive nursing training in Europe. After accepting the position, a distraught Rosensohn, sitting at a table in Achtel Stetter's Restaurant on Broad Street, publicly proclaimed that a Beth Israel physician, Saul Rubinow, had broken off their relationship. She then swallowed strychnine and morphine in an failed attempt to take her own life. Rubinow told the police that Rosensohn had imagined the relationship and she was committed to a mental institution. An investigation revealed that Rosensohn had never possessed nursing credentials, although she had been caring for Beth Israel Hospital patients.[34]

A succession of replacements for Ward proved unsatisfactory; the most troubling appointment and resignation was that of a Miss McKenzie, who was charged by the other nurses with making anti-Semitic remarks to the staff when she was conducting bedside teaching demonstrations for the student nurses.[35]

Finally, in 1912, Sarah Van Gelder was promoted from chief operating-room nurse to nurse superintendent.[36] Her paramount goal was to raise the entire hospital's deteriorating standard of hygiene to the level she had maintained in the surgical rooms. Her priorities may have been encouraged by a report from Danzis, who had noted to his colleagues that jars of dressings and salves in the clinics were not covered properly and that receptacles for soiled dressings were left uncleaned. Another physician reported that pillowcases in the children's ward were covered with spots. Mosquitoes were entering the patient wards through cracked panes and windows that lacked screens. Van Gelder's second priority was to impose order on the chaotic clamor in the hospital's halls, caused by well-meaning friends and relatives attempting to help with patient care. One physician reported seeing a patient's brother cooking for him in the hospital kitchen and another visitor emptying a full urinal into a sink. Visitors were promenading through the halls at all hours, talking loudly, and even smoking near post-operative patients and areas with highly flammable anesthesia drugs.[37]

The rapid turnover of women who held the nurse superintendent position affected the reputation of the Beth Israel Nurses Training School, whose strength lay in the quality of its nurse instructors and a cadre of in-house diploma graduates who rose from their student-training positions to positions of authority. In 1909, while the supervisory hierarchy was in flux, the board had purchased the Weston estate adjacent to the hospital and relocated the nurses to this residence in order to convert their quarters to ten additional private patient rooms. When the number of student and graduate nurses increased, the board purchased a large house at 646 High Street, converting it to dormitories and classrooms.

The move did nothing to improve the working relationship among the nurses and physicians.[38] Some senior physicians refused to make rounds with nurses they regarded as incompetent. Their behavior was echoed by interns, who clashed frequently with graduate nurses, many of whom possessed more experience treating patients than they had. To assert their authority, some interns refused to accept reports on patients over the telephone, insisting that nurses deliver written reports to them in person. When nurses responded by chiding them for avoiding the use of a modern convenience, the interns countered that the nurses were intentionally sabotaging the proper operation of phones on the upper floors of the hospital by muffling their rings with thick wads of paper so that they might take their tea uninterrupted.[39] When graduate nurses hired their own chiropodist to care for their feet, the interns complained that the chiropodist was not a member of the medical staff. The nurses countered that the chiropodist did more good in their weekly clinic at Beth Israel Hospital than most of the interns did for medical care.[40]

The nurses who graduated from the Nurses Training School and chose to continue as members of the hospital's nursing staff had trouble receiving payment for their services. The hospital bill presented to patients upon discharge itemized the cost of the room and the fees for physicians and nurses; as in other voluntary hospitals of the era, patients were expected to pay the doctors and nurses directly and separately from the hospital bill. While hospital administrators made some effort to collect what the nurses were owed, nurses often had to go to the homes of discharged patients to collect their fees.[41]

Limited resources and lax administration placed undue stress on those charged with the seemingly endless task of caring for patients who were unable to pay either the physicians' or nurses' bills. One episode was so memorable that it appeared in the medical staff minutes and became a Beth Israel Hospital legend. On April 19, 1916, a nurse came to the main kitchen to request four eggs for her breakfast, but the pantry waiter would give her only two. Their rude words escalated into screams, gestures, and finally, pushing. When the waiter pushed the nurse against the door, she retaliated by slamming the door and inadvertently smashing his finger. Infuriated and now wounded, the waiter approached the nurse with a menacing look, and they both picked up frying pans and began to brandish them. They were finally pulled apart and the waiter's wound bandaged by a physician.[42]

There were nurses who were devoted completely to their vocation, and others who fell in love and left the hospital. One such young student nurse left two months shy of receiving a Beth Israel nursing diploma when her beau, an ardent Zionist, came to the hospital with the news that they were departing for Palestine. Parsonnet and Danzis both pleaded in vain with David and Paula, the young idealists, to defer their trip until the young woman got her degree. Years later, Paula Ben Gurion, the wife of Israel's first prime minister, confirmed the story when she welcomed Danzis on a visit to Hadassah Hospital in Israel.[43]

Junior Medical Staff

In addition to assuring the hospital and outpatient clinics of competent physician and nursing coverage, Parsonnet and Danzis also sought to resolve the chronic problems that arose in the supervision of the interns.

The Beth was hardly alone in facing such difficulties. In 1916, A. B. Tipping, superintendent of New Orleans's Jewish hospital, the Touro Infirmary, noted that unpaid interns who were required to live on a hospital's premises soon resented the inconveniences of that lifestyle and the indignity of walking behind an attending doctor or performing endless laboratory tests. Interns initially brimming with enthusiasm for medicine began to lose their ambition; complaints and excuses became the order of the day.[44]

Medical staff minutes suggest a high turnover in the men who were hired to fill the junior staff positions. These young physicians hoped to affiliate themselves with hospitals approved by the American Medical Association for internships, which would enrich their medical experience and serve as a springboard for their careers. Lacking the idealism that motivated many of their senior colleagues to found the hospital, junior staff found it difficult to cope with the inconveniences of a charitable institution with limited resources. Some gave notice and departed, but others simply abandoned their positions and suffered no adverse professional consequences.

In September 1911, when a clinical assistant, Dr. Chasan, ceased appearing at the hospital, the medical staff declared his position open and Dr. Flowers was hired to replace him. Seven weeks later, Flowers resigned, complaining that he was not notified when urine specimens were ready for the laboratory, so that they had become contaminated; that the notices he posted in the laboratory were torn down; and that some junior physicians would not work with him, while members of the senior staff "were making things 'warm' for him." His resignation was quietly accepted.[45] Another intern was fired when he informed a patient's parents that their son's condition was deteriorating because, in his opinion, the hospital surgeon had not performed the right operation.[46]

The senior staff made efforts to provide closer supervision, requiring clinical assistants to complete patient charts and to sign a register upon entering and leaving the premises. By 1914, clinical assistants were notified that their failure to attend a clinic would result in loss of hospital privileges.[47]

Suicides, Illegal Operations, and Poorly Managed Births

On October 1, 1905, a frantic Louis Lesser summoned Parsonnet to his home. Lesser had attended the Rosh Hashanah High Holiday morning service at the synagogue and returned home to find his twenty-year-old daughter, vice president of the Newark Beth Israel Hospital Auxiliary, "stretched on the bed, dead, the pungent odor of carbolic acid telling the story of suicide all too plainly."[48]

Young women and, in rare instances, men chose suicide in the face of life's pressures, by poisoning themselves. A vial of carbolic acid, sold in drugstores for a variety of cleaning tasks, could be purchased for two cents and became the means whereby many distraught took their own lives. A mild anesthetic quality likely made the drinking momentarily painless, but no amount was too little to effect nausea, vomiting, convulsions, and suffocating death due to the acid's ability to dissolve the esophagus. The scene was heart-rending to witnesses, who would see a young person lift the glass vial to her quivering mouth and then almost immediately collapse on the street in paroxysms of agony from the chemical burn, clutching at her throat in an effort to breathe. Inevitable death throes followed in a few minutes.[49]

In a time of virtually no alternatives, a young woman who discovered that she was pregnant might choose suicide to avoid her shame and to spare her family. By 1911, Newark had restricted the sale of carbolic acid to individuals, but the choice of suicide had already been supplanted by the practice of "illegal operations" (abortions), which consisted of the insertion of a dilation device and a curettage instrument to scrape the lining of a pregnant woman's uterus. Women sought those who possessed the instruments and claimed to have the skill to perform the operation. But, these operations posed grave risks for the patient: incomplete abortions, lacerated cervixes, and lacerated perinea were the price of patients' desperation and of the incompetent procedure performed in a septic environment. The *News* ran articles, reporting that male interns and female nurses in New York City, in need of income and willing to take chances, at times crossed the Hudson and Passaic Rivers to carry out these operations. Some were caught in Newark's hotels and rooming houses, often with surgical instruments spread out on the rented bed. An investigation by the Newark Health Board concluded that many midwives were also performing "illegal operations" and related procedures for which they were not qualified.[50]

Correcting the mistakes made by abortionists often fell to Beth Israel's surgeons. The surgeons continued performing appendectomies, repairs of hernias, the removal of tumors, and minor surgeries for lacerations and hemorrhoids, and the skilled surgical draining of lung abscesses as a complication of rheumatic fever and bronchitis. (This was one of the first surgical procedures that young Eugene Parsonnet observed, standing nearby, as he watched his father perform it.)[51] But, those who had earned reputations as good general surgeons also began to specialize in the correction of female complications. The 1909 Beth Israel Hospital Annual Report listed female surgeries that included excising ovarian cysts and uterine fibroids, hysterectomies, lacerations of the cervix and perineum, as well as repairs of vaginal wall and uterus.[52] By 1911, appendectomies were outnumbered by female surgeries, which constituted almost half of all procedures performed at the hospital.[53]

A physician could be arrested on the charge of a death caused by massive hemorrhaging or postoperative septicemia attributed to an illegal operation. In 1913, such an indictment directly involved the Beth Israel Hospital. On January 13, 1913, a city clerk issued a marriage license to Rose Leibowitz, who lived at 240 Prince Street in the heart of Jewish Newark, and to her fiancé, Herman Goldstein. A week later, the blank form was returned to the clerk. The boy's father testified that Goldstein had tired of the girl and had left town, severing their engagement. On January 27, Dr. Nathan Shapiro, a physician from Brooklyn who had joined the Beth Israel Hospital staff, summoned an anesthesiologist, Dr. Silverstein, to the girl's home. The emergency surgery performed there did not improve her condition, and the young doctor sought permission from Dr. Armin Fischer, a senior member of the medical staff, to admit her to Beth Israel Hospital, where she died five days later of septicemia.[54]

Shortly before she died, Leibowitz made a deathbed statement for the county medical examiner, William McKenzie, charging that Shapiro had performed an illegal operation on her and that her illness was the consequence.[55] At the trial, Silverstein testified that he and Shapiro had been presented with an illegal operation gone wrong and had tried to save the girl. Shapiro was convicted of manslaughter; the jury rendered two verdicts, one for performing the illegal operation and the second for her death.[56] Newspaper accounts do not report the response of the Beth Israel hospital staff, board, and physicians to the Shapiro conviction, and his name does not appear in the official ledger of the medical staff.[57] However, the legacy of that court trial and the attendant bad publicity can be extrapolated from a later incident reported in the medical staff's meeting notes. In 1916, Dr. Jacob Polevski was severely reprimanded for attending a case that he diagnosed as placenta previa with a stillborn child because he had not sought out a senior physician to witness the case.[58] The Shapiro trial may have struck a cautionary note: the physicians needed to be prepared for litigation related to maternity and gynecological cases; the hospital's reputation was too precious to be put at risk.

The decision to carry a pregnancy to term and give birth was fraught with risks, too. Labor and delivery were generally left in the hands of midwives, and close female relatives and friends.[59] Of the 11,107 babies born in Newark in 1914, some 5,471 were brought into the world by midwives.[60] Of the 99 midwives practicing in Newark in 1915, 17 were not licensed, 50 failed to register births or did so belatedly, 20 did not apply silver nitrate to newborns' eyes, 9 carried illegal drugs in their bags, including arsenic and strychnine, and another 16 carried hypodermic syringes, uterine forceps, hard rubber catheters, specula, and other instruments.

Nearly three-quarters of Newark midwives admitted that they would not consult with physicians even in emergencies. Beth Israel Hospital physicians Nathaniel Price and Parsonnet attempted to reduce this number by giving lectures to midwives about the modern methods of hygiene that must be observed in deliveries. The doctors lectured in English, their words translated into Yiddish by Polevski.[61] But the victims of the midwives' diagnostic and procedural errors continued to be admitted to the Beth Israel Hospital as cases of postpartum hemorrhages, placenta previa, eclampsia, perineal lacerations, and endometriosis.

In 1912, a group of Newark Jewish women founded the Jewish Maternity Hospital, a specialized hospital under Jewish auspices, offering antepartum and delivery services to all women.[62] The name, "maternity

hospital" connoted among many the image of abortion shops where unfortunate girls were sent to have their illegitimate babies, administrators black-
mailed purported fathers, and the girls were passed along to the underworld
for immoral purposes. But, the Jewish Maternity Hospital, located at 750
High Street, was dedicated to improving the health of birthing mothers. The
work of the women founders and others in other cities was to redefine the
purpose and goals of these specialized hospitals: "so that they can live down
the reputation of the past and so that they can provide the best possible care
for the most dependent, helpless, and valuable classes of people."[63]

Frank Liveright

In 1914, Frank Liveright succeeded Philip Krimke to become the president of the Newark Beth Israel Hospital, a position he would hold for nearly
twenty years. The thirty-nine-year-old Liveright's father had been president
of Jewish Hospital in Philadelphia, among the earliest Jewish hospitals in the
country, founded in 1866; his uncle was the late Louis Frank, a Bamberger
Department Store partner. Frank Liveright began his work by attending the
medical staff meetings to report on the financial condition of the hospital and
to listen to the issues raised by the staff. He approved the expansion of the
medical staff to include adjunct specialists such as Dr. P. H. Federman, who
managed the surgical suite, and Dr. William Reich, who specialized in the
new field of X-ray services. Dr. Philip Hood was hired for the newly created
position of hospital superintendent along with two young physicians, Charles
Robbins and Vera Schechtman, the first female physician appointed at the
hospital.

In his 1915 annual report, Liveright demonstrated that he understood
how hospitals operated. His financial review and summary startled the Newark
community as he stated that the hospital had always operated with a deficit:
"Our finances are very much improved, though far from satisfactory, yet at
the beginning of the year our deficit for 1914 was $3,700, and it is now
reduced to $1,470. Our deficit for this year amounts to $3,431.13. Practically
$3,000 of this is due to the unprecedented increased cost of drugs and surgical
supplies due to the war in Europe. As former years always showed $7,000 or
$8,000 deficit, I considered this very remarkable." He singled out Hood and
Van Gelder for their efforts to make the hospital internal administration
better—"while of course, not perfect"—and stated that the cleanliness of the
institution was now above reproach. In 1915, there was cause for optimism:
some 2,106 patients were admitted, an increase of nearly 412 patients since

1914. Liveright praised the volunteers in the Ladies Guild, who had continually raised funds for linens and new laundering equipment.[64] By 1915, the guild had six officers, led by Jennie Reich Dansiz, the president; twenty-nine board members; and a membership roster of 150 women volunteers, including Dr. Schectman.

The 1915–1916 Beth Israel Hospital *Annual Report* offers evidence that membership subscriptions had increased nearly 30 percent, and charity-box collections had tripled. Judicious management had enabled the retirement of one loan. In addition, the hospital was receiving nearly $2,500 annually from the Newark city government for treatment of the indigent. However, half its total expenditures were for salaries and for feeding the patients, physicians, nurses, and staff. Building repairs totaled $2,373, suggesting that along with extensive service to the community came high wear and tear. Some statistics raised concerns, as the hospital had negotiated a new loan to pay the previous year's operating expenses.[65] The board members appealed to the community to donate a one-time sum of $15,000 to wipe out "the old standing indebtedness," the loan and interest, which would relieve the institution's leaders of "considerable embarrassment."[66]

Under the leadership of Liveright, Parsonnet, Danzis, Hood, and Van Gelder, the Beth enjoyed a period of stability between 1915 and 1920 as its facility underwent expansion. The hospital increased its beds from 85 to 110 by relocating departments and services into adjacent properties on High and West Kinney Streets, as well as Quitman Place. An additional operating room would take care of minor surgical cases. The laboratory expanded, and a record room was equipped for the systematic filing of histories and charts of individual cases. The medical staff established a night clinic for the treatment of venereal diseases, the first in Newark.[67] An air of pride and confidence pervaded.

The Crucible of Medical Care—For Hospitals

The 1910 Carnegie Foundation publication *Medical Education in the United States and Canada* by Dr. Abraham Flexner has been lauded as the report that transformed the U.S. medical education system. Flexner's intensely critical evaluation of 148 medical schools in the United States and Canada was instrumental in almost one-third of them closing by 1915. New Jersey did not fare well in Flexner's report. The state did not have a medical school in 1909 when Flexner was compiling his research, and he saw no need for one. In his view, New York State "must in the first place produce most of its own physicians and a considerable share of those who practice in the neighboring states, which like New Jersey, are without medical schools."[68] The recommendation would remain unchallenged for the next half century.

Flexner divided hospitals into three categories: teaching hospitals, large hospitals in great cities, and all others. Regarding the role of the hospital in the medical education curriculum, Flexner believed that medical schools would do well to establish their own teaching hospitals for the training of third- and fourth-year students, offering the Johns Hopkins Medical School, the Manhattan Eye, Ear, and Throat Medical School, and Philadelphia's Jefferson Medical College as excellent examples. He opposed merging existing teaching hospitals with large urban general hospitals, arguing that this would result only in a scramble for faculty positions on the part of hospital physicians hoping to enhance their reputations. The only redeeming feature of such mergers, according to Flexner, was "the amount and variety of clinical material that their students see."[69]

Newark's five official charitable hospitals all fell into Flexner's third category. Such institutions were "mere boarding houses for the sick," with medical staffs appointed "through favor, pull, or bargain" and superintendents with various inappropriate backgrounds—"a newspaper reporter, a ward boss, various clerks, and a varied assortment of clergymen." Flexner disparaged the appointment of women to hospital committees, "their only claim to knowledge being that of the 'born housekeeper' supposed to be inherent in every woman." He also offered a scathing description of U.S. voluntary charitable hospitals under religious auspices. His report briefly noted a few Catholic hospitals that provided clinical material for some medical schools but did not mention a single Jewish hospital.[70]

In September 1913, a new journal appeared that offered a different image of American hospitals: the monthly periodical *Modern Hospital.* Its cover of heavy coated-stock paper featured the new Brigham Hospital in Boston, Massachusetts. Its readers learned that the United States had 6,665 institutions for the care of the sick, with a capacity of 600,000 beds and an investment of nearly $1.5 billion in land and buildings, plus another $250 million invested annually in maintenance. In the nation's hospitals, nearly 65,000 physicians treated 9 million men, women, and children annually.[71]

The editor and founder of *Modern Hospital,* Dr. Otho Ball, would almost single-handedly give the voluntary and public hospitals a positive image in his monthly publication. Like Flexner, Ball had been commissioned to complete a cross-country survey of hospitals, learning that there was no organized body of data on hospital construction, equipment, and administration. Shortly after he returned from his survey work, his son became critically ill and lingered for months at Chicago's Michael Reese Jewish Hospital. Ball's daily visits to his son's bedside were eased only by his frequent conversations with Dr. John Allen Hornsby, the hospital's superintendent.

From these discussions, Ball decided to create a monthly magazine to collect and disseminate information and reports to the hospital world that would improve its common service to humanity. He enlisted the assistance of three colleagues: Dr. S. S. Goldwater, superintendent of New York's Mount Sinai Hospital; Michael Reese's Hornsby; and Dr. George H. Simmons, editor of the *Journal of the American Medical Association* (*JAMA*) and secretary of the American Medical Association.[72]

In 1913, Ball told his readers that hospitals were no longer a charitable storage facility for the impoverished sick and dying. The modern hospital "had become a powerful influence on Society, . . . now the chief factor in a process of remolding and remaking the modern social fabric." Taking a line from Israel Zangwill's play *The Melting Pot,* Ball wrote in his first editorial: "Social Science is the new human melting pot . . . and the process must bring forth a new humanity, a new moral code, a new religion. These are the appointed works of the hospital of the future." He proclaimed that the time had come for the prevention of disease and that "the hospital must show the way by the aid of the sciences and the arts, directed along the lines of hygiene, sanitation, pure living and right thinking." It was this sort of hospital that Ball envisioned for a "hospital year" of training for physicians before the granting of licensure.[73]

Every month, *Modern Hospital* provided readily available educational material on hospital administration. Superintendents, nurses, dietitians, housekeepers, pharmacists, social workers, and all other staff members concerned with the smooth running of a hospital and effective patient care studied each issue as if it were required reading. In its pages, they found commentary on the latest advances in hospital construction, nursing, dietetics, and labor-saving equipment, as well as homespun hints on making soap and using figured rag rugs to make a waiting area cheery. Ball, a meticulous editor, even reviewed the text of advertisements because he realized that his readers would soak up information even from the ads about new equipment.

Headquarters for *Modern Hospital* was, aptly, a converted nineteenth-century Chicago mansion, where Ball rented rooms on the first floor to the American Hospital Association (AHA) and devoted an issue to publicizing the city that would host the AHA annual convention, as well as abstracts of the AHA convention presentations. When he learned that the nuns who managed the Catholic hospitals did not attend AHA conventions, he was instrumental in urging for the establishment of the Catholic Hospital Association. Ball featured American hospitals that were models of innovation, design, and efficiency; and many of these innovators were the Jewish hospitals. Readers soon became familiar with the names of Jewish hospitals such as Michael Reese in Chicago, Illinois; Mount Sinai Hospital in Cleveland, Ohio; Mount Zion Hospital in San Francisco, California; and Mount Sinai Hospital in New York City.

Dr. Charles Craster and Epidemics, 1916–1918

In 1916, *Modern Hospital* was being read by thousands of hospital superintendents and their staff members, learning about the emerging issues in modern hospital management. They could not anticipate that they would be about to face in the next two years, waves of emergent infectious and deadly diseases that would reach epidemic proportions across the United States.

Dr. Charles Craster was the Newark chief health officer, charged with combating these epidemics. His credentials included an M.D. from the University of Edinburgh, a Ph.D. in public health from Cambridge University, work as a research pathologist at Columbia University, and three years' service at the Quarantine Station on Staten Island, at the entrance to New York City's harbor. In 1915, Mayor Thomas L. Raymond and Dr. William Disbrow, president of the Newark Board of Health, had agreed that Newark needed a physician trained in the best schools who would also possess a "Doctor of Public Health."[74]

In early autumn of 1915, Craster began his career in Newark with a campaign against the use of common cigar cutters, drinking cups, and roller towels as potential spreaders of contagion. A virulent form of influenza, or "grippe" had emerged in Newark; in one of his first public announcements concerning the outbreak, he said that contrary to the general belief that disease is spread by weather conditions, "human actions" are responsible. Craster advised people suffering from the symptoms of the grippe to be careful not to communicate it to their fellows, as "we are just beginning to realize how easy it is to communicate."[75] He was going to need all his knowledge and acumen to battle the city's next two epidemics.

The following spring, 1916, spirits soared as Newark launched a five-month-long anniversary celebration of its founding by Robert Treat and his Puritan coreligionists, the first Europeans to dwell on the banks of the peaceful Passaic River. The city government awarded a thousand-dollar prize for a commemorative poster, and celebrations included historical pageants, carnivals, conventions, and athletic competitions. Financial support came from $250,000 in philanthropic pledges plus private donations; the city expected visitors to generate another $4 million.[76]

But by early summer, young children were complaining of headaches and became restless and irritable; these symptoms rapidly progressed toward fever and paralysis.[77] All East Coast cities were menaced by an acute infection called infantile paralysis or poliomyelitis.[78] Some New Jersey public health officials likely read with alarm the editorial in the July 1916 issue of *American Medicine* warning that "the disease could never be controlled until the course and mode of infection are definitely determined." Meanwhile, under the current conditions, "no possible avenue of infection should be neglected"; parents should "keep young children from all public gatherings."[79]

The Newark Board of Health became locked in controversy with the Newark Board of Education over how best to protect schoolchildren. Newark operated an all-year school curriculum and a communicable epidemic could wreak havoc in classrooms, lavatories, and playgrounds. The Board of Education insisted that keeping schools open was preferable to closing them as the facilities offered a clean, medically supervised environment that they considered far safer for the children than being turned loose on Newark's steamy streets. A meeting of twenty-six doctors divided evenly on the question of the schools. Parents made their own decision: those who could, sent their children out of the city.[80]

During this same period, Liveright had temporarily closed the Beth Israel Hospital children's ward because of its dilapidated floors and beds, as well as the lack of sunlight and other amenities in the children's rooms.[81] The ward remained closed throughout the summer and so could not receive young patients crippled by the strange new illness.

Across the Hudson River in New York, the polio epidemic ran rampant. In July, New York City health authorities restricted children's travel to prevent the spread of the epidemic. Beginning July 18, 1916, those sixteen years old and under were placed in a restricted category and could not leave the city without a health certificate—a kind of traveler's identification card—saying that their homes were free of poliomyelitis; the measure was lifted on October 3. Parents were not always cooperative. When one couple denied that their child had polio and refused to isolate the youngster, the courts intervened and removed the child to Queensborough Hospital.[82]

In Newark, Craster placed guards at infected homes to enforce the quarantine when he learned that neighbors were visiting the stricken children, often with their own children in their arms. The Free Public Library of Newark and all but two branches barred children that July.[83] The Harry Lukens Wild Animal Show, which had pitched its tent in downtown Newark, was ordered out of town before its first performance for fear that any large gathering that included many children would spread the disease. The city's superintendent of schools postponed the summer spelling bee.[84] Because no one knew how polio spread, and everyone knew that mosquitoes carried malaria and yellow fever, children were told, incorrectly, that flies were possible carriers of the infantile paralysis germ. The *News* described a panic that ensued on a street when a decomposing dog attracted flies, and the children "saw the swarm of flies spiral upward and sail away in their thousand directions" and "fled in terror."[85]

By mid-August, physicians had reported 1,740 polio cases in New Jersey, which paled in comparison with the 6,653 cases across the river in New York. In both Newark and New York City, approximately 80 percent of those stricken were under five years old. Twenty-six states reported 27,000 cases of polio with 6,000 deaths. Improvements in personal hygiene and public sanitation had largely eliminated epidemics of diseases such as typhoid and cholera by the early twentieth century, with the ironic result that milder, immunity-giving strains of the polio virus were killed off. The more potent, crippling viral strains survived.[86]

Only with the cold days of autumn did the epidemic abate. In a superb analysis of the epidemic's impact on Newark, Craster noted that the primary area of infection had a population of Russians, Poles, and Polish Jews, along with a secondary area of Russian and Polish Jews, in the most congested part of the city. Perhaps because of his precautions, the epidemic was contained and fewer than 2,000 Newark children had contracted the infection.[87] They would need specialized care. Physicians ensured that the pediatric orthopedic cases being admitted to Beth Israel Hospital were referred to an appropriate member of the medical staff.[88]

As the winter took hold in the city, Craster and other health officers braced for the annual onslaught of the airborne influenza. The previous two years of influenza outbreaks had steadily increased in intensity and ease of transmission. An outbreak of influenza or in the winter of 1914 in New York City had been especially deadly for the aged. The influenza that swept through Newark in December 1915 was both virulent and easily transmitted among individuals; its incubation period was less than twenty-four hours.[89] The next winter affected far more individuals: by January 1916, nearly four hundred thousand Chicagoans were suffering from the grippe.[90]

The winter of 1917 brought influenza to Newark that was similar to the outbreak that had menaced the city in 1902.[91] The disease initially presented flu-like symptoms, but quickly became a bronchial illness. Boston reported forty-two cases of a "strange juvenile malady, described as both influenza and acidosis [an abnormal increase in the acidity of the body's fluids]."[92] In December 1917, the Newark Health Department reported 975 cases of the disease, 287 more than in November. The cases were largely bronchial pneumonia, with 94 fatalities. The report blamed severe weather and noted that "the increasing number of Negro laborers from the south easily became victims of the disease."[93]

The Beth Israel Hospital medical staff attributed the increased number of infections to the aging sterilizers. Every staff member was asked to contribute to a fund for new sterilizers in a campaign that raised almost $600 by February 1917.[94] Buying new sterilizers instead of repairing the existing ones may have saved lives, as a reservoir of pathogens coated the surfaces of the old equipment.

The March 1918 issue of *Modern Hospital* featured an article on the design of the new Michael Reese Hospital isolation wards for the care of young patients suffering childhood diseases and of the puerperal fevers common among adults. The wards replaced the isolation hospital building adjacent to the main hospital building. Editor Ball noted the timeliness of the article, as "a great number of communicable diseases in the military camps scattered over the country have made the isolation and care of the communicable diseases a very live topic."[95] Military camps regularly housed almost 120 men in some rooms and crowded thousands into mess halls.[96] Airborne infections such as measles and chicken pox could ravage entire camps.

In April 1918, a young recruit in a Georgia military camp died of influenza, an incident that was inconsistent with what was known about the disease.[97] Influenza was an infectious disease that was known to attack the very young and very old. The 1918 influenza, like the previous waves of contagion circulating in 1916 and 1917, was airborne, quickly incubated and targeted to the respiratory system, but it was unlike its predecessors in the fury it unleashed on healthy people in the prime of their lives. The 1918 wave of influenza struck soldiers in camps, between the ages of twenty and forty with greater virulence than it did younger or older victims. It would later be estimated that influenza killed 32,165 soldiers in U.S. camps and 18,136 in Europe's trenches.[98]

U.S. cities close to military installations thus became epicenters of epidemic disease. Newark, relatively close to Fort Dix and home to a military shipyard, was especially hard hit. One of the first young men from Newark to die was twenty-one-year-old Harry Schectman, Dr. Vera Schectman's nephew, who had traveled from Williams College to Fort Dix in August 1918 after being drafted. He became ill in New Jersey and in September died of the pneumonia that felled most of those infected with influenza.[99] On the day of his death, the army reported 9,313 new cases of influenza; by mid-September, whole divisions at Fort Dix were quarantined.[100] In a single ghastly day, September 28, 1918, more than thirty-one thousand U.S. Naval personnel ashore were stricken.[101] Although conditions at Fort Dix demonstrated that the influenza was transmitted by close contact, thousands gathered for a liberty-loan rally in front of Newark's city hall.[102] Two days later, the number of reported cases in the city jumped, including the first woman to die in Newark. Craster assembled a team of physicians, nurses, bacteriologists, and pathologists, who traveled to Fort Dix to draw blood specimens from the survivors. In hopes of creating a vaccine, he planned to prepare a serum from this blood, heating it to kill the germs and suspending the serum in a solution. The experimental vaccine did not work.[103]

On October 7, 1918, the New Jersey State Department of Health ordered every public place of assembly closed, including schools, churches, saloons, department stores, dance halls, movie houses, and soda fountains.[104] Statistics on the spread of the epidemic were staggering. Newark's Mayor Charles P. Gillen tried to prevent panic by underreporting the number stricken at 11,000. When Craster told *News* reporters that the Newark Board of Health estimate was nearly double the mayor's number, Gillen forbade the release of statistics except through his office and banned *News* reporters from city hall because he thought they exaggerated the situation.[105]

All Craster could do was quarantine the sick and minimize any gathering or assembling that could expose the uninfected to the germs. He ordered City Hospital to admit the sick men and women whom physicians expected to die shortly in order to quarantine them. Ten days later, he set up a second location only for those who stood a chance of recovery, converting the Hahne and Staff building on Broad and Central Avenue to a 750-bed emergency hospital.[106] By the time the hospital opened, the pandemic had subsided, and the Hahne building instead held hundreds of newly orphaned children.[107]

There are no statistics available on the number of Beth Israel Hospital medical staff who died as a result of the epidemic in 1918.[108] But from the 1921 annual report and other sources, we can identify some who survived: Danzis, Rogers, Polevski, Parsonnet, Price, Bernard H. Greenfield, David Gershenfeld, Louis Reich, P. H. Federman, Herman Kussy, and L. H. Fuerstman. Schectman went into private practice but remained a physician with courtesy privileges. Van Gelder continued as head of the nurses. Older men who survived included Morris Rachlin, Meyer Augenblick, and Edward Ill. Augusta Parsonnet became president of the Newark League of Women Voters; an ardent Zionist, she died a year after the creation of Israel in 1948. Craster continued to serve as Newark's health officer until 1951, when he retired at the age of seventy-six and died shortly afterward. Rabbi Solomon Foster served as a chaplain in both world wars and died at eighty-nine in 1966. Frank Liveright died in 1971 at the age of ninety-six.

A conference of public health officials reported in the December 21, 1918, issue of the journal *Survey* found that nothing they had done during the flu epidemic's few months had made any impact on its course. They could agree only that those who had felt the first rush of the illness and were able to go to bed and stay there for more than a week had the best chance of surviving.[109] The disease dealt a blow to the body's entire system, weakening victims for months afterward, some permanently. One postepidemic victim was Polevski, who would become an associate professor of cardiac research at the Graduate Medical School of the University of Pennsylvania, only to die at the age of forty-nine in 1936.[110]

Those who survived the influenza epidemic never escaped the memory and remained cautious, especially at the first sign of illness. In 1951, Danzis, scheduled to speak at a Beth Israel Hospital ceremony dedicating a new X-ray facility, felt the first rush of influenza and immediately took to bed, knowing the toll taken of his colleagues thirty years earlier.

Heart of the Hospital

Victor Parsonnet had worked through the epidemic, often taking twelve-hour shifts during its most virulent two months. He had already had his gallbladder removed and suffered bouts of angina, and he had exchanged his beloved cigarettes for Charms, the hard candy that he carried in his pockets. He also suffered some long-term discomfort after breaking several ribs in an effort to keep his Pierce Arrow from rolling forward when the brakes failed. According to his son Eugene, by 1919 he was physically weakened by the stress he had undergone during the influenza crisis.[111]

In 1920, Eugene and his brothers, Tom and Marion, were enjoying summer camp in Maine while their mother spent a few days at the family's summer house on the New Jersey shore. The Parsonnet home in Newark was empty except for Victor, who followed his morning routine, walking across the street to the Beth Israel Hospital to spend some hours in the laboratory after seeing patients. On July 20, the forty-eight-year-old doctor was found at his laboratory bench, dead of a sudden and massive heart attack.

Price, the secretary of the medical staff, eulogized Parsonnet in the 1921 Beth Israel Hospital Annual Report: "it was in his ordinary daily contact with people that his characteristic qualities stood out most vividly; . . . on his visits to the sick, his coming was hailed with exultant delight by the young hero-worshipper of the household, whilst the older ones would greet him with beaming visage and hushed expectation. His very presence so full of buoyant vigor and vitality brought cheer and comfort, whilst his optimistic viewpoint acted as a potent tonic to the weak and afflicted."[112]

Truly, Victor Parsonnet had personified the caring character of Newark's Jewish hospital and in his forceful dynamism, had established the hospital medical staff as a modernizing force in the city. By 1919, Beth Israel was a respected Newark medical institution. In the decade after Parsonnet's death, his legacy would help propel it into the forefront of modern hospitals.

CHAPTER 3

From Little House on the Hill to Modern Institution

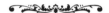

On Friday, May 30, 1924, the *Jewish Chronicle*, Newark's weekly Jewish newspaper, printed a full-page advertisement that proclaimed a new era for the Newark Beth Israel Hospital. The advertisement was a drawing of a young woman wearing a nurse's uniform whose short hemline revealed her legs, a nurse's cap atop her flapper bobbed hair, her smile made more alluring by lipstick. The young woman held out a tray that supported an architectural model of a skyscraper with four symmetrical towers and a central arched entrance. Inscribed behind her in the heart was the statement: "My heart is with the hospital," and the accompanying caption asked, "Will you help to build the new Beth Israel Hospital?" After almost a quarter century, Newark Jewry had an image that embodied their hospital: the lovely 1920s flapper would become known as "Miss Beth Israel."[1]

Miss Beth was a potent image: a modern woman campaigning for a modern hospital. By the 1920s, embracing modernity included the pursuit of good health. Municipal governments appropriated enormous sums to ensure pure water and clean streets. On the front lines of the domestic war for health and hygiene, Americans were expected to consume nutritious meals and to scour their homes until they were germ free.[2] Healthy, robust bodies were productive bodies, and membership in the middle class depended upon an affluence that only healthy individuals could attain.[3] Nativist literature was crammed with comparisons of sickly immigrants who wilted under the stress of economic competition against the robust physiques of the "pioneering breed" celebrated by Wisconsin sociologist E. A. Ross and others.[4] In communities with large numbers of poor immigrants, such as Newark, hospitals were especially critical outposts of health and hygiene. Repairing bodies efficiently and keeping them healthy so that they might resume productivity required state-of-the-art facilities and well-trained physicians and nurses. But modernity cost money and required effort.

A new generation of Newark Jews would resonate with Miss Beth's image of good health and hygiene. In the span of four years, 1924–1928, they would pledge nearly $3 million to erect a third hospital structure, and the hospital would move from its aging, overcrowded 120-bed facility to a modern 350-bed skyscraper that towered above the highest point in the south Newark neighborhood of Weequahic. Miss Beth not only transformed the image of their hospital but would prove a potent magnet to draw a generation of Newark Jews from the Hill to the streets around their new hospital.

The Need to Be a Class A Hospital

The 1921 Beth Israel Hospital Annual Report suggests that at the beginning of the decade, the administration was engaged in improvements to the physical structure of the building. The laundry facility was finally removed from the main building and in its place stood a new $10,000 X-ray room with modern apparatus, purchased by the ladies' auxiliary and dedicated in memory of Dr. Victor Parsonnet. Under chief of the medical staff Max Danzis's leadership, Drs. Polevski and Wolfe created a clinic to treat heart diseases; Dr. Charles Rosewater was encouraged to create a clinic for nervous disorders. The report noted that the medical staff was finally using the International List of Causes of Death to collect the hospital morbidity and mortality data. The report also noted that its thirteen-year-old operating rooms had accommodated 1,252 cases, most surgeries related to the genitourinary, respiratory, and circulatory systems.[5]

The previous two decades had been a formative period for the American hospital sector. The Association of Hospital Superintendents, founded in 1899 by eight hospital administrators, had renamed itself as the American Hospital Association (AHA) and in 1918, opened its membership to hospital institutions: "to form a body which can speak for the hospitals with all the power the institutions can assemble."[6] The AHA application blank was printed in *Modern Hospital*.[7] Church leaders formed sectarian hospital associations. In 1915, the Catholic Hospital Association of the United States and Canada was formed, promising to "bring about the endowment of beds, wards, and rooms to increase the efficiency for public service of Catholic Hospitals."[8] The Protestant Hospital Association was established in 1920 to "assist hospitals to become more efficient and to aid in the standardization and give such help as to possibly enlarge their facilities and equipment for the care of the sick."[9]

The Progressive movement had inspired the establishment of professional standards and methods of standardization by creating lists of those who met specific requirements. In 1906, the American Medical Association included in its American Medical Directory of state-by-state medical colleges and physicians a list of hospitals and sanatoria. In 1914, the AMA Council on Medical Education issued a plan for the state licensing boards to make mandatory a year of hospital internship training as the last year of medical school training. The council had determined that there were sufficient hospitals to provide internship positions for all American medical schools, whose numbers had shrunk by one-third as a result of Dr. Flexner's 1910 survey of medical schools. The first compulsory internship year would be in 1919, giving enough time for "a complete investigation of the hospital situation of the country" and to provide sufficient time for the state licensing boards to enforce this requirement.[10] The 1921 American Medical Directory included a list of 482 general hospitals approved for offering 2,962 internship opportunities; 17 general Jewish hospitals were on this list including the Newark Beth Israel Hospital. (See Appendix, Table 1 for the 1906 list of hospitals and the 1921 AMA list of hospitals approved for internships.)

The third and most powerful determining accreditation entity was created in 1913, by 450 surgeons who organized an American College of Surgeons (ACS) modeled on the Royal College of Surgeons of England, Scotland, and Ireland. The ACS mission was to address the training of surgeons by improving all teaching facilities, including hospitals. In 1916, the AHA formed a committee to cooperate with the ACS in its program of standardization.[11] In 1917, the ACS began a concerted drive for the standardization of all hospitals, asking 692 hospital superintendents to submit for review 100 case records of major surgical operations performed on their premises. According to one account: "These records were so incomplete and fragmentary that most [institutions] failed even minimal standards." In fact, the ACS committee was so concerned about the adverse reactions to their first, very long list of nonqualifying hospitals that at New York's Waldorf Astoria, where they had been meeting, they fed the papers and notes into the furnace. Out of the ashes of that first list, the ACS resolved to engage in a widespread campaign to standardize U.S. hospitals.[12]

The ACS established an initial requirement that hospitals desiring to receive accreditation organize their competent physicians into a "definite medical staff" that would abide by a formal set of bylaws and not engage in fee splitting. These hospitals would then have to meet a set of minimal standards for record keeping, autopsies, and other procedures, to impose order and supervision on how hospitals treated patients. The ACS then sent a trained corps of inspectors, all medical school graduates, who were instructed to inspect hospital areas, observe routines, and, following their on-site review, discuss their findings with the hospital superintendents. The ACS Report for 1919 demonstrated the progress quickly made by the standardization movement. The list of general accredited U.S. hospitals with 100 or more beds, included thirteen Jewish hospitals: Mount Zion in California; Michael Reese in Illinois; Touro Infirmary in Louisiana; Hebrew Hospital and Asylum in Maryland; Jewish in Missouri; Beth Israel, Jewish Hospital, Lebanon, and Mount Sinai in New York; Jewish and Mount Sinai in Ohio; Jewish in Pennsylvania; and Newark Beth Israel in New Jersey.[13]

By 1921, the second wave of general, specialized, and chronic disease Jewish hospitals had emerged in American cities, many listed in the AHA membership directory, fewer in the AMA Council on Medical Education list of approved hospitals for internships, and the fewest in the list of those that had achieved ACS accreditation as Class A hospitals. According to Dr. C. S. Danzer of the Brooklyn Jewish Hospital, those hospitals that did not meet Class A standards were "founded by physicians who desired to create departments in which they could specialize" and who "would not be admitted as department heads by hospitals of standing." Danzer was especially critical of some proprietary hospital administrations for refusing to award internships competitively, preferring instead to admit internship applicants who had "influential connections."[14]

Dr. Boris E. Greenberg, superintendent of the Boston Beth Israel Hospital in the 1920s, described his view of ACS accreditation: "In its survey, the college [ACS] looked at a hospital's laboratory facilities as well as its medical staff organization and case records. If excellence in these three factors were attained, the college stated, 'all other factors of a good hospital service will naturally follow.' " Thus, failure to receive ACS accreditation was devastating to an institution and disrupted morale. When the Boston Beth Israel Hospital fell short of the 1921 ACS standards, eight physicians, a dentist, and two members of the medical executive committee wrote to the hospital's board of trustees to protest what they regarded as the reasons for the rejection. "We wish to state that in our opinion the growth of the hospital is greatly hampered by its defective administration. A hospital should above all things be immaculately clean, orderly, with well-kept records, well-trained and disciplined nurses and interns; it should pay close attention to diet, ventilation, and general hygiene. In each of these things, the hospital is conspicuously lacking."[15]

In 1921, Newark Beth Israel Hospital barely passed its ACS inspection. That year, nearly 74 percent of all hospitals with a minimum of 100 beds achieved ACS accreditation. If the Beth could not remedy its shortcomings and pass the next ACS accreditation survey, the hospital would become mired at the bottom level of the less reputable hospitals. President Frank Liveright's first initiative to prepare for the 1922 ACS survey was to hire a new superintendent, whose professional training would guide the efforts for achieving accreditation.

Dr. Paul Keller, the Beth's new superintendent, met the hospital community at the November 24, 1921, opening ceremonies for a renovated children's ward. Other notables that spoke before the crowd of three thousand included Dr. Charles V. Craster, Newark's chief public health officer, and Dr. Herbert Schwartz of New York's Mount Sinai Hospital. Keller, a serious-faced young man with dark wavy hair and round, black-framed glasses, possessed a medical degree from Philadelphia's Jefferson Medical College and had served in the navy as a senior medical officer during World War I. He had initially prepared for the Presbyterian ministry and his brief remarks to the Newark Jewish community bore the crisp cadence of his Philadelphia origin as he told his listeners that he had "a keen perspective of what he wanted to do for the betterment of the hospital."[16]

Soon after Keller's appointment, on December 16, 1921, the hospital announced that Lillian Rafter was assuming the position of superintendent of nurses.[17] She convinced Keller to recruit students to the Nurses Training School with the offer of a monthly stipend, as well as a tuition-free, three-year course with room, board, and laundry in the new Nurses' Home. The board also approved the hiring of Paula Marx as Keller's assistant. In 1922, when the ACS hospital survey corps walked past the tenements of West Kinney Street and climbed the steps to the Beth Israel Hospital entrance, they would be met by not only Danzis, whose accent and bearing spoke to the institution's roots in the Jewish immigrant community, but also by Keller, whose voice, appearance, and style reflected the institution's commitment to competence and expertise, and next to him, Marx and Rafter, two well-trained young modern American women.

The 1922 ACS requirements for accreditation included a functioning X-ray Department, documentation that the hospital held regularly scheduled staff conferences to discuss morbidity and mortality cases, and review of the "deaths, infections, complications, and unimproved cases" at the institution. Keller prepared for the inspection by developing a system of case records that included the patient's history and the diagnosis of the

attending physician. This third requirement for ACS accreditation was performed by a new class of clerks described by the ACS as "historians." They
were to preserve patient records in a separate record room equipped with
standard filing cabinets and card indices for names and diseases so that each
record could be made immediately accessible.[18]

The ACS inspection would perform an intense review of the Beth's
clinical laboratory, to ensure that it provided clinical bacteriological, sero-
logical, and pathological services.[19] The ACS maintained that "even in hospitals with complete laboratory facilities, one frequently finds laboratory
services markedly deficient, due to the insufficient quantity of tests performed." It required every hospital to perform a basic battery of laboratory
tests that included hemoglobin, urinanalysis, and leukocyte count, and to
charge a flat-rate fee for all hospital tests to "allow the hospital to assume
the responsibility of having each patient receive adequate laboratory
aid." Moreover, the ACS required proper pathological analysis: "Every
specimen from the operating room should be sent to the laboratory automatically; this should be as rigid a part of the operating room technique as
the sterilization of instruments." The ACS insisted that every specimen
examined by the pathologist be accompanied by a report of a histological
examination, because the data from these examinations of tissue under
the microscope were becoming useful in determining the etiology and
pathogenesis of a disease.

In 1921, the Beth Israel Hospital laboratory was housed in the Weston
home, a wood-frame nineteenth-century contemporary of the Pennington
mansion. In 1909, the house had been acquired for the nurses, and a year
later, when the nurses were able to move to a larger home, it was renovated
for laboratory work. In 1921, it had presented poorly and received a failing
grade from the ACS inspectors. Danzis took it upon himself to raise funds
to remodel and upgrade the Weston building into a modern facility. In his
February 10, 1922, report to the board, he announced that the hospital
annex with a laboratory was in operation and that the hospital staff performed up to ACS standards all procedures for the care and treatment of
newborns, blood transfusions, and compulsory laboratory tests.

Their efforts succeeded and the name "Newark Beth Israel Hospital"
appeared in the November 1922 issue of *Modern Hospital* on the list of hospitals receiving ACS accreditation. In the fourth annual ACS review, 1,012—
approximately 62 percent of the 1,623 hospitals across the country with fifty
or more beds—met ACS requirements. The number of accredited Jewish hospitals had doubled from 12 in 1919.[20] (See Appendix, Table 1.)

Momentum for a New Hospital

In 1922, *Modern Hospital* launched a golden age of hospital construction by initiating the first nationwide architectural competition in hospital design. The editors proclaimed that this competition would recognize that modern hospitals needed to be designed differently than in the past, with attention to simplicity and utility. Hospital architects of the 1920s, freed from the nineteenth-century pavilion style often used for isolation hospitals and the early twentieth-century "Greek cross," now experimented with colonial, English Tudor, and Italian and Spanish renaissance designs. Hospitals soon began to look like skyscrapers or office buildings. And their interiors were modern as well, featuring sound-absorbing materials, incinerators for destroying infectious materials, telephone systems, and artificial electric illumination in the operating suites rather than natural light and skylights.[21]

Although Newark Beth Israel had achieved Class A status by the ACS and the Council on Medical Education, its 1908 physical facility was aging and outmoded. When the Twenty-fourth Annual Conference of the American Hospital Association met in Atlantic City in November 1922, less than twenty miles south of Newark, the Young Pier's huge exposition hall displayed state-of-the-art hospital equipment: building and construction equipment, general furnishings, clinical and scientific equipment, laundry equipment, and food service equipment. The convention sponsored day trips to Philadelphia and New York City to visit modern hospital facilities. Visitors passed autoclaves, laundry mangles, electric ovens, dishwashers, operating-room lighting, and laboratory equipment that demonstrated to many, including the Beth personnel, that their hospitals were inadequate.

At the December Beth Israel Hospital board meeting, a month after the AHA convention, Liveright obtained approval to convene a special January meeting to discuss the future of the hospital and permission to invite twenty-five of Newark's prominent Jewish leaders to join them. And so, in January 1923, nearly fifty men finished supper in the banquet room of Newark's Progress Club and settled into their chairs to listen to the hospital president's presentation. Liveright tried to help his audience envision what he had seen in Atlantic City that autumn. New standards for modern hospital construction, everything from flooring to walls and room design, made renovating the Beth's facility impractical. They needed a new building. These very men had just finished raising the funds to construct the Young Men's and Young Women's Hebrew Association community building, directly across the street from the Beth Israel Hospital.[22] Liveright made the speech of his life, as the men voted almost immediately to appoint a committee to raise $1.5 million for a new Beth, to be constructed adjacent to the 1908 building.[23]

And these men were not surprised when after accepting their approval, Liveright immediately described the preliminary architectural plans for a pavilion of buildings designed by Frank Grad's firm (the only Jewish architectural firm in Newark) that would cover the entire block of the present site.[24] Grad envisioned this modern 275-bed hospital as a seven-story building on the corner of High and Baldwin Streets with an open roof garden. His later drawings showed the 1908 hospital building as one of a pavilion of buildings with a center walkway.[25]

That spring, Danzis would be quoted in the *Jewish Chronicle*: "Our work is just begun. We are still in a transitional stage; there is still a great many tasks to fulfill and many a problem to solve. All our efforts ought to be directed for one common purpose—to make Beth Israel a model hospital in this city."[26] Almost every Friday for the next two decades, Jewish Newarkers could count on at least one article in the *Chronicle* about the new hospital.

To Raze or to Relocate?

The proposed additions to the 1908 hospital facility were innovative and exciting, but the most controversial proposal was yet to come—not to raze surrounding buildings and build an addition, but to relocate the hospital to another area of Newark.

World War I had brought unanticipated demographic change to Newark, as to many northern cities, which directly affected the Jewish neighborhood on the Hill. The Great Migration of African Americans out of the South begun in the 1890s had accelerated during the war as the sons and daughters of impoverished sharecroppers and tenant farmers sought new lives and higher wages in the North. In one month, May 1916, two trainloads of African American students from private institutions in Georgia came to northern cities for summer jobs. Not long afterward, railroads and steel mills sent labor agents to the South to scout for workers.[27]

By 1918, nearly seven thousand African Americans (nearly six thousand were male) from the South had settled in Newark, for the extensive and varied industries that needed wartime labor.[28] Many of the migrants worked in munitions plants for an average wage of $2.60 per day, far higher than they could have made in the South. Others performed unskilled labor in chemical factories, leather factories, or iron foundries, on construction sites, or behind teams of horses navigating the city's streets. Women worked in clothing factories, glue factories, tobacco factories, or manufacturing plants that turned out celluloid, leather bags, or trunks. Their average wage, eight dollars per week, was generally higher than they might have made doing the domestic chores for which they were often hired. In shell-lading plants (where fully armed artillery shells were assembled for loading onto ships) and other armament industries, wages could be even higher.

The newly arrived migrants needed housing. The neighborhood surrounding the main streets of High and Kinney, such as Broome, Montgomery, and Charleton, had some of the oldest, most dilapidated buildings in the city. Lacking kitchens, lavatories, baths, toilets, and heat, the buildings had been closed as undesirable; now they were reopened for rent again and quickly filled by the newly arrived laborers from the South.

The congested urban neighborhoods sometimes exploded in violence. A dispute among several men in September 1917 escalated into a melee that lasted several hours. Bricks, knives, beer bottles, blacksmith tools, and even parts of bed rails became weapons; the resulting injuries sent dozens to the emergency room at City Hospital. According to the *News*, a fight had broken out about 4:00 P.M. over how much money had been bet on a roll of the dice. The white men involved were winning until one of the African Americans fired a shot that attracted more than a hundred others, who ran to the assistance of their friends. The white men retreated "to the Polish and Jewish district, where they organized a gang to meet the oncoming Negroes." After 150 police officers separated the two groups, small throngs of men remained; two hours later groups of white men began to hurl bricks and other objects at black men. Police from four stations were required to restore order. Later that day, yet another battle broke out among an estimated crowd of 350 youths and men, resulting in many injuries. The Newark police inspector ordered all reserves to remain on duty; a curfew was issued for an area "occupied by 4,000 Southern Negro munitions workers and 100 saloons within a radius of ten blocks of the two districts [white and black] were ordered to close for the night." Had the violence continued, there were plans to summon the first New Jersey Infantry, preparing to go South for training before shipping out to Europe.[29]

The same *News* article that detailed the riot, however, noted: "The Negro colony in the Third Ward is not of long standing, at least in its present proportions. Several buildings at this point which house Negroes impinge upon the dwellings of whites, for the most part Jewish. Relations between white and black have in some cases been friendly and in nearly all cases tolerant."[30]

As the Hill streets became increasingly crowded and tense, Jewish businesspeople studied the newest section of the city, two miles to the southwest, beyond Clinton Avenue on which stood the private homes of wealthier, more assimilated German Jews and the Hebrew Orphan Asylum. Newark had in 1902 annexed the area adjacent to Lake Weequahic, once part of Elizabeth County.[31] This high ground above the lake had belonged to the large Lyons Dairy Farm, the site of the Newark City Open Air School for Tubercular Children, and the lodging houses where boarders such as the late Esther Newman had sought some rest in the hot summer of 1901. Gradually, streets divided the farm fields and orchards, named for those who once owned the lands—Schley, Nye, Meeker. In 1903, the trolley line from Newark was extended toward Elizabeth Avenue, the orchards gave way to rows of detached homes with neat front lawns and sidewalks, and Pot Pie Lane became Chancellor Avenue. In 1912, paving replaced Bergen Street's wooden planks set on beer barrels. An ad in the real estate section of the *News* for April 27, 1912, declared the Weequahic Park tract the most beautiful residential section for people of "artistic temperament who want desirable restricted residential property"—that is, no rentals or sales to African Americans or Jews. Developers' claims that Pennsylvania Station would put the neighborhood scarcely twenty minutes from metropolitan New York met with mixed success among New Yorkers moving north and east of Manhattan. By the 1920s, some individuals in the area had become willing to sell their land to Jews.

Thus, when the question was raised as to whether the hospital should remain where it was or move to a location where a bigger, modern facility could be built, the business minded thought of the two-family houses and the affordable still-vacant lots in Weequahic for a new hospital building.[32] In May 1924, readers of the *Chronicle* learned that Miss Beth Israel was presenting the city with a new hospital, to be located at the intersection of Lyons Avenue, Osborne Terrace, and Irving Place in the Weequahic section of Newark.[33]

A New Hospital in a New Neighborhood

The decision to construct a new Beth Israel Hospital and to transplant it from the Hill, a teeming immigrant neighborhood, was consistent with the effort to provide modern medical care in a modern facility. The process required forceful leadership at the hospital, leadership from within the Newark Jewish community, and the efforts of the ambitious editor of the *Jewish Chronicle*, Anton Kaufman, who would fill the newspaper's pages with the hospital's publicity and advertising.

The Beth's transformation was undertaken by board president Frank Liveright; Max Danzis, chief of the medical staff; Israel J. Rachlin, chair of the building committee; and hospital superintendent Paul Keller. In Liveright, the hospital had a dynamic president with strong community ties and access to funding; in Danzis, an articulate and forceful chief of the medical staff; in Rachlin, a physician whose father was in the construction business; and in Keller, an administrator with a knowledge of the social sciences and of public health priorities, as well as other tools cherished by progressive-minded professionals. Keller could envision what was best for a community's health and to formulate a rational plan for making it a reality.

The cadre of businessmen who would lead the campaign was well-grounded in Newark. Felix Fuld, Louis Bamberger's partner and brother-in-law, was one of the leading philanthropists of the city who attributed his financial success to one concept: "looking ahead to see what people want; then giving it to them."[34] Beth Israel Hospital board member Michael Hollander, the son of Newark furrier Adolph Hollander, took a leave from the international family business of fur dressers and dyers to run the campaign; as he told Newark Jewry, he had found "a better business than the fur business."[35] Fuld and Hollander were joined by the diminutive Michael Stavitsky, who held a graduate degree in social work and had acquired extensive experience in fund-raising campaigns for Jewish charities while developing his own real estate business interests in Weequahic.[36] Stavitsky had previously directed fund-raising campaigns in Nashville, Kansas City, St. Louis, and Philadelphia, and may have been responsible for the creation of the image of "Miss Beth Israel" and its slogan.[37]

The editor of the *Chronicle*, Anton Kaufman, joined these seven leaders in centering Newark Beth Israel Hospital in the community's consciousness. Kaufman had come to Newark after his first paper, the *Detroit Jewish Chronicle*, had failed. A short man with poor eyesight, he rushed around the city selling advertising and conducting interviews, returning to his tiny office at 156 Market Street, where he would light cigarette after cigarette as he wrote copy—"features of Jewry the world over, editorials, society, and other news."[38] Kaufman wrote with a passion and exuberance that the English-reading Jews of Newark had never seen. If his language had a florid lilt and a flourish of the grandiosity typical of the Yiddish press of the era, Kaufman's content was increasingly different from the nostalgic treacle that all too often passed for Jewish journalism. His stories were less about the quaint Russians buying chickens at the Prince Street markets or the Purim balls held to raise money for charity and more about Newark's generation of Jewish men and women whose reputations as leaders were based on their involvement in institutions that melded modernism with Jewish values. Typical of Kaufman's inspirational pieces was a profile of Dr. Israel Rachlin's father, "Morris Rachlin, Master Builder," describing his modest beginnings as a cigar maker, his suffering through the economic panic of 1893, and his eventual success as the builder of the first apartment houses and homes on Clinton Avenue.[39]

The Groundbreaking

Even with the fund-raising campaign launched, a year elapsed before the hospital's negotiators could persuade Weequahic landowners to sell their plots for a Jewish hospital, a total of 450 feet by 680 feet. What was the difficulty? *Chronicle* articles obliquely suggested that some of the landowners were resisting a Jewish presence in their midst by declaring that the new hospital would demonstrate "the folly of anti-Semitism" and that the Jewish hospital was likely to be "a finer more tangible proof of the Jew's devotion to altruism . . . than a thousand speeches or printed arguments."[40] The Daughters of Israel attempted in January 1925 to buy a 5.5-acre lot on the northeastern side of Chancellor Avenue, two blocks south of the Lyons Avenue site, an even deeper incursion into Weequahic, but inadequate funding forced the women to abandon their plan to erect a million-dollar home for the aged near the new hospital.

The hospital negotiators eventually struck a deal; there would be a Jewish hospital in Weequahic after all.[41] But, Frank Grad's pavilion hospital design, used in the 1924 campaign, would not fit on the land plots acquired. Now Grad and Keller sought the advice of Dr. S. S. Goldwater, associate editor of *Modern Hospital* and the director of New York's Mount Sinai Hospital. The collaboration of Grad and Goldwater was expected to yield, according to the March 7, 1925, *Chronicle*, "something entirely new in the hospital field, and eminent authorities claim that it is the most wonderful layout for the hospital building." The revised plans that appeared in the hospital's 1926 annual report presented one tall skyscraper tower with stepped-back levels for solariums, flanked by smaller buildings and a tall smokestack for the hospital furnace.[42] The six-building complex would consist of the tower, a service building, an operating pavilion, a powerhouse, an outpatients' department, and a nurses' home.[43] The main building was set at an angle that made it look as if the "arms" of the nurses residence and service building encircled or embraced it. The rear of the tower would cast a shadow over a parcel of land covered with weeds and rubbish at the corner of Osborne and Lyons Avenue whose owner would not sell it to a Jewish hospital. Nearly twenty-five years later, when the Beth finally bought that lot, one board member commented: "While the hospital has no particular need of it, it was felt that we should purchase it for its nuisance value."[44]

Poking fun at the groundbreaking festivities on the rainy afternoon of August 17, 1926, attended by 150 of Newark's most prominent citizens, Anton Kaufman published a cartoon in the *Chronicle* and, under the pen name "D.S.," and an amusing pastiche of the ceremony. The attendees were a "Noah's ark of slick-clad, rubber-shod and umbrella-breaking amphibians," who looked on as Frank Liveright lofted a shovel full of presifted mud after a few brief words. Department-store owner and philanthropist Louis Bamberger, a "New Jersey merchant-prince," raised an U.S. flag three times to accommodate newspaper camera men. The mix of Jewish and Irish notables comprised an assemblage of "the Cohens and the Kellys," a reference to a popular radio program that dealt humorously with ethnic stereotypes and emphasized tolerance.[45]

The Beth was the first "Jewish" building in Weequahic, but would quickly be joined by other "Jewish" structures. As the hospital steel framework began to define its signature tower building, two blocks away, ground was being broken on Bergen Street between Lyons and Weequahic Avenues for a two-story building that would house thirteen ground-floor stores and four professional apartments on its second floor. Each ground-floor store would have an individual storage cellar, black and gold marble steps, and mosaic tiles in the vestibules. Stavitsky, the real estate investor, was convinced of the bright future for Jews in Weequahic, and in addition to building the shopping center, was erecting four special streetlights on the street corners to attract foot traffic from the hospital staff and visitors.[46] When the *Chronicle* began to run advertisements for the stores under the banner "In the Weequahic Section," they implied that Jewish customers were welcome and would not be treated disparagingly: "There is an air about the section that makes the visitor, bent on shopping or just looking around, feel comfortable and at ease. In its stores one senses that one is welcome to stay as long as one wishes and to purchase as much or as little as one chooses."[47]

Modern Medical Care for the Modern Hospital

Superintendent Keller had his own vision for the new Beth Israel to be an efficiently operated modern hospital that would marshal broad support to solve the health problems that affected Newark, especially its poor, working, foreign-born population. At a 1925 educational forum on hospital and welfare work held in Bayonne, New Jersey, Keller told his audience: "The hospital is to my mind, the most important agency in the public health program of a city. Hospitals are no longer isolated buildings for only the care of the sick, but the center of a community health program working and co-operating with the family doctor, the specialists, the schools, the recreation facilities, educational publicity, and all other health groups."[48]

Keller advocated a division of labor of professional, medical, and service personnel, using a business model as the way for a modern hospital to serve the community: "Hospitals in recent years have been gradually assuming many of the characteristics of a successful business enterprise and the board of managers are taking over complete executive control, so the doctors may devote all of their hospital time to the professional aspect of their patients." Paying homage to the progressive value of systematic and rational procedure, he continued: "In order to have systematic work done in a hospital, there must be some centralized responsibility and a proper gradation of authority of the men in the various departments. Physicians realize the value of such a procedure and are cooperating with the board of directors toward the perfection of this new business plan of management. This is what Newark Beth Israel Hospital is doing."[49]

As construction of the new Beth building continued, Keller made personnel changes that reflected the commitment to modern first-rate medical care. He hired two graduates of the Columbia University Teachers college: Sophia Morris to be supervisor of the dietary department, and Lenore B. Rubinow to head the newly created social service department. He elevated administrative staff positions, including housekeeping, engineer, pharmacist, and laundry supervisor, to executive status. Anticipating the demands of a 350-bed facility, Keller hired generously—porters, maids, waitresses, yardmen, plumbers, steamfitters, engineers, an iceman, and numerous watchmen for security. The hospital's revamped organization and employees increased expenditures almost 75 percent between 1922 and 1927.

The senior, adjunct, and associate medical staffs were all increased as well. It was an open staff, with new members admitted regularly. Senior medical staff served on committees addressing the examination of interns, nurses' training, social services, record keeping and standardization, and publications. There were now separate divisions: surgery, orthopedics, physiotherapy, anesthesia, genitourinary and proctology, medicine, obstetrics, gynecology, pediatrics, otolaryngology, phthisiology, dermatology, serology, ophthalmology, bronchoscopy, neurology, roentgenology, roentgenotherapy, dentistry, and metabolism. Keller singled out for special treatment those departments where demand was greatest, such as physiotherapy under Dr. Kessler, and orthopedics, under Dr. Szerlip. These divisions were temporarily located in a separate bungalow next to the soon-to-be-closed hospital, equipped with machinery for treating physically handicapped children and adults, the victims of polio or wartime injuries.[50]

The hospital also established a follow-up clinic managed by the social workers, so that patients could be assessed after discharge to ascertain if their treatment had been successful and if they were following doctors' instructions for postoperative regimens. Such clinics that extended the hospital's relationship with patients were a hallmark of modern medical practice. By the last years in its Hill site, the most impressive statistics were reported by the Beth's laboratory, where clinical pathology tests increased from 4,288 in 1922 to 13,174 in 1926, owing to the acquisition of state-of-the-art equipment.[51]

Campaigning and Construction

Such medical proficiency could be sustained only in an improved facility. Department-store magnate Felix Fuld had begun the first campaign in June 1924 with a soft-pedal appeal to key businessmen to match 60 percent of the contribution he had pledged for the hospital construction. His strategy was to approach "preferred prospects" first, more than a hundred Newark businesspeople and professionals, to solicit "the larger pledges" before embarking upon a general canvass. The Newark Jewish community embraced the campaign, officially launched with the image of Miss Beth Israel, making nearly $1.8 million in pledges by the end of the first month. Throughout the summer and into the following fall and winter there were special events to raise funds. At one such event, for which 500 tickets were sold, the Beth nurses cheered the young physicians who challenged the city's senior physicians to a basketball game at the Young Men's Hebrew Association. And as often happened in those days, everyone crowded onto the hardwood floor after the game for a dance.[52]

Early on in the 1924 campaign, Fuld publicly expressed his concern that the $1.5 million goal was too modest. At a fund-raising banquet, a surprised audience heard him predict: "That hospital can never be built for a million and a half. They want 300 rooms in that hospital and it costs $8,000 a room to erect a model hospital. That means $2,500,000 so that if they do not get more than a million and a half in this drive they cannot accomplish what they set out to do."[53] Fuld's data were on the mark. When the Beth's officers and Starrett Brothers, Inc., finally contracted for the erection of the new hospital, the cost was projected at $2,725,000. If the outpatient department was postponed, the cost could be capped at $2.5 million.[54]

Construction had to proceed through late December 1927, whether or not the campaign goal was achieved. Unlike the controversy in 1907, the contractors never halted construction, working with Dr. Rachlin as the construction site clerk-of-the-works, who in turn sought the advice of his father, "master builder" Morris Rachlin. The senior Rachlin, who had chaired the Building Committee in 1907, remembered well the financial problems that had halted the completion of the High Street hospital. It was the father-son team, with their practical knowledge of building problems and ability to interpret plans and specifications, that made progress run smoothly in the 1920s. Many of the subcontractors publicized their involvement in the *Chronicle*, such as the L. Del Turco and Brothers Company that had tiled twenty-seven New Jersey hospitals and had recently completed tiling the Holland Tunnel that connected New Jersey with Lower Manhattan. The companies completed their work with the pragmatic goal of doing what could be done with the cash in hand, and left the hospital site in late January 1928.

A 1928 photograph of Fuld, Stavitsky, and Hollander captures them on the brink of an effort to obtain funds to complete construction.[55] Fuld pledged $250,000; Bamberger, $100,000; and Michael Hollander, $60,000—all contingent on a successful campaign. Dr. Victor Parsonnet's widow, Augusta Parsonnet, used her considerable prestige in the community to chair the campaign's women's division.[56] When Miss Beth Israel reappeared on 250 posters throughout the city, the largest on a billboard at the corner of Broad and Market, the *Newark Star-Eagle* quipped: "After an absence of almost four years, 'Miss Beth Israel,' a charming young woman whose complexion is the kind gentlemen prefer, and a marvelously successful gold digger will return. . . . She returns with the smile of victory. She is now in a position to show Newark more than a promise. She has the completed buildings to show."[57]

February 1928 passed in a frenzy of fund-raising. Pledges soon reached $632,000 as promises came from every corner of the community. The campaign became a series of local dramas; for instance, a reporter noted tears in Michael Hollander's eyes when he announced that a Beth

Israel nurse had donated five dollars, her entire savings.[58] At the end of the month, nearly two weeks after the new tower building had admitted its first patient, the campaign was completed; the Newark Jewish community had pledged more than $2 million.

The Dream Realized

Prior to the formal dedication ceremonies, the new hospital was opened for a Public Inspection Week coordinated by the Ladies Guild, whose members dressed in nurse costumes as embodiments of Miss Beth. The public viewing days created a de facto procession, as nearly thirty-five thousand men, women, and children walked the two miles from Prince Street, through the streets of Weequahic, forming a queue outside the main entrance that stretched for blocks. The crowds produced the hospital's first admission when one woman fell on the steps to the front entrance and broke her collarbone.[59]

The February 18, 1928, dedication ceremony of the new Beth Israel Hospital in Weequahic was heard throughout the New Jersey and metropolitan New York area as a special radio program broadcasted by WOR, the Bamberger radio station.[60] Some traditional ceremonial rituals were repeated from the 1908 dedication. Rabbi Foster gave a speech, the Hazomir Society of the YMHA sang Handel's "Hallelujah Chorus," and Dr. Rachlin presented the symbolic key to the hospital to board president Frank Liveright, who then presented the key to Newark's mayor, Thomas L. Raymond, as a symbolic gift from the Jewish community of Newark to the city.[61] Mayor Raymond praised the spirit of toleration that brought together Americans of every race, religion, and creed. Edward D. Duffield, president of the Prudential Insurance Company, one of the most important institutions headquartered in Newark, told the assemblage and the radio audience that the true value of the building would not be measured in bricks and mortar and that Newark should recognize that the Beth Israel Hospital "is a civic effort carried out by a community that wants to render a service to all."[62] The *News* published a celebratory article, "Great Hospital Replaces Little House on the Hill," in admiration of the great modern hospital, but bidding a fond farewell to the first era of the Jewish hospital that had provided so many colorful stories for its readers.[63]

The last patients were moved from the High Street hospital to the new building on February 21, 1928, via a convoy of automobiles that traveled west on Kinney Street and turned left onto Clinton Avenue. In a few minutes, the patients would be carried into a skyscraper so new that the paint on some walls was still drying.

But the old Beth did not remain empty. Mrs. Henry Tepper, president of the Daughters of Israel Association, had gained permission to move seventy elderly patients into the building while the association prepared to buy the property.[64] A quarter century earlier, in 1904, sixteen women had met in the home of Blume Hollander to create a *moshav zekenim*, an old-age home, naming themselves the Daughters of Israel Association in honor of the women's group that had been so successful in establishing the hospital.[65] By 1907, they had raised sufficient funds to purchase the Eye and Ear Infirmary on Sterling Street. The next generation of the Daughters of Israel had replaced their shirtwaists and long skirts with the styles of the 1920s and would make their home at the corner of West Kinney and High Street.[66]

The first surgery in the Turco-tiled operating suite of the new Beth Israel Hospital was performed by Dr. Eugene Parsonnet, with the assistance of his father-in-law, Dr. Max Danzis. The procedure was a routine gallbladder removal, but the symbolism was critical. The memory of Dr. Victor Parsonnet was palpable to physicians in the gallery and the personnel, volunteers, and board members nearby. When his son made the first incision, the heart of the modern hospital in Weequahic truly began to beat.[67]

CHAPTER 4

A Modern Hospital Surviving Depression and War

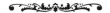

*I*n the 1920s, the skyscraper epito-
mized modern urban construction. In his 1929 report to the Newark Beth
Israel Board of Directors, President Frank Liveright informed his colleagues
that the opening of the skyscraper hospital tower in Weequahic marked the
beginning of a new era for Newark's Jewish hospital as a modern institution.
The tower not only spoke to the future but also created space for contemporary needs, increasing the number of beds from 120 to 350. And along with
growth came other aspects of modernity: increasing costs and administrative
complexity. A larger medical staff would be engaged; board members and
hospital supervisory personnel would have increased responsibilities.

The Beth was built during the golden age of hospital construction,
one of the 960 new hospitals completed in thirty-seven states in 1927. In
1928, nearly $300 million would be spent on hospital construction in
the United States.[1] In the week before the hospital was in full operation,
crowds of Jewish men and women from the Hill traveled to Weequahic to
see the new Beth. The *Newark Star-Eagle* offered a glowing description:
"Towering above the city, the great building stood like a sentinel in the
afternoon sun, as if challenging death and disease, its roofs of Spanish tile
glistened with the warmth of friendship; its buff-colored brick rising almost
200 feet from its foundation, became almost golden as the sun's warm rays
poured upon it."[2] The new Beth seemed to beckon patients to the hills of
Weequahic for care and cure.

In April 1928, the Newark Beth Israel Hospital was accorded the
highest honor that could be bestowed by those concerned with hospital construction: it was selected as the *Modern Hospital* "Hospital of the Month."
A full-length article describing the hospital was written by architect Frank

79

Grad and Dr. S. S. Goldwater of the New York Mount Sinai Hospital, who had been an adviser to the architect during the planning.

Grad and Goldwater's sentences sketched a structure geared to efficiency, yet aesthetically pleasing to the eye. The buff-colored brick building, a modified T-shaped structure, was placed diagonally across the lot to maximize sun exposure in all rooms. The edifice was set back from the street on high ground, so that the upper solarium offered a vista of the surrounding country. The main building windows "have wrought iron grills; the tower and patios red tile roofs reflecting a Spanish influence." A Spanish-style tower, specially constructed for wind bracing due to its height and elevation, housed the elevator machinery and water tanks supplying the hospital.[3]

The ground floor of the three-story outpatient building would be used for employee quarters, a central record room, a detention room, a pharmacy social services office, central waiting halls, and a large dental clinic. The design of this building allowed for the construction of a separate maternity building at the northern corner of the site. The main service kitchen was designed with multiple sinks and other facilities so that Jewish dietary laws could be observed should the board decide to mandate a kosher kitchen. The raw ingredients for meals would be assembled in the main kitchen and receive final preparation in the dietary kitchens on each hospital floor.

The medical service building included an ambulance entrance, emergency room, and receiving wards on the ground floor, as well as a separate operating suite and hospital ward for tonsil and adenoid surgeries.[4] A three-room isolation ward nearby had a separate entrance for the emergency care of contagious cases. The top floor of the medical building was devoted to four operating rooms, each with a sterilizing and scrub alcove.

Visitors to the new Beth would approach the south end of the hospital building, climb ten steps, pass through the office section, and cross the first floor to a bank of elevators. The impressive entrance lobby carved of Tavernelle marble with arches and decorative spiral columnettes and molded keystones would greet the patients and visitors; the reception room would have a large fireplace; and the floors of terrazzo, a composition of marble chips set in mortar and polished to a high sheen, lined the corridors and solariums for noise abatement. The first floor also had laboratory rooms, a medical library, meeting rooms, and a museum display room.

The seventh floor with its sun porches and roof promenades was reserved for children, "since sound hospital procedure requires that children be kept entirely apart from adult patients as a sanitary safeguard and for the comfort of the adults."[5] Upper floors were designated for semiprivate and ward patients, with a separate floor for private maternity patients. Delivery rooms were on the tenth floor, with separate suites for ward and private patients. The eleventh floor included another convalescent solarium and a roof promenade. Hallways were painted a calming light buff color; metal equipment was finished in a utilitarian gray. A two-pipe vacuum-steam system kept the patient rooms at 70 degrees Fahrenheit and the operating room and maternity sections, five degrees warmer. All rooms and wards would have telephone, radio, power outlets, nightlights, and nurse call buttons. Plans provided for a separate refrigerating plant with ice-making capacity that would circulate brine to all kitchen and utility room refrigerators throughout the building.

Why did Grad and Goldwater offer *Modern Hospital* readers such details? Like a sailing ship of old, the urban hospital building was a physical presence that allowed those who walked its halls to serve their patients efficiently and well only insofar as the building's design and capabilities permitted. Architects and hospital personnel who were designing their own new buildings wanted to know every detail of the modern hospitals being designed for physicians and surgeons at the frontier of medicine and celebrated in *Modern Hospital*.

From Visionary Blueprint to Cost-Cutting Reality

But the new Beth Israel Hospital complex that opened in February 1928 was not the hospital so extensively described and lauded in *Modern Hospital*. Nor was it the structure that hospital superintendent Keller had in mind when he considered administration and staffing of the new colossus. Grad and Goldwater had written an article that envisioned the new Jewish hospital; but the cost of their vision far exceeded the funds raised by the Newark Jewish community in 1924 and 1927, and even the pledges made in 1928. While the Newark newspapers focused on the drama of the campaigns, Dr. Israel Rachlin, clerk-of-the-works, and his father, Morris, instituted cost-cutting measures that affected the hospital's every detail in order to complete the items essential to the building's structural integrity and remain within the estimated budget. There are no reports of what Grad said when he toured the completed building for the first time, but when Goldwater inspected it, according to newspaper reports, he chose his words carefully, commending the building for "its cleanliness."[6]

The extent of the cost-cutting measures quickly became evident. Keller wrote to the Beth's board in April 1928 that the paint was peeling off the walls due to the poor ventilation of the tower building.[7] The hospital's engineers and maintenance crews themselves had to finish constructing pasteurizing rooms, laundry facilities, and storage areas.[8] Soon both boilers needed to be replaced.[9] Liquids in the garbage settled in the bottom of the incinerator, producing noxious fumes.[10] The plan for the main kitchen and diet kitchens did not work, so the hospital had to construct separate food services, one to prepare kosher meals under rabbinical supervision and the other to prepare meals for staff and nonobservant patients.[11]

In addressing the deficiencies of the building, the needs of the patients came first and improvements for the benefit of nurses and staff were postponed. The heat and noise generated by the mangles in the laundry room and the lack of ventilation made it difficult to retain workers. When Keller recommended the purchase of a hood to alleviate the problem, the Administrative Committee postponed the purchase, pointing out that the need for a hood would not be as great during the winter months.[12]

The building that suffered most from the economies of construction was the Nurses' Residence. Keller had likely envisioned that the Beth Israel Nurses Training School would have many of the features of the Michael Reese Hospital nurses' residence: a seven-story building that offered its student nurses a well-furnished reception lobby with a Tudor fireplace, laboratories, a library, an auditorium, a gymnasium, and a rooftop garden.[13] In contrast, Beth Israel's Nurses' Residence was a bare, cold, sparsely furnished building with painted cement floors instead of linoleum, and an asphalt roof. With no covered walkway, the women daily battled rain, snow, and cold as they trod the muddy pathway from their quarters to the main hospital building. Five years after the hospital opened, the Ladies Guild finally finished furnishing the rooms and had raised the funds to cover the walkway.

The employees' quarters were entirely eliminated in the final construction plans, with devastating results. Had the hospital remained on the Hill, this economy would have had negligible impact; most of the employees lived in that neighborhood, and many rented rooms in nearby buildings the hospital owned. The move from High Street meant that employees could no longer walk to the hospital, but were dependent on streetcars and buses that did not run at regular intervals. Along with the nurses and nurse trainees, employees who needed to be readily available soon filled the Nurses' Residence, including dietitians, the night admissions clerk, and assistant director Paula Marx. There was no room for Adelaide Goldbeck, the nurse supervisor, who moved to an apartment near the hospital.[14] Hospital housekeeping and dietary employees who depended on the public bus and trolley system discovered that not only did the routes not run near the hospital but also the schedules were incompatible with their workday, which began at 6 A.M. In the first three months after the hospital opened, many of the employees stopped showing up at work. By May 1928, the Administrative Committee assigned a new member, Abraham Lichtman, to assess the new neighborhood for rental possibilities or the purchase of a property to house nearly seventy-five affected employees, but he was unable to succeed at either effort.[15] Meanwhile, other Newark hospitals took advantage of the Beth's problem and actively recruited the hospital personnel whom Keller had carefully hired and trained.[16]

Liveright's 1929 annual report to the board, which addressed these mounting problems, was overshadowed by the loss of the hospital's great benefactor. On January 20, 1929, sixty-year-old Felix Fuld died of the twin scourges of influenza and pneumonia. In downtown Newark, the flags were lowered to half-mast, the Bamberger Department Store closed, the radio station WOR observed a silent hour, and the Jewish community YM-YWHA center covered his portrait in mourning drape.[17] That evening, 4,000 spectators at the Max Schmeling–Pietro Corri boxing match stood silent for a moment in tribute to Fuld. Liveright even proposed to the board that the name of the hospital be changed to Fuld Memorial. The *New York Times* estimated that Fuld had contributed more than $2.5 million to institutions and causes.[18]

The Impact of the Depression

Ten months later, the economic burdens of sustaining a modern hospital, difficult to bear in the best of times, grew even heavier. On October 24, 1929, security prices on Wall Street collapsed in a wave of frenzied selling. Despite the efforts of J. P. Morgan and a group of other New York bankers who pooled their resources to avert a panic, during the next several weeks the market and the nation slid down a slope of despair. By November, the securities listed on the New York Stock Exchange lost $26 billion, more than 40 percent of their face value. By July 1932, the *New York Times* average of industrial stocks had fallen from 452 after Labor Day 1928 to 58.[19]

Across the nation, more than a hundred thousand businesses would fail between 1929 and 1932. In 1929, 659 banks with total deposits of about $200 million closed their doors. In 1931, 2,294 banks with deposits of almost $1,700 million were failing at a rate of 200 per month. Industrial production plummeted, falling by the middle of 1932 to 51 percent of its 1929 level. Middle-class families saw their incomes shrivel, then their savings; finally, unable to pay their mortgages, many lost their homes.

In Newark, by mid-1930, "more than 7,500 families—about 37,500 persons—were on direct relief." The poor queued up to see the city overseer of the poor, whose office was in the basement of City Hall. Reports of "indifference and incompetence" led to his dismissal, with his desk still laden with unprocessed applications for what was popularly called "home relief." Between 1925 and 1933 more than six hundred factories in the city closed; payrolls dropped from $90 million to $40 million. As elsewhere in the nation, Newark men sold apples in the street, shoveled snow for pennies, and begged passersby for alms. In July 1932 alone, 38,000 Newarkers signed up for relief work; by the following January, 45,986 had registered as unemployed.[20]

Journalist Benjamin Kluger recalled, years later, "a long line of hungry men stretching across the downtown Military Park, moving slowly toward a soup kitchen where food was being doled out; a huge crowd of job seekers gathered in front of the *News* building on Market Street, waiting for the first edition, snapping up the papers when the newsboys appeared with them and then breaking in all directions with the Help Wanted sections flying in their hands: Oh for a job at the 'Pru' [Prudential Life Insurance Company, one of Newark's biggest companies], New Jersey Bell or Public Service!" Describing the plight of Jewish shopkeepers such as his father, Kluger recalled: "Customers who had always paid in cash pleaded for shoes for their children on credit and got them. Others wore their shoes to a pulp. The tenants who lived in the building my father owned could no longer pay their rent."[21]

The Great Depression opened up a huge gap between hospitals supported by tax dollars and those supported by fees and charitable donations, yet the American College of Surgeons 1931 report on hospital accreditation noted that "the economic crisis seems to have acted as a challenge to these hospitals to keep their standards higher than ever in order to give safe care for the many persons needing medical aid in time of financial stress."[22] Indeed, the United Hospital Fund in New York City reported that in the first seven months of 1931, hospital visits increased 25 percent over the same period in 1930. Data indicated that public hospitals were fuller, though paying patients many fewer in number. These tax-supported public hospitals were thriving, "besieged by people asking for free care because they cannot incur the expenses which usual incomes could meet."[23] By 1932, the country's public hospitals were overcrowded; beds were set up in their solariums, the open, sunny spaces being hastily enclosed.

The Newark City Hospital improved its service thanks to its thriving internship program, nursing school, and emergency room. The interns wanted to serve at the hospital because of the wide variety of "clinical material" they could observe during their twenty-month rotation; riding the ambulances broadened their experience even more.[24] During the Depression, one of Newark's city commissioners briefly considered securing a federal loan to replace its overcrowded City Hospital with a 1,200-bed facility, utilizing Frank Grad's original pavilion design for the expansion of the Beth Israel Hospital.[25] The plans were set aside when all the voluntary hospitals banded together "for the purpose of considering the extent of the effect which the increased capacity of the proposed new hospital would have upon the status of our private charitable hospitals."[26]

No major hospital closed its doors in the Depression.[27] In contrast, a survey of ninety-one voluntary general hospitals revealed that from January 1929 to December 1932, their average bed census dropped from 72 to 52 percent.[28] In some of these institutions, entire floors were vacant. New buildings were left uncompleted or unopened when funding dried up. However, mounting utility bills forced smaller voluntary hospitals around the country to shut down, including the Bronx Jewish Hospital, which was unable to pay for food, coal, or electrical lighting.[29]

The Impact of the Depression at the Beth

Keller informed the board in October 1929 that in less than eighteen months of operation, the hospital had treated more than 25,000 patients, "most of whom live in Newark and of this number, more than 10,000 were bed patients, of which 4,942 were operative [surgical] cases." Keller estimated that the free ward service in 1929 had averaged $17,379 per month or approximately $208,548 per year. In addition, free clinical service would be $25,000 per year, bringing the total free service to $225,000. The payment of these charitable expenses would be covered by the annual allotment of $180,000 he anticipated receiving from the Newark Community Chest, and the balance of $45,000 from paying patients in private and semiprivate rooms.[30]

But within a year, evidence of the impact of the Great Depression began to appear. The 1930 Laboratory Department report, while glowing and optimistic, contained a cautionary note that research begun in 1930 was halted because of the change in the economic climate.[31]

The board "held in abeyance" the hiring of additional professional social workers, which greatly delayed the process of admission to the hospital. Professional social workers performed the important preadmission financial interviews, reviewing with each incoming hospital patient both the initial diagnosis and prospective treatment during the hospital stay and the financial means of the person, based on income and family situation. Thus, the social workers had to possess a knowledge of medical terminology and of the scope of medical services that might be performed, and the skills to assess the ability of the individual and family to pay for services. The Social Service Department developed a sliding scale of payments for patients who were not able to afford private or semiprivate rooms at the time of admission, ranging from full ward rate to gradual reductions to free admission. Some patients were initially admitted to semiprivate rooms, then transferred to wards as their ability to pay diminished.[32] The social workers also served in the outpatient clinics, where they assessed the ability of individuals to pay for private medical care, eyeglasses, dentures, medications, and burials. At the Beth, the social workers received clerical assistance from the Ladies Guild Auxiliary members.[33]

The Depression-era experiences of hospital social workers were aptly described by Bessie Glassman, head of the Department of Social Work at Jewish Hospital in St. Louis: "The head of the family . . . begins to worry, cannot eat or sleep, grows nervous and irritable, suffers from indigestion, loses weight, and finally is persuaded by his equally worried wife to go to the clinic. While the doctor may relieve insomnia and indigestion, he cannot remove the real causes of the illness, which are unemployment and financial insecurity."[34]

The Beth, like many other voluntary hospitals, charged its patients an "all-inclusive" rate, that is, one rate covered room and board, nursing service, diagnostic X-rays, laboratory tests, electrocardiograms, physiotherapy, hospital formulary drugs, and surgery, including the administration of anesthesia. To be admitted, a patient was required to pay in advance for twelve days for surgical cases, and seven days in medical cases. A patient was separately billed for special therapies, including oxygen, radiation, intravenous pyelography, bronchoscopy, vaccines, and both blood transfusion and the services of the blood donor. The schedule of all-inclusive service for maternity patients was the same as medical, for both mother and child. T and A (tonsils and adenoids) patients paid an extra five dollars for the services of the hospital anesthetist. Bone fractures were an all-comprehensive cost of fifteen dollars, with additional charges for plasterwork.[35] Each patient was required to pay a portion of the charges in advance of admission based on the physician's diagnosis of the condition for admission, but once admitted, treatment could encompass more than this diagnosis and quickly become very expensive for the hospital.

The Compensation Bureau of the Newark Beth Israel Hospital filed liens upon discharge if patients' bills were not resolved during the hospital stay, following up "systematically for collection, turning over such accounts as necessary to the collector or to an attorney for legal procedures."[36] In January 1931, the bureau reported an accelerating debt in unpaid hospital charges: $3,846.08 from 1928, $23,447 from 1929, and $32,489.69 from 1930. The most troubling drop showed up in the monthly collections, from $3,457.25 at the beginning of 1931 to $803.90 by the end of the year—unpaid bills were growing exponentially.

The economic downturn spurred consolidations or amalgamations of hospital operations. Dr. Lee K. Frankel, a health-care expert and vice president of the Metropolitan Life Insurance Company, contributed this caveat in the introduction to the Beth Israel Hospital Annual Report of 1930: "Changes are taking place. Those of you who have watched have seen that, following the example of business and industry, there has been a tendency toward consolidation or merger of hospitals."[37] Frankel's observation of this trend, which had begun in 1929 at the onset of the Depression, coincided with the 1930 publication of Dr. Joseph Chapman Doane's survey of Newark hospitals that had been commissioned by the late Felix Fuld.[38] Doane criticized the city's small specialty hospitals and recommended their melding or amalgamation into the newer modern general hospitals. In 1929, New York City had consolidated twenty-two hospitals into a single organizational municipal department, while Columbia-Presbyterian Hospital had absorbed Babies Hospital, New York Neurological, Herman Knapp Eye, and New York Orthopedic.[39]

Many amalgamations merged smaller maternity hospitals into the large general hospitals erected in the 1920s. A month before Doane's report came out, the Jewish Maternity Hospital in Philadelphia was absorbed by Mount Sinai Hospital, which offered within its new building state-of-the-art maternity facilities.[40] Doane's report had especially harsh criticism for Newark Jewish Maternity Hospital, "a specialty hospital inadequately housed and improperly organized, its superintendent having harmful limitations of authority and prerogatives and its scientific atmosphere depressed by the need of radical improvements in research work."[41] The report concluded that the Jewish Maternity Hospital and the Hospital for Women and Children ought to be merged with Newark's general hospitals.[42]

Mrs. Abraham (Ruth) Schindel, the president of the Board of the Jewish Maternity Hospital, denounced the Doane report for serving the interests of Newark's general hospitals, whose beds were only 54 percent full, while the Maternity Hospital was operating at 90 percent of capacity.[43] In 1930, the Maternity Hospital had the lowest maternal and infant mortality rate in Newark. Schindel feared that moving maternity cases to a general hospital would unnecessarily increase the risk of infection to mothers and babies. But the Great Depression was bearing down on the Newark Jewish community, and the Maternity Hospital's all-female board faced the inevitability of amalgamating with the Beth. As the agreement plans were prepared, Schindel continued to insist that "maternity cases should be separately housed and managed to avoid the spread of infection."[44] The Beth's architectural plan as described in *Modern Hospital* had provided for the future construction of a separate maternity building, but the economic downturn precluded new construction. Instead, one floor of Beth Israel Hospital's main building would be designated as the Newark Maternity Hospital Department. The 1931 merger included the appointment of the Maternity Hospital physicians to expand the Beth's obstetrical service. Sadly, Schindel's concerns were realized in 1937, when an outbreak of diarrhea in newborns shut down the Maternity Hospital floor for three weeks to be completely emptied, painted, and renovated.[45]

In September 1931, a special committee of the Beth Israel board recommended reducing the operating expenses of the entire hospital "with the least possible detriment to patient care." The committee proposed eliminating routine laboratory procedures whenever possible, all laboratory research, all special diets for patients unless directly related to their health, and the number of resident house staff and social workers.[46] These recommendations were carried out, along with more curtailments, which included closing the hospital's second floor, thereby eliminating thirty-six ward beds, one operating room, and an isolation ward.

The Ladies Guild and the Maternity Auxiliary

While the Beth's hospital committees focused on reductions and curtailments of services, its two women's volunteer groups focused on generating income. The Ladies Guild members volunteered to assist the professional social workers; a special course was created for them, taught by hospital staff, so that they could competently perform duties on each ward floor and in the admissions office, work that raised their awareness of the specific needs of nurses and patients. The Ladies Guild also initiated a pension fund for disabled nurses and raised money to buy specific items for the hospital, including an infant respirator, a multitherm machine for cancer treatment, textbooks for student nurses, new furniture and linoleum for the Nurses' Residence, and ultimately the covered walkway to the hospital. They formed a transportation corps to bring patients to the hospital, provided a weekly movie for the children's ward, and supplied a nursemaid for families whose mothers were hospitalized. In 1931, three sewing groups churned out 12,000 linen items: patient gowns, linens, operating room materials, and uniforms.[47]

In March 1931, the former board of the Maternity Hospital reorganized themselves as the Beth Israel Hospital Maternity Auxiliary, toured their new venue, and then regrouped for a planning session at the Kresge Department Store tearoom, where ex–board president Ruth Schindel's husband, Abraham, was a general vice president and superintendent.[48] Shortly afterward, the Maternity Auxiliary sent a brief and modest proposal to the Beth Israel Hospital Board that granted permission to the women's group to open a little gift shop in a vacant room next to the first-floor elevator bank.[49] Opening day, November 16, 1931, every patient received an advertising flyer; every hospital staff member saw the advertising signs atop the lending library bookcarts that continuously circulated through the hospital corridors. Every person waiting for an elevator or exiting onto the first floor could admire displays of layettes for newborns, small toys, and special Christmas gifts that were positioned carefully to be seen through the shop's open door. The Maternity Auxiliary had already made sure that photographs of the shop were published in the *Newark Sunday Call* newspaper. They hired an experienced saleswoman to give the shop a professional quality for the customers. The Maternity Auxiliary would focus on negotiating agreements with wholesalers—who welcomed the free publicity—to display their donations.

Within a few months, the Maternity Auxiliary presented a second modest proposal to the board: to sell sandwiches wrapped in paper donated by the Kresge store (with its name displayed) and coffee brewed in an urn donated by the Washington Coffee Company. The Maternity Auxiliary convened again in the Kresge tearoom to evaluate the results of selling light refreshments and presented a third proposal to the board: could the hospital allow them to convert a vacant room near the gift shop into a separate tearoom where visitors and staff could pause during the day for refreshment and encouragement? Yes, it could. The tearoom met a need in the hospital that Schindel beautifully described:

> There the doctors and interns enjoy lunch, a refreshing drink or perhaps
> only a cigarette with their friends, and often a round table discussion

lasts for more than an hour. The nurses come in for a bite and a few moments of relaxation, and the members of the office staff too enjoy a short recess from the humdrum of typewriters and figures. . . . But those who are most grateful for our service are the weary, worried families and friends of patients, who are glad for the opportunity to enjoy a meal or perhaps only a cup of excellent coffee within the hospital building.[50]

At each monthly Newark Beth Israel board meeting, the Maternity Auxiliary presented a check from the steadily increasing profits generated by the gift shop and the tearoom. The women were gaining a reputation for transforming ideas into action, so when Rebecca Hoffman wrote to Liveright suggesting that the hospital create a Babies Alumni Club whose membership would be open to every child born in the hospital, he brought the idea to the Maternity Auxiliary. Hoffman proposed that each baby born at the Beth should receive an annual birthday card from the hospital, which would include a request for a one-dollar donation to mark the occasion and help support medical efforts for new babies born at the Beth.[51] Thus, the campaign "Born at the Beth" was launched with the hope that Beth "alumni" might develop into a large band of boys and girls who would grow up with a feeling of affection and responsibility that would translate into sustained financial support. The Maternity Auxiliary reinforced the theme with an annual June Babies Day in a nearby park, where the children could enjoy pony rides, Dixie cups of ice cream, and free examinations by the Beth's pediatric staff. The annual campaign event offered innovative preventive care: diagnosing and treating emergent problems presented by the young Beth "alumni" who were less fearful of the doctors and nurses in the nonhospital setting.

On the Brink of Bankruptcy

By 1932, the Golden Age of hospital construction and expansion had been reversed or obliterated by the Great Depression. The president of the American Hospital Association warned that there might be a complete breakdown of the voluntary hospital system in the United States.[52] Dr. B. C. MacLean, superintendent of the Touro Infirmary, the Jewish hospital of New Orleans, wrote in the *Bulletin of the American College of Surgeons* that before the stock-market crash "philanthropy became a business and, too often, business a philanthropy in hospital administration." He declared that in an era of overdevelopment and overexpansion, the boards of voluntary charitable hospitals had themselves to blame, for "the hospital machine, like a motor car with high power and no brakes, was traveling at a speed which inevitably would end in disaster. . . . The blatant voice and perverted genius of the advertising expert had captured the imagination of the country. . . . Individual vanity, misguided public sentiment, and myopic group patriotism responded to the appeals for funds. . . . Hospital economics sneered at hospital economies."[53]

The Beth, like other voluntary hospitals that had undergone expansion, now teetered dangerously on the brink of bankruptcy. The Beth Administrative Committee minutes suggest that the hospital could not pay routine bills. A produce dealer presented unpaid invoices in the amount of $10,000.[54] There was no choice but to reduce the ward capacity of 125 beds to 90 beds and to designate that 40 be partly self-sustaining, to limit the number of free patient beds to a maximum of 50; this policy meant rejecting a patient who requested free hospitalization when the 50 allotted beds were occupied, even if one of the other 40 was vacant. Only if the social worker and the patient could construct a budget so that payment of a portion of the daily rate of four dollars was feasible would a referral to City Hospital be averted.[55]

On May 4, 1932, Liveright invited the board members to a special meeting to discuss the lack of support for the hospital from Newark's Jewish Welfare Federation.[56] The Jewish hospitals that were able to be designated as a component entity of a Jewish community's philanthropic associations were able to weather the economic depression of the 1930s with a smaller, but steady operating budget. Thus, Pittsburgh's Jewish Montefiore Hospital, founded as a constituent part of the Pittsburgh Jewish Federation, continued to receive annual allotments. In Newark, Jewish organizations had functioned independently, joining together only in 1924 in the new Conference of Jewish Charities, under the Jewish Welfare Federation. The conference had pledged extensive financial support to the Beth during the first building campaign, but the increased costs of the new hospital had never been matched with increased contributions from the conference.

When the Beth's 1932 budgetary request to the conference was not approved, the response of the hospital Administrative Committee was furious:

> We the Administrative Committee of the NBIH express to the Conference of Jewish Charities our great displeasure with their apparent antagonistic attitude toward the Hospital and maintain . . .

that the Hospital is being operated efficiently as has been verified repeatedly by those who are in a position to know. . . . That we, the Administrative Committee of NBIH, desire a definite assurance that the Conference approves of the hospital management as presently constituted. If not, then one of two courses must be pursued—either the present Hospital administration must resign or the NBIH must be withdrawn from the Conference of Jewish Charities.[57]

The internal politics of Newark's Jewish community that forced Jewish organizations to compete with each other for limited funds threatened to injure the hospital at an especially vulnerable moment. By April 1933, the conference announced that it had to cut the May, June, July, and August allotments to the hospital by 50 percent, and then transfer the funds on a monthly basis only when cash was on hand.[58]

Touro Infirmary Superintendent MacLean's ideas for economies had included centralizing services, curtailing training for nurses, and cutting out care for World War I veterans, whom the federal government should send instead to private hospitals. But such measures would fall far short of solving the Beth's problems. By 1933, the hospital was borrowing from Newark banks each month to remain in operation. The crisis for the Beth was exacerbated by two major problems, apparent from the beginning of its move to Weequahic but still unresolved nearly four years later.

The first problem was the mismanagement of the Beth's properties near the old hospital. Liveright had made clear that in 1930, "we must get rid of our old property and put our financial house in order." But since the stock-market crash, the properties on High Street and West Kinney had remained vacant, unrentable, and unsold.[59] Their value plummeted, but the mortgages remained at the same high level. Instead of focusing on selling the properties, even at a loss, the board ultimately abandoned to foreclosure many of the homes on West Kinney and High Streets.[60] It was fortunate that the women of the Jewish Maternity Hospital had sold their building to a hospital for chronic diseases and merged with the Beth unfettered by a mortgage.

The largest unsold property was the old hospital building, occupied by the Daughters of Israel's Hebrew Home for the Aged. The Daughters had moved into the building almost immediately after the last hospital patient had been transferred to Weequahic, promising that they would purchase the building. And there they remained. In 1930, while a special committee was appointed to "thresh [sic] out the matter" of the sale price, the hospital paid the interest on the mortgage against the property, while the

Home was generating income. The original price had been set at $125,000, and the final negotiated sale price in 1931 was lowered to $85,000, with the Daughters of Israel managing to get agreement on a deposit of only $4,000, ironically the same sum an earlier generation of Jewish women had negotiated as a down payment for the Pennington mansion.[61] Two months later, the Daughters announced that they had sufficient funds to modernize and expand the old hospital building.

The second problem and the crux of the Beth crisis was the outstanding balance of unpaid pledges from the 1924 and 1928 campaigns. In the heady days of the 1920s, many members of the Newark Jewish community were swept up in the frenzy of the campaigns and made pledges based on a false optimism about the economy and the stock market. Between 1926 and 1928 the board had used financial campaign pledges as collateral to secure the building construction loans it needed to proceed with the 1928 structure. These loans totaling hundreds of thousands of dollars were further secured by the guarantees of a handful of financially able businessmen. Such a course was not at all unusual, but a method created in the 1920s and frequently used by charitable institutions for fund-raising.[62] The board did not seek the services of a professional collector for unpaid pledges until 1930, and even then, the method was simply a letter reminding those who had pledged of their commitment. By 1933, the pledges still unfulfilled totaled $789,000. In the midst of the Depression, prospects for full collection were dim.[63]

Now the board discussed consolidating loans, negotiating loans against the building fund, and approaching banks outside Newark for new loans. The absence of precise records makes figures uncertain, but the amount owed by the Beth to various banks and creditors by 1933 was such that the banks, also pressed by the Depression and the fear of failure, began to demand repayment.

As the crisis worsened, one board member emerged as a leader—Abraham Lichtman. He was the "son" in the Lichtman and Son Tannery, which specialized in making glove leather and whose factory was located on Frelinghuysen Street, at the bottom of the hill that ran up to Beth Israel's hospital tower on Lyons Avenue. Lichtman had quietly joined the board in 1927 at the behest of Fuld, who saw his business skills as an asset that the board ought to tap. Many decades later, Abraham Lichtman's son, Cecil, would recall his father's spending every day in the "dirty business" at the tannery, where hands, arms, and faces were stained brown, and then driving up the hill to partake of the "clean business" of the hospital.[64]

In May 1928, Lichtman had joined in the search for housing for hospital employees near the Beth. By 1932, he was a member of the special committee to inspect the operations of each hospital department, which issued a report in spring 1933 recommending possible reductions in force and consolidation of services. The committee suggested, in addition, that each worker take several weeks of unpaid furlough and a permanent 5 percent salary reduction. The savings of $4,500 per month realized from these measures helped, but not enough. Lichtman was firm in opposing any further reductions because they would compromise hospital care and threaten the institution's reputation.[65]

Lichtman's trips up the Lyons Avenue hill became more frequent, and the evening meetings longer. In 1933, he and the other members of the board learned that unpaid tradespeople who did business with the hospital had appealed to the banks, that their casualty company had canceled the hospital's compensation and liability insurance, and that the hospital had defaulted on its interest payments.[66] The Hebrew Maternity Aid Society, which paid twenty-five dollars toward the hospital bill of indigent Jewish mothers, began to refer these cases for admission to City Hospital. In the face of such crises, petty bickering erupted; board members could not agree whether to meet at the office of Louis Bamberger or at the Progress Club.[67]

Bank officers of the various banks to which the Beth owed money had met to discuss whether they should acquire the lists of pledges that remained unpaid and engage in direct collection tactics, as it was on the basis of these pledges that the banks had made the loans.[68] To stave off this assault, the Ladies Guild and the Maternity Auxiliary offered to collect outstanding pledges of less than $200, while board members went to donors who had pledged above that amount. When Lichtman was elected treasurer in 1934, he recalled, the Beth's financial position was critical; "in addition to the mortgage on the Hospital, we owed approximately $465,000 to the banks for loans and interest, and some $90,000 to our vendors for hospital supplies. The total owed was $1,664,000."[69]

The Great Depression was not the only enemy that the Beth and the Jewish community faced. In 1933, with German anti-Semitism on the rise, the Beth would no longer purchase goods manufactured in Germany.[70] In 1934, Friends of the New Germany held a rally a mile north of the hospital, at 717 Lyons Avenue. A "vicious attack" on seventy-five "friends" who arrived from New York dressed in bright blue Nazi uniforms swelled to a riot of a thousand, with "fists swung right and left, missiles flown, and men, grappling in individual contests, rolled in the streets."[71] Only two men were taken to hospitals for treatment—the New Jersey man was transported to the Beth Israel Hospital emergency room, but the man from New York City did not want to be taken to the Jewish hospital.

Early in 1934, the banks to which the hospital owed money contacted the guarantors, those who had agreed to secure construction loans with their personal assets. These twenty-two individuals, some of whom were also members of the board, had signed their names to ensure the loans, some without fully realizing the extent of their personal liability.

While Lichtman and Liveright were grappling with the implications of the liens being placed on the guarantors, they were simultaneously staving off an effort by Vice President Michael Hollander to take over the administration of the hospital and reorganize the hospital board. In early July 1934, Hollander drafted a letter outlining his plans for the reorganization in which he designated himself as the new president. Former treasurer A. H. Puder and Dr. I. J. Rachlin would be elevated to vice presidents, and Dr. S. I. Kessler would be treasurer. In Hollander's list, Lichtman's name did not appear. At the end of his letter, Hollander imperiously announced that he was leaving for a three-week trip to Europe and that he had designated Samuel Leber, president of the Conference of Jewish Charities, to deliver his letter to the board. Several days after Hollander sailed, Liveright received letters from four banks "demanding payment of our indebtedness within ten days under threat of bringing action against the guarantors." Convening an emergency meeting of the Beth's board for July 20, 1934, Liveright then contacted Leber and learned of the Hollander letter that had been left "in escrow" until his return from Europe. Wisely, Liveright refused to receive the sealed envelope when Leber offered it to him at the emergency meeting.[72]

With the Beth's future hanging in the balance, the board room crackled with tension. Meyer Augenblick, one of the guarantors, stood and addressed all: "I have received a letter and so far as I am concerned the letter means what it says. Either you gentlemen of the board will present a plan whereby we guarantors are protected or we guarantors will take over the hospital."[73] Mrs. David Laskowitz's warning of such a takeover twenty-seven years earlier in the Columbia Hall had proved prophetic. What could the guarantors do to save both the Beth and themselves? One solution proposed was to persuade their insurer, Mutual Benefit Life Insurance Company, to lower the interest rate from 6 percent to the range of 3 to 5 percent. Such a renegotiation would require all guarantors who signed the original agreement to sign a new one. However, the guarantors were anything but united on the issue. Some made clear that they would sign only if they could bring suit against any guarantor who refused to sign. And, indeed, one guarantor did refuse to sign: Lichtman.[74]

Lichtman believed it was possible to collect the unpaid pledges and put the hospital's finances in order. He ordered that the bank securities in the vault be checked and inventoried, that the deed to the hospital be examined, and that there be a new and detailed report on the state of uncollected campaign pledges. He then revealed to the board and guarantors the content of a supposedly confidential conversation with an official of fidelity Union Trust. Louis Bamberger had assured the banks that the board management was sound and that they would get payment on their loans.[75] A month later, Lichtman succeeded in negotiating an agreement with the life insurance company both to freeze the interest that had accrued in 1933 and to lower the interest on the mortgage, as long as the hospital was "carrying itself." An immediate $40,000 payment was made to reduce the principal owed the banks, the collateral securities held by the hospital were liquidated to pay off another note, and the stocks owned by the Beth were distributed to the creditor banks.[76]

On January 31, 1935, six months after the July crisis, Newark Beth Israel Hospital installed its first new president in twenty years. When Lichtman stepped forward to acknowledge the applause, he praised the Ladies Guild and the Maternity Auxiliary as the Beth's two "greatest assets" because of their tireless efforts to sustain the hospital in its time of crisis.[77]

Abraham Lichtman and I. E. Behrman

The change in leadership of the board and the high regard in which Lichtman was held yielded a cooperative response from the banks. By May 1935 all had agreed to reduce the outstanding balance of the hospital's debts by $250,000, nearly 25 percent less than the amount owed. To assist in reducing its debt, the Mutual Life Insurance Company would accept an amortized mortgage on the hospital's furniture and equipment. The hospital's building-and-loan stock would be sold, and a new group of guarantors contributed $23,750 that Lichtman promised to pay back from outstanding pledges. Bamberger also quietly contributed $30,000. By December, the hospital was up to date in paying its vendors and all bills were fully liquidated.[78]

That very month the small boxes (*pushkes*) installed throughout the new hospital in 1928 were removed; a card on top of each box, which had an opening large enough to accommodate coins of all denominations, had read: "Contributions for the Newark Beth Israel Hospital." The hospital would no longer solicit charity from those visiting their family and friends.[79]

The nearly two thousand individuals who had not completed their payments received letters explaining that the hospital, while not unmindful of the conditions that affected all Americans, trusted that those who had heeded the hospital's call in its time of need would not fail the Beth. A new policy enabled individuals to make monthly installment payments on their outstanding pledges that recognized the impact of the depression.

Lichtman also insisted that the 118 physicians with outstanding campaign pledges fulfill their promises. Many came forward with apologies for their delinquency; however, he also encountered some resistance and acrimony from physicians who had made sacrifices and had suffered during the Depression. Danzis, after assuring the board that "the general character of our professional work has kept pace with the most modern scientific methods of medical practice," referred obliquely to the physicians' discomfort: "Parenthetically I may state that regardless of the disturbed tranquility that is usually the result of sudden administrative changes in any hospital, and which is necessarily followed by some professional friction, the medical staff never lost sight of its main objective, which is to give the best possible medical services to our patients."[80]

An attorney employed by a collection agency contacted the subscribers who did not respond to the letter, but Lichtman and his colleagues on the board decided to absolve others from their pledges—businesspeople whose personal fortunes had been wiped out and individuals who had been associated with the hospital from its founding and were now quietly suffering in poverty. Lichtman personally took charge of one outstanding pledge to ensure that few members of the Jewish community would ever know that Frank Liveright, who had served the Beth for a quarter century, had suffered a tremendous financial loss and was nearly destitute.

Years later, when he reflected upon his first term as hospital president, Lichtman recalled that "for the next nearly two years I spent a considerable portion of each day in the hospital. It was then that I received a real education in hospital operation. . . . There wasn't a single administrative department of the institution that didn't need correction. . . . It was only by constant application of time and effort by a few members of the board that the financial picture slowly changed for the better and the administrative functions of the hospital improved."[81]

In February 1935, Lichtman invited Joseph Baker, president of Brooklyn Jewish Hospital and chair of Long Island College Hospital, to be the guest speaker at his first board meeting as president. Baker, an attorney and not a physician, made clear whom he thought best able to run a modern hospital: "You are the trustees of the money that has been put into the hospital—you have no right to lose money." He urged the board to pay attention to two reliable sources of income, "surgical and obstetrical cases," because "if private services on these are off, you will run down hill." He urged the Beth board to create a separate medical board, composed of both doctors and lay persons, that would have final approval of physician appointments. Baker also recommended that the hospital discontinue the practice that enabled certain physicians to operate their own businesses in the hospital, presenting separate bills to patients for procedures and treatments not covered under the all-inclusive billing system. Specifically, he recommended that the Beth Israel department heads for Pathology and Anesthesia cease billing patients separately for their services; instead, they should become members of the Beth Israel staff and their services should be included in the hospital operating-room bill.[82]

As one scholar has characterized the situation, "The American hospital was grounded in the local marketplace of volunteers and physicians."[83] Baker was proposing that hospital boards insist that the heads of hospital departments be hospital staff and not operate a de facto monopoly in the hospital. When Beth board members asked Baker what they might say to a surgeon or physician who refused to comply, Baker replied: "I would say: The Board of Directors is making the rules. If you don't want to conform, leave."[84] When laboratory director Dr. Asher Yaguda refused to change his financial relationship with the hospital, Lichtman replaced him with Dr. William Antopol, a full-time pathologist for the hospital.[85]

The Beth board was galvanized by Baker's talk, recognizing that he was offering them a new way of thinking about medical services as revenue generators to sustain the institution. They needed to apply to the governance of the hospital the same standards of financial administration they exerted in their own businesses. Lichtman's appointment of Ira Schwarz, in March 1935, to reorganize the hospital pharmacy was consistent with this desire to effect economy and efficiency. Schwarz, who owned a chain of nine retail drug stores, promoted the assistant pharmacist to chief pharmacist and hired a new registered pharmacist. The new staff completed a careful inventory that in one year saved the hospital $3,300 in pharmacy purchases.[86] Even before Baker's talk and his own installation as president, Lichtman had initiated a major change in the hospital administration, quietly accepting Keller's resignation from the position of superintendent in late 1934.[87] The hospital superintendent left the Beth only when Lichtman had begun to steer the institution toward fiscal recovery, and he moved on not because he disagreed with the new president, but because he saw the future of health care in a fledgling New Jersey prepayment insurance plan that called itself Blue Cross.

In 1931, Keller had been president of the Essex County Hospital Council when it authorized the initiation of the insurance plan, which copied the Baylor University Plan.[88] Frank Van Dyk, the executive director of the council, had worked in a compensation bureau like the Beth's and recognized that most people who were not paying their hospital bills would pay them if they could. Van Dyk investigated the Baylor plan, which was designed only for university employees and collected actuarial data on pre-payment, and, along with similar plans, had been approved by the American Hospital Association. In 1933, the AHA Board of Trustees adopted a resolution approving of "the principle of hospital insurance as a practicable solution of the distribution of hospital care, which would relieve from financial embarrassment and even from disaster in the emergency of sickness those who are in receipt of limited incomes," and the AHA distributed a booklet, "Essentials of an Acceptable Plan for Group Hospitalization," that listed the seven characteristics of a good plan.[89]

In 1933, Van Dyk convinced the Essex County Hospital Council to launch a pilot insurance plan that offered employees of companies the opportunity to enroll. They would be eligible for up to twenty-one days of semiprivate hospitalization for ten dollars a year, not including maternity or dependents. The plan enrolled employers throughout the county, who could then choose their hospital. The following year, Van Dyk became executive director of the Associated Hospital Service of New York to enroll residents of New York City within a radius of fifty miles with no restrictions to occupation or income. One hundred hospitals that participated in the "three-cents-a-day plan" included Newark Beth Israel.[90] By 1934, Keller, who had encouraged Van Dyk, now wanted to work for his organization.

Lichtman did not immediately replace Keller but made assistant director Paula Marx acting superintendent and assigned her an apprentice on executive loan from Bamberger's Department Store, Isadore Ellis (I. E.) Behrman. Behrman joined the House and Plant Committee, gradually increasing his hours at the hospital under Marx's tutelage until he became superintendent in January 1937. A trained engineer and an experienced supervisor, he inspired loyalty in his employees; some worked under his leadership for a quarter century. The Maternity Auxiliary minutes recorded that Behrman and his department heads often had lunch in the hospital tea-room, where their table resounded with laughter.[91]

But all the skilled management of Lichtman and Behrman, and all the efforts of Beth physicians, could not save Dorothy Lichtman.[92] In 1939, the hall outside the women's ward displayed a new bronze plaque in her mem-ory. Her husband, who had saved the hospital, learned the limits of medi-cine and the need for medical research. By 1939, the institution, Beth Israel Hospital, had survived the U.S. Depression and its own financial disaster. Nor was Lichtman the only one of the Beth's benefactors to suffer a per-sonal loss after laboring long and hard to save the hospital. Maternity Auxiliary head Ruth Schindel was widowed that same year when her fifty-three-year-old husband suffered a heart attack and died in Beth Israel.[93]

The Beth during Wartime

Shortly after his wife's death, Lichtman embarked on his first vaca-tion in many years: a trip to Europe in April 1939. The trip was both a heal-ing and sobering experience for him; what he saw overseas hardened his resolve to prepare the hospital for wartime conditions.

For U.S. hospitals, preparations for war began nearly a year before the December 7, 1941, attack on Pearl Harbor. In October 1940, the American Hospital Association held a symposium on the role of the civil-ian hospital in the preparation for national defense. East Coast hospitals were urged to make their operating rooms bombproof, to increase the reserve in their blood banks, and to train volunteers to replace the staff who would be drafted.[94]

The Beth had forged ahead in its preparations. At the January 1940 annual meeting, Lichtman placed the hospital in national context: "While all hospitals have detailed problems particularly their own, national and state policies are likely to loom large in the coming year and hold broad significance for the entire field. No individual institution can hope to be immune from their far-reaching consequences." In May, the Beth was des-ignated one of seven New Jersey hospitals to begin preparation in case of a "national emergency."[95]

Throughout 1940 and 1941, the New Jersey Examining Board used hospital facilities to examine military draftees.[96] Senior medical staff began to rotate into periods of service at military installations; Dr. Aaron Parsonnet served for a month at the Naval Base Hospital, Philadelphia.[97] As for the junior medical staff, internship at the Beth was reduced to one year

to be consistent with the Selective Service policy to issue one-year defer-
ments to medical students to "enable them to complete one year of internship."[98] By January 1941, Lichtman told the board that in addition to
serving the sick of the Newark community, "our hospital has prepared to do
its share in the country's defense program and has arranged to handle any
emergencies caused by increased industrial activity."[99]

By March 1941, the doctors who held reserve commissions reported
for active duty. Almost as quickly, Newarkers learned that influenza had
broken out at Fort Dix, as well as scarlet fever and spinal meningitis. There
were also concerns about sabotage. In August, more than fifty persons in
Kearny, New Jersey, were overcome by chlorine fumes and the most seriously hurt workers were hospitalized at the Beth. Three FBI agents were
dispatched to investigate but, fortunately, traced the fumes to a leaky pipe
used to pump liquid.[100]

In the board minutes, there are no direct references to the U.S. declaration of war; but the December 22, 1941, minutes refer to Lichtman's
action to secure bomb insurance because the federal government would
reimburse a maximum of only $100,000 for damages from bombardment,
and the hospital was located scarcely a mile north of the Newark airport,
now leased to the military as a training field.[101] The Beth was designated in
1943 as a depository for frozen blood plasma to be used in case of an enemy
attack.[102] And it would become in May 1944 one of the thousand hospitals
selected by the War Production Board to serve as a depot for the limited
civilian distribution of the new drug, penicillin.[103]

Nearly 160 Beth doctors and dentists enlisted in the medical corps,
untold numbers of Beth hospital staff and technicians enlisted or were
drafted, and the Beth's bed census was nearly 100 percent. How could the
hospital care for all these patients? It is estimated that one thousand Newark
Jewish men and women stepped into the positions vacated by the enlisted
and the drafted, volunteering hours of work in addition to their own jobs
during the war years. Red Cross volunteers were able to assume some of
the nursing duties, but in 1943, the chief relief for the Beth graduate nurses
came from a grant to create a Cadet Nurse Corps, which guaranteed a steady
supply of student nurses on site.[104]

Superintendent Behrman fought the battle of peeling paint in a poorly
ventilated building that was beginning to show its wear and tear. In
December 1941, the House Committee had presented a three-page list of
needed physical improvements and repairs to superintendent Behrman,
who directed his staff to complete them despite dwindling resources.[105]

He spent nearly four thousand dollars in 1942 to repair and repaint the interior walls, as the hospital's costs skyrocketed and inflation drove prices ever higher. Sophie Morris, the director of dietary, fought a daily battle of pennies per serving to provide 1,000 meals to 350 patients as the cost of food increased nearly 19 percent, and her dietary workers were drafted into military service.[106]

By the end of 1943, admissions had dropped at the Beth, as at other hospitals. November admissions had decreased 15 percent, with a drop of 21 percent in private room occupancy and 24 percent in ward admissions. The birth census fell for the obvious reason that men were away at war. In Behrman's opinion, elective surgeries and treatments were being delayed because few wanted to forgo even a week of the high salaries they were earning during wartime.[107]

Despite a lower bed census, the Beth realized in 1943 a $90,750 net profit from operations, including capital and endowment income, a substantial increase over 1942's $74,172. By January 1944, Lichtman could report that 1943 had been the hospital's most economically successful year in its history. He also noted that a greater percentage of patients were assessed by the social workers to b e able to pay the full all-inclusive rate "because of the general improvement in economic conditions."[108]

Civilian Casualties

Anton Kaufman was unable to sustain the *Jewish Chronicle* by 1942, informing his readers that the war had increased the cost of printing paper and that the dailies and weeklies were not receiving news of social and fraternal organizations. Later that year, he resorted to selling family grave plots to pay publication costs. His wife, Fanny, had died; three sons were serving overseas; and in December 1942, his fourth son enlisted in the army. The last issue of the *Chronicle* appeared on January 8, 1943, its borders framed in black. The official story, as reported in his newspaper and the *News*, was that sometime during the early hours of New Year's Eve, when the more fortunate were still making their festive rounds, the editor, in his home on a high floor of the Robert Treat Hotel, had mistaken the bay window for a door and fallen eight stories to his death. The Beth and the Newark Jewish community had lost their chronicler.

Nor was the newspaperman the only friend the Beth lost during these years. In December 1943, a pale man in pain, fifty-two-year-old Paul Keller, hailed a taxi on Madison Avenue in New York City, and asked the driver to head for the nearest hospital. Keller died of a massive heart attack in the back seat as the cab sped through the streets.[109] Louis Bamberger died in 1944, followed shortly afterward by his sister, Caroline B. Frank Fuld, the widow of both Louis Frank and Felix Fuld. Newark mourned these distinguished individuals, renowned for their generosity to the community. A bachelor, Bamberger reserved his largest single bequest for the Beth—an unrestricted $200,000.[110] His sister's bequest to the hospital was $100,000, and with their combined legacies, the board in December 1944 paid off the Beth's mortgage.[111]

"Now Is the Testing Time"

The successful Allied landing on Normandy Beach in June 1944 meant that the restrictions for hospitals would be relaxed. More hospital facilities would be needed to care for returning wounded and civilians suffering industrial accidents as the push to victory escalated. The Beth began the construction of a three-story addition that would create a lower-level space for central supply and storage rooms and a top-floor lecture hall.[112] In the next year, the ninth floor and two wings of the third would be converted to private and semiprivate rooms, as veteran nurses returned from military service to attend inpatients.[113] The Beth, a voluntary nonprofit hospital, would finance the construction of its addition solely with its own funds and loans, without federal government assistance. However, hospitals increasingly were turning to public funding for their expansions, a trend that would continue over the coming decades.

In 1945, the American Hospital Association issued a special report, *The Individual Hospital*, noting that "as the avalanche of war against our enemies has come to an abrupt halt, we find ourselves facing into that dreaded and desired era, 'The Post War World.' " The report contended that in the later years of the Depression and during World War II, the years 1935 to 1945, a startling change had taken place in the structure of health care in the United States. Blue Cross plans that had covered a hundred thousand Americans in 1935 covered nearly 19 million in forty-three states in 1945. It was time to recognize that a shift from the local community to active planning at the local, state, and national levels had taken place in other institutional arenas, and to expect the nation to show "an increased appreciation of the value of state-wide planning, stimulated, assisted and even guided from the national level." The AHA report described the impact of the impending legislation that would come to be known as the Hill-Burton

Act, the startling prospect of nearly $1.2 billion in federal funds allocated for new hospital construction, which should create nearly a hundred thousand new jobs, facilitate the purchase of $40 million worth of new equipment, and increase the number of U.S. hospital beds by an estimated 40 percent.[114]

Dr. Joseph Chapman Doane, who had surveyed the Newark hospitals in 1929 and served as president of the AHA, declared in the report: "Now is the testing time for the hospital. Now decisions must be made that will determine whether it will choose to use wisely the contributions which wartime science has placed before it or whether it will be content with the traditions of the past."[115]

Doane compared the typical architecture of prewar hospitals—Tudor, Gothic, Spanish, and art deco, with ornate solariums and marble entrance lobbies—to the nautilus, a mollusk with a pretty shell that hid an ugly body. In the future, the function of the hospital would dictate its form, and new hospitals would be built based solely on regional need; neither a new hospital nor an expansion of an existing hospital should be motivated by the desire to preserve a family name or to propagate a religious belief. Future state or federal authorities should reject such motives; only proven community need should justify hospital construction.

For Doane, the founding of voluntary hospitals by associations, legacies, and religious orders was over. Provision of health care in the second half of the twentieth century would be accomplished through regional planning, which would take into special consideration the needs of rural areas lacking hospitals, as well as of cities that often had many hospitals but few of high quality.

During the period between 1928 and the end of World War II, Lichtman and Behrman had navigated the hospital past the Scylla and Charybdis of financial ruin during the Great Depression and years of wartime privations, including the reduced personnel and redirected resources required of a nation fighting foreign foes. They could rightly take pride in the hospital's recent past. But, Doane warned them, they would be judged on their future, not on their past, and the problems of the second half of the twentieth century would be far different than the ones that had been faced in the Beth's boardroom during the previous decades.

CHAPTER 5

Medicine at the Beth, 1928–1947

*A*t noon, on May 15, 1929, the switch-board of Sinai Hospital in Cleveland, Ohio, lit up with frantic telephone calls, alerting the Jewish hospital that its staff was about to receive the victims of the worst disaster "in the annals of hospitals." Within a few minutes a caravan of ambulances, taxicabs, delivery trucks, and drays converged at the emergency room entrance. "Men from all walks of life, in gray and blue business suits, overalls, even rags . . . butchers, grocers, sailors, brokers, and clerks" carried the injured and dying into the hospital. Teams of nurses, interns, physicians, janitors, and scrubwomen worked at each bedside to treat the burns and administer artificial respiration. Interns rushed from other hospitals to Sinai, which had received nearly all the victims and was depleting the city's oxygen supply.

In the basement of the Cleveland Clinic, sometime early that morning, an exposed light bulb began to heat a stack of X-ray films in a storage room already piled high with more than seventy thousand nitro-cellulose X-ray films. At 11:30 A.M., the film ignited and exploded, shattering the inner walls and floors and sending upward plumes of fire and "instant death" as nitrous oxide, bromine, and chlorine gases filled the building. Eyewitnesses reported that, "Physicians, chemists, and nurses fell with instruments, charts, and test tubes in their hands . . . screaming figures on the roof were dimly seen through rolling orange-hued fog . . . piles of bodies were crammed into the stairwells and the elevator shaft . . . the faces of the dead and the walls were the same dark yellow color." More than 123 patients and hospital staff died that day "as the very instrumentalities of advanced science turned against their users."[1]

Two weeks later, Dr. Paul Keller entered the meeting room of the new Newark Beth Israel tower and knew from the anxious expressions of the

Administrative Committee that he had to allay their fears. The Cleveland Clinic tragedy had been a wake-up call to hospital administrators across the United States. Keller reassured them that because the Beth was a new hospital, there were no old films in storage, the current films were safely stored in steel cabinets in ventilated rooms, and plans were under way to construct a fireproof vault to meet the requirements of the Newark Fire Department.[2]

Keller then turned to the agenda for the meeting: the results of the May 6 survey for the American College of Surgeons completed by Dr. Fritjof H. Arestad. He announced that Arestad had recommended full accreditation for the hospital. Dr. N. P. Colwell, secretary of the ACS, had written to Keller, thanking him for extending his courtesy to Arestad and adding that Newark Beth Israel Hospital would remain on the AMA Council on Medical Education approved intern list.[3]

While the new hospital building did not match the architectural vision of Frank Grad and Dr. S. S. Goldwater, neither its structural integrity nor its medical facilities had been compromised; all had been built to meet the increasingly stringent standards of the ACS. In 1929, Arestad, a twenty-four-year-old graduate of the University of Minnesota Medical School, did not address the peeling paint and smelly incinerator, but the well-equipped and organized medical departments. His report began with an overview of the Beth, a 360-bed institution consisting of a "central eleven-story hospital building, an adjoining six-story nurses' home and a three-story outpatient department," as well as "excellent facilities available for the treatment of patients" and "excellent equipment."[4]

Increasingly, those who judged the quality of medical institutions expected fine laboratory facilities, critical for diagnostic testing and additionally important to those physicians engaged in an active program of research. Arestad found the laboratory "built and organized so as to offer the best type of service to the patients and to be of the highest educational value to interns, residents, and staff members." The lab was equipped for the standard medical diagnostics of the day, including urinalysis, blood tests, Wasserman tests, sputum examinations, and gynecological smears. There was ample facility for tissue examination, and the lab handled all blood transfusions from donors to recipients and basal metabolism tests.

Arestad judged the facilities for autopsies well equipped, and the number of autopsies performed in 1928 (320 patients had died at the Beth and 230 autopsies were reported) indicated that "the hospital is interested in scientific medicine and in the teaching function which it has assumed."[5] The Radiology Department had upright and horizontal fluoroscopes, a separate room for bone work, and cystoscopic X-ray facilities. Arestad noted that preparations were under way to initiate a radiation-therapy clinic in November 1929.

As Arestad reported, the Beth medical records system and its admissions records for its first year in Weequahic demonstrated that there was sufficient "teaching material" (patients with various illnesses and injuries) to approve the hospital for the training of interns. Internships were set at eighteen months and consisted of rotating services in surgery, medicine, obstetrics, specialties, and X-ray, and two months in the laboratory. Interns were allowed to give anesthesia under the supervision of staff. They also got hands-on experience in surgery and obstetrics.

Medical, Nursing, and Laboratory Services

Arestad's glowing report was due, in part, to the medical and professional staff Keller had hired. When Newark Beth Israel Hospital had opened its doors in February 1928, its 405 staff members were among the nearly 1.5 million persons in the United States engaged in the care of the sick: 143,000 physicians, 200,000 graduate nurses, nearly the same number of practical nurses, and nearly 191,000 midwives, physician's attendants, dental assistants, and pharmacists caring for patients in hospitals; and more than 500,000 individuals who provided supportive services, including the skilled engineers, painters, plumbers, and workers who maintained hospital facilities, as well as those in dietary and housekeeping.[6]

But although the ACS reported that the hospital had provided excellent facilities for postgraduate medical education for physicians, and dentists, Keller encountered the same housing shortage for these staff that other hospital departments were experiencing. Five years after the American Medical Association Council on Medical Education had initiated the medical education requirement for a one-year hospital internship, the 1919 publication of "The Essentials of an Internship" initiated the requirement for hospitals that interns should be accorded living quarters within the hospital and provided meals, laundry, and uniforms. By 1928, there were firm standards in place for the New Jersey State Board examinations for licensing of physicians and dentists, which included the criteria for housing. The architectural plans for the Beth had provided intern quarters on the third floor of the domestic service building, but the house staff subsequently "took over" the top floor of the tower building and trekked down the stairs to the wards and surgical floors.[7] The inadequate living quarters for interns, medical supervisors, and nurses also affected the dental interns. In New Jersey, dental students who had graduated but not yet passed the state board examinations could practice as interns in a hospital dental clinic—provided that they resided in the hospital. When two dental interns rented rooms in homes adjacent to the hospital building, the State Board of Registration and Examination in Dentistry asked Keller for an explanation of the infraction of the dental intern amendment to the New Jersey Dental Practice Act.[8]

Meanwhile, throughout 1928 and 1929, Keller had made modifications in response to the doctors' requests for changes in the new building that from their perspective might improve the quality of medical care. One early request was to convert a solarium into a patient recovery room, as it was important to supervise patients until they had recovered from anesthesia.[9] A first-floor staff room and library were merged to create a conference meeting room for physicians. A room on the third floor was outfitted with eight beds for those injured in industrial accidents. By November 1930, the increasing number of injuries requiring surgery led to the emergency purchase of an operating-room autoclave and to relocating the plaster, orthopedic, and splint rooms adjacent to each other for the combined staff of these departments.[10]

Well-organized hospitals needed well-trained nurses, and Keller knew the Beth Nurses Training School needed improvement. The uneven quality of U.S. nursing was a matter of considerable concern to the nursing leadership and many others in the health-care field in the 1920s. Were the hospital-based nurse-training schools capable of providing an adequate curriculum of education and clinical bedside training, or would an academic curriculum offered in a college setting produce better-qualified nurses? In 1923, a committee of experts chaired by Yale's distinguished professor of public health, C.-E.A. Winslow, and supported by the Rockefeller Foundation, shed fresh light on the entire issue. The Goldmark Report, named for its author, Josephine Goldmark, RN, included data on forty-nine community agencies and twenty-three nursing schools. The report's conclusions, ranging well beyond the data amassed, called for requiring a high school diploma for admission to nursing school and for focusing the nursing-school curriculum on education rather than on service on the hospital floor.[11]

On February 23, 1928, Adelaide Goldbeck, who had served as super-intendent of nurses for Brooklyn Jewish Hospital, became the fifth director of the Beth Israel Nurses Training School and Director of Nurses, embarking a year-long reform campaign to make her school a first-rate training program, in preparation for the 1929 ACS inspection.[12] As she surveyed notes, folders, and reports left by her predecessors from 1901 to 1926, she was appalled at the disorganization and incomplete notations, especially in student records that did not include classes completed, ratings, and service performed while in training. Hospital orderlies were instructed to take the stacks of worthless materials to the incinerator, thus destroying the history of the first twenty-six years of the nursing department and the school.[13]

Goldbeck increased the hours of weekly classroom instruction to meet New Jersey requirements, culling out the students who had not graduated from high school (nearly half) and those of insufficient caliber to complete the course work and qualify as registered nurses. Nearly two-thirds of the students were required to repeat classes. In her January 1929 report to the board members, Goldbeck promised that the Nurses Training School would accept two classes each year so that the hospital would always have a staff of student nurses, who could provide better service than some of the poorly trained graduates preceding them and whom they would gradually replace.[14] Over the next two years, she met this goal: the student nurses, all high school graduates, made up the majority of bedside nurses in the hospital.

Many of Goldbeck's reforms received praise, but she clashed with the Administrative Committee over benefits and vacation scheduling. In 1928, each department hired its own employees and determined salaries and vacations. By 1930, the standardization of salaries with graded scales for increases had finally begun, and the committee learned that Goldbeck's staff was receiving a more generous benefit package than were those of other departments. The Administrative Committee had decided that all hospital employees would work a full year before being eligible for vacation benefits of three weeks for nurses, teachers, and dietitians; and two weeks for student nurses and other employees. Goldbeck had instituted four-week vacations for nurses and other staff under her supervision, contending that nurses were medical professionals and so entitled to a different level of benefits.[15] The nurse scheduling left large gaps in supervisory coverage, especially during the summer months. Complaints mounted. In April 1930, Goldbeck resigned, taking with her both her administrative assistant and the furniture from her apartment; the Administrative Committee complained about the loss of furniture.[16]

Goldbeck's departure produced two positive changes. The Administrative Committee set up a chain of command for the hospital that guaranteed that, day and night, a single person would be in charge of the hospital.[17] The second change was generated by Goldbeck's criticism of the increasing amount of record keeping and other clerical tasks burdening nurses. The Ladies Guild, working with Adele Zweiman, the sixth nursing director, and Lenore Rubinow, the director of social work, created a training course that taught them to be "History Takers," perform secretarial work on the ward floors, and assist in the Admissions, Outpatient, and Social Work Departments.[18] Dr. Max Danzis, chief of the medical staff, praised these volunteers for supportive work that was invaluable to the overburdened medical staff.[19] The Ladies Guild volunteers who worked side-by-side with the nurses became their staunchest supporters.

By 1930, the Departments of Roentgenology (radiology), Obstetrics, Otolaryngology, and Physical Therapy had all grown substantially. Roentgenology now provided immediate emergency service and had initiated a new technique of intravenous injection for the visualization of urinary tracts and gallbladders. Misadventures occasionally occurred. When three radium platinum slivers, each worth $1,000, were mistakenly tossed into a wastebasket, a frantic search began through the hospital. Finally, four days later, the radium was found by painstakingly sifting through the incinerator ashes.[20] The Oxygen Therapy Unit operated a special oxygen chamber for the treatment of pneumonia. A new centralized Surgical and Sterilizing Supply Department supported the new Departments of Radiation Therapy and Plastic Surgery. A Department of Mental Hygiene to care for the psychological needs of patients was established under the direction of the New Jersey Department of Institutions and Agencies. The Physical Therapy Department initiated a nine-month training school, which was accredited by the American Physiotherapy Association. The Social Work Department was collaborating on studies with the American Association of Hospital Social Workers and served as a center for the New York City Training School for Jewish Social Work. There were also new clinics for asthma, hay fever, and sterility. The services of these departments were covered in the all-inclusive hospital bill.

A Scientifically Conducted Health and Hospital Institute

In his introductory essay for the 1930 *Annual Report of the Beth Israel Hospital*, Dr. Lee K. Frankel wrote that the hospital personnel should revise their perspective on the role a modern hospital could perform in the care of a community. He noted that the modern hospital personnel must think of "medical care in terms of modern thought, . . . in terms not merely of curing but of preventing disease and that the well-organized hospital with trained staff and with adequate facilities not only to cure, but to prevent disease . . . the nucleus around which much of our life-conservation work of the future will center."[21]

Keller put Frankel's words into action. He promoted the creation of twenty-five outpatient clinics for those who could be "treated in the early stages of their illnesses so as to prevent their becoming bedridden."[22] Chief among these clinics was the Michael Hollander Dental Clinic, opened on February 24, 1928, and named in honor of the fund-raiser and now vice president of the hospital, who had made the clinic the focus of his family's contributions. With its own X-ray section and specialists in anesthesiology, prothodontia, orthodontia, and periodontia, it was hailed as unique on the East Coast. The clinic offered artificial teeth at cost or, in urgent cases, free, for adults, and free orthodontia for children of poor parents. The staff also was committed to research, maintaining rounds for hospital patients, as they considered infection around the teeth to cause systemic infection.[23]

The American Hospital Association committee on post-mortem examinations reported at the October 1930 AHA convention that Newark Beth Israel was one of only thirteen hospitals in the United States and Canada not connected to a university that offered the proper opportunities for the study of post-mortem pathology. In addition, the department had created a one-year laboratory technician training school program approved for membership in the American Society for Clinical Pathologists; the program accepted only college graduates and preferred those with theoretical work in the biological sciences. More than ninety thousand laboratory analyses were completed, including for the first time quantitative urine analysis, a revolutionary change from the qualitative reports. The purchase of a lab-auto-technicon machine that mechanically performed the chemical preparation of tissues reduced the running time for analysis by a full day. Delays in transmitting reports were now the result of the stenographers' inability to keep up with the reports dictated by the technicians and the students.[24]

Felix Fuld's Legacy

The January 1929 death of Felix Fuld led to speculation about his legacy. In the early summer of 1930, a *New York Times* article reported that Louis Bamberger and Caroline Fuld, his sister and Felix Fuld's recent widow, would establish an educational institution to be known as the Institute for Advanced Study with an initial gift of 5 million dollars. The institute "will be established in Newark or its vicinity, exclusively for post-graduate work and scientific research. The institute would be coeducational, accepting members of all races and creeds and will provide facilities for research by eminent men of learning."[25]

The first director of the institute would be Dr. Abraham Flexner, the author of the 1910 *Carnegie Report on U.S. Medical Schools*, fueling speculation that the institute might ultimately include a medical school for Newark. Newark's *Jewish Chronicle* announced that the institute would initially be located on the Bamberger estate in South Orange, with its permanent home to be in Newark.[26] *Chronicle* editor Anton Kaufman added to the speculation when he interviewed Flexner and asked whether the institute would be a teaching institute for medical teaching and research. Flexner's responses were vague; he mentioned Dr. William Welch's work to establish a world-renowned medical institution at the Johns Hopkins University in Baltimore and then coyly noted that "he himself is not trained in medicine."[27]

As late as December 1931, Kaufman still thought the institute would be in Newark.[28] But in August 1932, it was announced that Albert Einstein, who had fled Germany, would be the first faculty member of the Institute for Advanced Studies, to be located in Princeton, New Jersey.[29]

The Medical Staff during the Great Depression

The physicians at Beth Israel found their professional work severely affected by the measures that were taken to respond to the exigencies of the Depression. In 1931, Drs. Aaron Parsonnet and Jacob Polevski, who would shortly leave the Beth to join the University of Pennsylvania medical faculty, could continue to operate their nighttime cardiac clinics only if they supplied their own drugs, nurses, and social service worker; the hospital would supply a cabinet for their medications.[30] The medical staff approved consolidation of services, and where no further staff reductions were possible, there were reductions in salaries. The Laboratory Department reduced salaries for its director, stenographer, chemist bacteriologist, tissue technician in hematology, and mortician. After promoting a round-the-clock, twelve-month program of service, the Beth now furloughed employees for at least one day a month and enforced a compulsory two-week vacation without pay for all.[31]

The Nurses Training School cut back to one incoming class, beginning in 1934. Zweiman, continued as the director of nurses, and also assumed the duties of clinic supervisor and obstetrical supervisor. All Nursing Department personnel took a further salary cut of 5 percent.[32]

The financial crisis was exacting a toll on physicians, who had many fewer patients, but "notwithstanding the limitation of hospital admissions, the character and quality of the professional work had not suffered," Danzis said at the January 1934 annual meeting. The physicians were publishing articles in respected journals, and a spirit of collegiality prevailed to the point that senior staff permitted junior-staff representation at their meetings. Keller, equally upbeat that January, said that although the economic stress was unrelenting, "the Hospital had managed to survive in a relatively good position" because of the "special effort on the part of the personnel," who had "maintained the standard of treatment." However, while praising the efforts of those who had sacrificed to keep the quality of care high, Keller cautioned that "any further cuts in service, salaries, or supplies would make it impossible to maintain the present standard of work."[33]

Dr. Eugene Parsonnet, Victor Parsonnet's son, recalled that in 1925, he was "lucky to have a guaranteed income of $300 per month" as a surgeon, half of which came from "assisting at surgery and the other half from caring for all the medical needs of 3,000 Italian, Portuguese, Spanish, and Polish employees of the Hollander Fur-Dyeing Company." In 1931, Parsonnet qualified as an ACS fellow and made the critical decision to devote himself to surgery at the hospital. His income was nearly halved, and his wife supplemented his salary with private piano lessons.[34]

In resolving the hospital's financial crisis, board president Abraham Lichtman had antagonized the physicians by dunning them to carry through on their pledges. Many, like Parsonnet, whose salaries were reduced sharply and who paid for materials and equipment out of their own pockets, did not feel that their new president fully understood their problems.

But the medical staff underestimated the dedication to quality medical service of Lichtman, the businessman from Freylinghuysen Street, and I. E. Behrman, the engineer manager who succeeded Keller. When Behrman officially assumed the position of executive director, his first report to the board members concerned the completion of a new animal house, necessary for research work; his second, increased funding for the Radiation Department.[35] Both Behrman and Lichtman realized that if the Beth was to survive and prosper as a medical institution, they must minimize the financial exigencies' impact on patient care, medical performance, and clinical research.

In July 1935, Lichtman carried out the advice of Brooklyn Jewish Hospital's Baker, and hired medical staff for an Anesthesia Department and, in December, approved a new recovery room with five beds.[36] His first concern in his 1936 annual report was the continuing problem of mortgages and pledges, but his second was patient care; he wanted additional funds for the Pathology Department and the Cancer Clinic, which were both receiving recognition in New Jersey.[37]

Research and Publication

The researcher who needed a new animal house in the 1930s was Dr. Rita "Ricka" S. Finkler, a petite woman with dark hair and expressive eyes, who described herself as a "small woman in a hurry."[38] In 1928, Finkler became the head of the Department of Endocrinology, with the title of associate in the Biology Research Department, assisted by Mrs. Friedlander, a full-time a laboratory technician, and Drs. Rose D. Bass and Zelda Marks. Medical research at Beth Israel was Finkler's third career. Born in Ukraine, she completed two years of law school at the University of St. Petersburg and then lived in anarchist and revolutionary communes in Turkey, Greece, Italy, France, and England, supporting herself as a tutor, waitress, and chambermaid. In 1910, she arrived in Philadelphia, completed a medical degree at the Women's Medical College, and in 1916, drove a horse-drawn ambulance through the city. Finkler combined her internship with postgraduate education at the University of Pennsylvania and began a thriving obstetrical practice, first in Philadelphia, then in Newark.

In 1927, her husband, an ardent Zionist, left for Israel. Newly divorced and mother of a four-year-old, Finkler gradually shifted her focus to the science of endocrinology as in the 1930s, "in the field of endocrinology rapid progress was being made and one was almost breathless trying to keep up with the new ideas and discovery sprouting here and there." Finkler was excited by the new studies of the effect of hormones on puberty, ovarian function, sexual gender, and hypertension. She first studied the effect of male sex hormone changes using capons: "I caponized roosters and later injected them with extracts of blood and urine of hypogonadel males. I sweated over the hypophysectomies until I could not straighten out my back or open my eyes. The work was precise, delicate, and often discouraging." Finkler was forced to discontinue this work after the cries of hormonally created roosters began to reverberate throughout the hospital at dawn.

Finkler then studied with Dr. Bernhard Zondek in Germany, assisting him and Dr. Selmar Aschheim in developing the first hormonal test for pregnancy. When she returned from Berlin, she immediately gave lectures on the endocrinology of early pregnancy. Her section of the Beth Israel Laboratory Department received a deluge of requests to perform the test. Sometimes, a female patient would bring a urine specimen to Finkler and say, "My doctor wants you to test it from A to Z."

As Finkler continued her work, she began to present exhibits at scientific meetings and acquired a camera, floodlights, and a screen so that she could take pictures to illustrate her presentations and articles. She was joined by a young Beth resident, Dr. George M. Cohn, who had also become interested in endocrinology, and they worked together to plan and organize the materials.

The excitement of bringing in the exhibit charts to the exhibit hall the day before the convention opened officially, arrangements for the carpenter and electrician to set them up in the booth had to be made and to watch your colleagues do the same with their exhibits, as well as discuss with them the best technical arrangement and lighting effects, gave one such a feeling of companionship and belonging that it was deeply satisfying. . . Colleagues would come and if the exhibit was attractive technically and instructive scientifically, large groups would gather and you were in your glory . . . and the applause was exhilarating like heavy wine.[39]

When Lichtman hired Dr. William Antopol in August 1935 to head the Pathology Laboratory, succeeding Dr. Yaguda, he acquired both a full-time pathologist and full-time researcher. An indefatigable Antopol produced a steady stream of articles in peer-reviewed journals, almost all coauthored with Beth senior staff, among them Finkler, Robbins, and Schotland. He also encouraged those at the onset of their careers, including Applebaum, Goldman, Robinson, and Glick, to pursue research studies in conjunction with their clinical work.

In addition to Finkler's and Antopol's research, Dr. Leonard Morvay, an attending dentist at the Beth and a dental consultant to the Rehabilitation Commission in New Jersey's Department of Labor, completed studies to determine whether infections of the mouth were the source of systemic infections presented by hospital patients. In 1936, a dental intern and medical intern together examined ward patients on admission when a dental foci of infection was suspected. Morvay praised Newark Beth Israel, where "a service of continuous [dentistry] rounds has been conducted over a period of seventeen years [and] hundreds of patients have received dental examination."[40]

Antopol hired Dr. Philip Levine for the laboratory staff in October 1935 as a serologist and bacteriologist. Levine, like many other Jewish doctors of his generation, was a Russian immigrant. Antopol and he had graduated from New York City's tuition-free City College, attended different medical schools, and as interns their paths had briefly converged again. Levine went on to work at the Rockefeller Institute and the University of Wisconsin. He worked with Dr. Karl Landsteiner, the discoverer of blood types, and became an expert on blood subgroups. By the time he began to assist in the Beth Israel Pathology Laboratory, Levine had authored more than fifty papers. In 1936, he was elected to the Medical Control Board of Blood Transfusion Betterment Association.[41]

By 1937, the hospital had established one of the first blood banks in a voluntary hospital. Levine observed a woman who hemorrhaged after delivering a newborn child with jaundice, swelling, and a fatal anemia, *erythroblastosis fetalis*. Analysis of the mother's blood demonstrated that it lacked an Rh protein—termed Rh-negative. Her baby had inherited from the father a blood type that had the Rh protein, termed Rh-positive, and thus its red blood cells were Rh positive. The mother's Rh negative immune system would identify Rh positive red blood cells as an infection and mount an attack to destroy the infection. During the pregnancy, the mother's and baby's circulatory systems had not mixed, but during the birth process when her Rh-negative blood and the Rh-positive placental blood mingled, the mother's immune system had attacked and destroyed her baby's Rh-positive red blood cells. Levine demonstrated that if an Rh-negative mother was injected with Rh-positive antibodies prior to the birth process, her immune system would not attack the baby's red blood cells and the subsequent birth and delivery of an Rh-positive baby would be successful. The unraveling of this mystery at the Beth would save countless lives.[42] Levine published his initial findings on the Rh protein while working in the Beth Israel Pathology Laboratory, but shortly afterward left to continue his research at the newly established Ortho Research Foundation in Raritan, New Jersey.

Toward the end of the decade, Lichtman noted that "the scientific standing of any hospital depends in great measure on the quality of its Medical Staff and its Laboratories. It can be said that a hospital is as good as its Staff and its Laboratories. It is with pleasure that I can say that the number of scientific papers being published by our Staff is ever increasing."[43]

The Jewish Hospital as a Portal for Jewish Doctors

While Drs. Antopol, Levine, Finkler, and others were publishing scientific research, Dr. Max Danzis, chief of the medical staff, was writing extensively on the issues of medicine and Jews, as were other Jewish physicians who felt the need to speak out on matters other than bench science or clinical studies. In 1937, a group of Jewish physicians published the first issue of an annual, *Medical Leaves*. Many of them drew on medical history as their vehicle to address the future of Jews and the need to consider the building of a Jewish homeland. Danzis would publish two articles—one on the need for residency programs in Jewish hospitals, and the second, coauthored with Dr. Charles Robbins, on the early history of the Beth Israel Hospital.[44] But Danzis's focus remained the history of Jewish medicine and the anti-Semitism practiced against U.S. Jewish physicians, which he had experienced personally.

Jewish medical students were often met with hostility, subjected to admissions quotas in medical schools, denied residencies in non-Jewish hospitals, and, after graduation, even refused hospital privileges. U.S. Jewish hospitals were thus portals for many young Jewish immigrants who sought careers in medicine.

In 1923, the progressive journal *Survey* said that Jewish hospitals were needed "to obviate the discrimination against Jewish physicians in non-Jewish hospitals." In Hartford, Connecticut, Dr. J. J. Goldenberg, glancing at the photographs of men and women on the walls of Hartford's Mount Sinai Hospital, bitterly remembered the indignities suffered by Jewish physicians at the hands of non-Jewish hospital administrators: "Jewish doctors had to put their patients on a list for elective admission to the hospital. Usually a week or two would pass before a gentile colleague would admit your patient and turn over the care to you, if you were lucky!" Dr. Arthur Wolff, who became Mount Sinai's chief of staff, observed that since its opening in 1923, that hospital had been critical "for the younger medical men of our city who for years have been hampered in the accomplishment of their surgical work."[45]

Yet despite the hostility, Jewish immigrants and the children of newcomers poured into medical schools. Jewish immigrants to the United States, whether from Germany or Eastern Europe, held medicine in the highest esteem. Russian arrivals, especially, craved careers in medicine because of the prestige and mobility they offered; in Russia, physicians had been allowed to leave the Pale, where most Jews were confined, and migrate to cities. In the United States, young Russian Jews saw in medicine social advantages as well.[46] German Jewish medical school applicants met with little discrimination until the 1920s; however, with the arrival of millions of Eastern European Jews at the turn of the century, quotas were imposed upon admissions both to medical schools and, at many colleges and universities, to undergraduate programs. In 1934, the secretary of the Association of American Medical Colleges documented that more than 60 percent of the 33,000 applications on file that year were from Jews. Historian of medical education Kenneth Ludmerer quotes one Harvard Medical School officer who described himself as feeling "overwhelmed by the number of Jewish lads who are applying for admission."[47]

By the late 1930s, rigid medical school quotas were firmly in place. As historian of medicine Leon Sokoloff observes: "A variety of indirect methods were employed to establish the Jewishness of candidates in the first place."

An initial pass through the applications identified Jewish names, especially in geographic areas known to have high concentrations of Jewish residents. In some cases there were data from applicants' colleges. Personal interviews allowed admissions officers to see the faces behind the names, as they sought to identify those Semitic in appearance. Eventually, applications required a photograph and answers to questions concerning religion and place of birth of father and mother. When Jewish groups raised objections to the question concerning religion, the schools substituted questions about the "racial origin" of the applicant, the mother's maiden name, and whether the applicant had ever changed his or her name.[48]

At some medical schools, the "problem" was not the professed religion, but the manner and style of immigrants, for example, the son of a "recently immigrated" Russian Jewish family who is "intensively aggressive and presents other personality difficulties," or students "who were born in Europe, or whose parents have recently migrated from Europe" and who "are apt to be an entirely different type, sometimes radical, sometimes asocial, often unstable."[49]

In Newark, Dr. Arthur Bernstein recalled the hostility he encountered when being interviewed for medical school at the University of Pennsylvania in the early 1930s. The dean told Bernstein, who had been an undergraduate at the university, that he did not have a chance of being admitted because "we took in the ten Jewish boys that we always take in and that is our quota." The dean advised him to "go to Germany, France or Switzerland" if he wanted to go to medical school.[50]

By the early 1940s, three of every four non-Jewish students were accepted by the University of Pennsylvania, but only one of every thirteen Jewish students.[51] In New York City, where the concentration of Jewish applicants was highest, the restrictive measures produced the most marked change in admissions statistics. Between 1920 and 1940, the enrollment of Jewish students in Columbia University's College of Physicians and Surgeons declined from 47 percent to 6 percent of the class; at Cornell University Medical School, Jewish enrollment dropped from 40 percent to 5 percent. Even the City College of New York, known for its largely working-class Jewish student body, reduced admissions of Jews to its school from 58 percent in 1925 to 20 percent in 1941.[51] The historian Kenneth Ludmerer observes that even those who were themselves the target of quotas did not always practice solidarity. Women's Medical College of Pennsylvania, too, had a Jewish quota.[52] According to one study using data from 1933–1934, a decade after the end of the peak period of Jewish immigration, of 22,000 medical students enrolled at seventy-six "approved" medical schools, only 4,000—18 percent—were Jewish.[53]

Assimilationist Jewish leader Rabbi Morris Lazaron so feared an anti-Semitic backlash within the medical community that he conducted a survey to see how medical school deans felt about the influx of young Jewish students. He sent questionnaires to the deans of sixty-five medical schools. From the forty-four responses he received, he drew the somewhat problematic conclusion that "while there is limitation of Jewish enrollment [usually through quotas] there is no anti-Semitism involved in the admission of Jewish students to medical school." However, the deans' letters suggest that at least some had their doubts about admitting Jewish students to their schools.[54] Dean Burton Meyers of the Indiana University School of Medicine deplored the "anti-Jewish reaction in Germany" but thought it might be echoed in the United States if "forty percent of the Doctors of Medicine were Jews."[55] Dr. C. C. Bass, the dean at Tulane University, said their teachers thought Jewish medical students had a "disagreeable manner and attitude in their classes" and were "less acceptable to patients with whom they come in contact in their studies," though he conceded: "Some of the most distinguished members of our faculty are Jews. Some of our best students are Jews. Some of our most distinguished alumni are Jews."[56]

The perceived personality traits that were used as excuses for excluding Jewish students from medical schools were also used to exclude Jews from medical faculties, or at the least to curb their number. Before the 1910 publication of Flexner's Carnegie Report, Jewish doctors held appointments on medical school faculties in Midwestern cities such as Cleveland, Cincinnati, and St. Louis. In each city, senior physicians at the local Jewish hospital contributed their efforts to medical education. The Carnegie Report indirectly reduced the number of Jewish medical education faculty, as many of the medical schools were absorbed by large private Protestant-dominated universities with restricted personnel policies. By 1927, Dr. S. M. Melamed lamented that of the thousands of Jewish physicians in New York City, not one held a "full-fledged" professorship in any medical school that was part of a university.[57]

The same complaints about the manners and comportment of Jewish medical students were often leveled at Jews seeking faculty appointments or upward mobility as department chairs. As Leon Sokoloff observed: "A concern with personality can also be a cloak for prejudice."[58] Those with liberal or socialist political views were especially vulnerable, as were those not educated at an elite Ivy League university. A profession that had long valued gentility, according to the historian of medicine Gert Brieger, often used a scale that included a classical premedical education at an elite university to determine a student's suitability for membership.[59]

The handful of Jews who achieved prestigious appointments did not always pry open doors for others, for insecurities bred of discrimination left a residue of fear. Successful Jews who helped other Jews might become the targets of a backlash that would undo their accomplishments. Such is the explanation Susan Cheever offered on behalf of her grandfather, the brilliant pathologist Milton C. Winternitz, who was the dean of Yale Medical School from 1920 to 1935 but had a well-earned reputation as "almost a caricature of the American Jew striving to become part of Gentile society." Cheever believed that her grandfather, who prided himself on his ascent from working-class Baltimore, would not have prospered in his career if he had ignored the anti-Semitism that surrounded him and made it his mission to mentor other Jews.[60]

A voluntary hospital would admit hurt and sick Jews and provide them high-level treatment and care while at the same time refusing privileges to Jewish physicians to practice in the hospital. In Newark, the police officer did not hesitate to carry the smoldering victim of a bonfire through the emergency entrance of Saint Barnabas Hospital on High Street because she was Jewish, but its administration did not appoint Jewish physicians to training, staff, and attending positions. In 1936, Arthur Bernstein experienced this refusal himself when the Saint Barnabas Hospital administrator who interviewed the young Jewish doctor was polite but unequivocal: They "did not accept Jews on [their] staff." Bernstein recalled that Jewish physicians who could not find a hospital that would accept their patients often had to make a referral "to one of [their] Gentile colleagues."[61]

After Saint Barnabas rejected him, Bernstein applied for an internship at the Beth. He completed his training under the guidance of Dr. Aaron Parsonnet, who had had joined his brother Victor at the Beth in 1913.[62] No records suggest that Victor's fatal heart attack had motivated him, but his focus became the mechanics of the heart and the arrhythmias that caused sudden death; he proposed that the fluoroscope could be used to see the heart in action, and coauthored two books on heart pathology.[63] In 1937, Parsonnet founded an evening cardiac clinic for the poor, whose jobs prevented them from spending daytime hours in a hospital waiting room. Bernstein was willing to endure the privations of a financially troubled hospital for the opportunity to practice medicine in an atmosphere of dignity, but he had not been prepared for the multi-talented, intellectually restless doctor who, when not studying the mechanics of the human heart, rested by working through the night, painting, designing insignias, or bookbinding. That year, Bernstein often answered a telephone call after midnight from Parsonnet, who would say, "Hey, I've got a great idea, Arthur. Why don't you come over and we'll talk about it?" After an entire night of work and discussion, Bernstein had just enough time to shave before going to the hospital to examine the patients admitted at 8:00 A.M.[64]

The Medical Staff during World War II

In 1939, as Lichtman prepared the hospital for the war that he saw as inevitable, Danzis was advocating for assisting refugee physicians fleeing Nazi Germany. He later wrote: "The years 1938 and 1939 brought to New Jersey a number of refugee physicians who were trying to establish themselves in what they thought to be the provinces or rural sections." Many had started out in New York City, but when they arrived in New Jersey, "there arose serious doubt in the minds of a number of physicians as to the ability of this State, particularly the County of Essex, to absorb this new group of doctors." The issue was income. "Some medical men were extremely apprehensive lest a serious economic problem would be created by this medical mass immigration." Danzis was especially troubled by those who attacked the newcomers and their supporters, including himself, as "sob-sisters" who made their living " 'by drumming up pity for the down-trodden,' and by encouraging officials to be lenient with immigrants and by seeking positions for them." He objected to the characterization of refugee doctors as arriving in droves or as poorly trained.[65]

Danzis appealed to the Beth's board at the March 27, 1939, meeting to exert all possible influence on the behalf of these refugee doctors. He and the New Jersey Committee for Refugee Physicians that he helped form secured sixteen internships for refugee doctors in 1939, because the AMA had ruled that refugee physicians must not be placed in vacancies that could be filled by U.S. medical school graduates. In compliance with the AMA ruling, those who came to the Beth did not see patients but were often assigned to laboratory positions under Antopol's supervision.[66]

In January 1941, Lichtman presented to the board a proposal for the hospital to establish a Laboratory Research Foundation. There were many reasons for his decision. Certainly, he possessed an altruistic commitment to medical research as the legacy of his late wife. Lichtman, an astute businessman, also noted that increased scrutiny was being directed toward the tax exemptions afforded to voluntary hospitals. He believed that a Laboratory Research Foundation would attract the "larger pharmaceutical companies" to support it in the form of "subsidies or even endowments for research purposes because of the personnel of the Laboratory and the existing facilities."[67] Finally, the Welfare Federation was "insisting that income from endowments should go toward the operating expense of hospitals. Endowments made to Research Foundations, on the other hand," were "used only for the scientific work of the Foundation."[68] Six months later, the Newark Beth Israel Research Foundation was incorporated, its organization patterned after the New York Mount Sinai Hospital's research foundation; its trustees were the officers of the hospital, the chief of the medical staff, and the director of the laboratory.[69]

By December 1941, the medical staff at Newark Beth Israel Hospital was comprised of those who were enlisting, those who would be drafted, and those who were over the age of 45 or rejected for active medical service. Physicians in this third category were commandeered into service in October 1942 to form a medical unit of the U.S. Public Health Service. There were two such units in Newark, designated to triage and treat an estimated fifteen thousand civilian casualties in case of an enemy attack on the nearby port, Fort Dix, and the Newark airport. Fifteen doctors of the Beth Israel Hospital Medical Unit, of which Bernstein was the youngest member, were sworn into the Public Health Service.[70] Bernstein had attempted to enlist in the army but was rejected because of the curvature of his spine. For most of the war, he served as a volunteer physician at his local draft board, helping examine recruits.

If the casualty estimates proved true, a plan would be implemented to evacuate civilian patients from a hundred hospitals along the eastern seaboard, including the Beth, and convert the facilities to military installations to receive the wounded. To prepare for this possibility, the Beth Israel Unit reported to Halloran General Hospital on Staten Island for two weeks of full-day intensive and well-organized courses, which introduced them to the use of penicillin, an antibiotic available only to the military and rushed into mass production for U.S. troops in the South Pacific. (Soon after the unit returned, the Beth was designated one of the thousand depots for the civilian distribution of penicillin.) In the classes, the unit also learned about the traumas that the soldiers would be suffering and about new rehabilitation protocols. The physicians were required to learn to march in formation. Bernstein remembered the less than stellar performance of the unit's daily marching drills—one morning while marching across the field, several of the Beth Israel doctors collapsed in pain, suffering leg cramps, and were carried on stretchers back to the barracks.[71]

The Beth physicians who had served in the reserves were called to military duty first, followed by those who chose to enlist, and then those who were drafted. Lichtman petitioned the Newark draft board for a deferment for Antopol on the grounds that as laboratory director, he was indispensable to the hospital; Antopol made the difficult decision to enlist. The laboratory director's last presentation to the hospital board in December 1942 addressed the blood-plasma program for use in the event of enemy attack and concluded with a presentation to Lichtman of a bound collection of 72 reprints of the scientific work of the laboratory staff.[72]

Dr. Eugene Parsonnet, at the age of forty-two, also chose to enlist, recalling years later that "early in 1942 I felt I had to play a part in the fight against fascism and Nazism." He initially supervised the physical training of officer corps and then was assigned to the South Pacific, "the only experienced surgeon on an island with about five thousand naval personnel, including Marines. The Seabees built a little underground operating room for me, which was quite well equipped with jeep lights for illumination."[73] Dr. Samuel Diener, who would later become the Beth Israel's "surgeons' surgeon," gained skill and experience as a battalion surgeon, landing in North Africa at Casablanca and traveling with General George Patton and his troops up the boot of Italy. He worked in the field, receiving at his medical tent badly wounded young men "with their intestines in their hands."[74]

By early 1943, 150 of the Beth's medical staff had entered the armed forces. In 1944, of the 248 physicians on the active staff, 102 were in military service. The May 1943 hospital *Bulletin,* a mimeographed newsletter, published excerpts from their letters, which reflected exhaustion, a bit of homesickness, and, for those not yet overseas, anxious anticipation. Captain S. J. Soschin wrote from the Eighty-ninth Station Hospital, Camp Beale, California: "I have just finished a six-week course on surgery of the extremities at the University of California. My outfit had meanwhile moved out here. . . . My unit is fully activated and our stay here will not be long." A homesick Major Raphael Pomeranz wrote: "I shall treasure this first *Bulletin* and its future editions; read them over and over again."[75] The community erected a tablet in May 1943 engraved with the names of the physicians in service.

The war effort reduced the size of the nursing staff as well. From 1941 to 1943, the number of staff nurses decreased from 142 to 112, while in 1943 the U.S. Public Health Service approved the Beth Nurses Training School for the U.S. Cadet Nurse Corps; thirty-seven Beth students joined the corps to prepare in case of civilian casualties.[76] The shortage of nurses required curtailing some surgeries normally performed at the Beth. Behrman told the board in April 1943 that there were sufficient nurses to staff the two major surgery operating rooms, but not a third room used for minor surgeries. He predicted that even with the shortages, however, there would be 7 percent more surgeries at the Beth in 1944 than in 1943. The hospital's mortality rate in surgical cases was under 2 percent. Meanwhile, the Nurses Training School graduates did exceedingly well on the January 1943 state board exams, achieving some of the highest grades in diseases of children, *materia medica,* nursing arts, and obstetric nursing.[77]

The role of many female staff members changed at the Beth, much as the role of women changed in every other arena of U.S. life during the war. The May 1943 *Bulletin* sent to physicians in the service carried greetings from the Radiology Department and reported that "on the 20th day of May in the year 1943—*we have two female technicians,* and a prospect of a third as Danny Weinberg is taking the Army Signal Corps course evenings and will soon graduate and be on his way"—this despite the recollection by one writer that the head of the unit had often said in the years before the war: "I wouldn't have a female technician in the place; they're no damn good; haven't any technical sense; don't know anything about the physics of X-ray; just 'Button Pushers.' "

Even as it struggled with wartime's exigencies, the Beth continued to receive recognition for its medical expertise. In January 1943, the ACS designated Newark Beth Israel Hospital and Saint Barnabas Hospital as among the 386 cancer clinics approved to offer cancer diagnostic and treatment clinics.[78]

Postwar Planning

Before World War II, a hospital residency—a period of postgraduate medical education undertaken after an internship—was exceptionally hard to find, offered only at a few outstanding medical institutions. Boards of specialization certified the credentials of those who completed residencies, but who would ensure the educational quality of the residency programs? Initially, the AMA Council on Medical Education assumed responsibility for bestowing their imprimatur on these programs, but eventually the ACS and the surgical specialty boards assumed oversight for evaluating surgical residency programs.[79]

In the era when Jewish medical students and interns often had difficulty finding residencies, the need for such programs at Jewish hospitals was critical. In 1940, after retiring as medical chief of staff, Danzis clarified the problem in an article in *Medical Leaves*. He noted that the ACS had approved 158 accredited hospitals for residencies in surgery and its subspecialties: 117 were under university supervision through their medical schools, and 41 had no medical school affiliation. While 36 Jewish hospitals met ACS accreditation standards as Class A hospitals, only 6 appeared on this list as approved to offer graduate residency training.[80] (See Appendix, Table 1.)

Danzis wrote that many of the chiefs of staff of these Jewish hospitals thought the AMA approval for internships was equivalent to approval by the ACS and the surgical specialty boards. Furthermore, in Danzis's opinion, "a certain proportion of the medical personnel, being entirely occupied with private practice, is not very much interested in, in fact, is entirely indifferent to—most of the problems affecting the clinical and educational activity of the medical staffs," seeking hospital affiliation only to "find accommodation for their private patients." Danzis urged Jewish physicians to create ACS-approved residencies so that future generations of Jewish medical graduates could readily access postgraduate education in their fields without battling anti-Semitism where it still existed in non-Jewish institutions.[81]

In the wake of Allied victories after D-Day, the Beth in the autumn of 1944 began to engage in postwar planning, and the hospital's physicians wanted to include in such planning the establishment of residencies. Dr. Robbins, Beth medical chief of staff, observed that "young doctors are taking residencies in the large hospitals, spending two and three years in a specialty, after which they are qualified to take their boards as specialists," and that "the Jewish hospitals, with few exceptions, have taken no part in this residency program, making it almost impossible for the Jewish boys to secure residential appointments." However, Robbins said: "Under the G.I. Bill of Rights . . . the government is making provision for defraying the cost of resident training." The postwar medical staff finally heeded Danzis's advice and readied itself to create its own residencies in surgery, medicine, and orthopedics right after the war.[82]

In January 1945, Lichtman announced a goal of $2 million for the establishment of an endowment to fund new research. And with the end of the war in sight, the Lay Medical Committee recommended that to avoid penalizing the returning veterans, all medical staff promotions would be suspended in 1944.

In February 1946, Dr. Harry Comando succeeded Robbins as chief of the medical staff and announced to the board the good news that "most of the doctors have been discharged from military service and have resumed their positions on the Staff." The transition back to civilian life was not always easy or smooth; circumstances and people had changed during four years of war. But Eugene Parsonnet recalled: "In late 1945 I returned to private practice and relocated in my old office with my father-in-law. Within six months I became the busiest general surgeon in the community."[83]

Whatever personal readjustment difficulties individual physicians experienced as they reentered the Beth community, the larger picture of the hospital's growing medical reputation and development was bright. In February 1946, the report resulting from a recent ACS visit complimented the administration and facilities of the hospital and recommended that the Beth broaden its educational programs for physicians-in-training. Comando announced that he was instituting "monthly clinical conferences for the discussion of scientific aspects of interesting hospital cases" and that he had divided the staff into specialty groups so that there could be discussion of cases in weekly or bimonthly departmental conferences. These conferences, he said, would "provide a medical checkup of the work of the Hospital." There were plans to hire not only a secretary to take notes at these meetings but also a librarian.[84]

Although in the postwar period, the residency had become a key component of a U.S. medical education, change came slowly, even to Danzis's own hospital. Not until January 1947 was the Beth approved by the ACS for residencies in medicine and surgery; by 1952, the hospital would be able to increase the number of its residencies to six.

American Medical Research and Education:
The New Frontier

The Beth's increased focus on medical education and its attention to scientific research were entirely consistent with the broader national priorities of the 1940s. In 1941, President Franklin Roosevelt had appointed the brilliant engineer Vannevar Bush to the newly created position of Director of the Office of Scientific Research and Development, the major civilian organization to conduct scientific research on problems related to the war. Bush organized a Committee on Medical Research that invested $15 million in research programs. Its list of war-related accomplishments was impressive, including investigation of the therapeutic value of penicillin; the development of insect repellents and insecticide, especially DDT; a study of human blood plasma on the use of serum albumin as a blood substitute; and the use of immune globulins to combat infections, as well as fibrin foam to stop bleeding. Improvements were made in the prevention of malaria by atabrine.[85]

In 1944, Roosevelt asked Bush to address four questions in a report that would detail his vision of a peacetime role for science: (1) how can government promote and aid scientific research in public and private institutions? (2) how can the nation organize research programs to continue the major wartime advances against disease? (3) how can we better foster the education and training of scientific talent in America's youth? And finally, (4) within the bounds of national security, how should America disseminate the store of scientific knowledge developed during the war?[86]

The 1945 report, *Science, the Endless Frontier*, presented a continuing role for the federal government in funding science and advocating basic science as a critical and on-going endeavor in American life. Bush advocated the establishment of the National Science Foundation to fund basic research. He also urged that the federal government agencies should continue to perform scientific research after the war, such as that conducted by the Public Health Service at the National Institute of Health. He also wanted the federal government to support extramural research in the medical sciences, providing grants to medical schools and universities to conduct research.

Whereas the Bush report presented a macro agenda for postwar research programs, the returning veteran scientists and physicians were exerting their own changes in research institutes and hospitals. The veterans who resumed their positions on the medical staff at Newark Beth Israel Hospital included Eugene Parsonnet, who had learned that postoperative recovery from anesthesia could be accelerated; he had "performed a number of operations for acute appendicitis, hernias, and several splenectomies under sodium pentothal. . . . Almost without exception such patients would walk back to their tents after a short period of post-anesthesia recovery."[87]

Dr. Henry Kessler, who had served on the orthopedic service of the Beth, saw military service as a captain in the navy in the South Pacific and became a chief of orthopedic rehabilitation and amputee service for the Mare Island Naval Hospital.[88] He returned to Newark to found the Kessler Institute for Rehabilitation in West Orange.

The Beth's dedicated physicians, surgeons, and nurses had been pillars of its strength as the medical institution survived economic depression and war. The hospital had served as a haven for Jewish physicians unwelcome elsewhere because of barriers of prejudice. It had offered them an avenue of professional advancement. And they, in return, amplified the hospital's medical reputation with their clinical skills and imaginative research.

Ahead would be the challenges of postwar peace that would transform the viability of the health care sector. The interns of the 1930s had returned as veterans of World War II with voices deeper and hoarser from age and smoking to share their war stories with a new generation of interns who would serve in the Korean conflict. And among them would be the accents of European refugees and the occasional cadence of an Israeli. All would come to question whether the Beth Israel Hospital would continue to serve those for whom it had been founded.

CHAPTER 6

The Modern Institution at Midcentury

*In the historian Rosemary Stevens's introduction to her study of American hospitals in the twentieth century, she recalled a childhood memory of her hospitalization in 1945 for scarlet fever, seriously ill and unable to receive penicillin for treatment. In Great Britain, penicillin was rarely available for civilians, and in the United States, only available in 1,000 designated hospital depots, including Newark Beth Israel. In 1961, Stevens, having already distinguished herself as the youngest administrator of a London hospital (age twenty-five), came to the United States to pursue graduate studies in public health and the history of medicine. Examining the American hospital system from a transatlantic perspective, she was impressed by its mutable role in society.

Stevens observed, "Hospitals are characterized by change. They are affirming and defining mirrors of the culture in which we live, beaming back to us, through the scope and style of the buildings, the organizational 'personality' of the institution, and the underlying meaning of the whole enterprise, the values we impute to medicine, technology, wealth, class, and social welfare."[1]

The period 1945–1965 was one of tremendous transformation of the American economy, social systems, geographical distribution of population, politics, and health systems. Stevens notes that hospitals reflected these changes. However, the most critical change for hospitals during these twenty years was that "for the first time, the federal government became an important force in sustaining the hospital as a local institution," according to Stevens.[2]

The changes that Stevens observed, including the dramatic influence of federal legislation, is readily evident in the history of Newark Beth Israel. There were transformations in the population, social systems, and economy of the city of Newark in the twenty years of the postwar period. By 1966, these changes would create a cauldron of turmoil in Newark that would reach the boiling point one July night in 1967, when two policemen brought a man in handcuffs to the Newark Beth Israel Hospital emergency room and the city erupted in violence.

Newark, a City in Transition

At mid-century, Newark was an industrial city in decline. The 1940 U.S. Census preliminary report indicated that the city's population had decreased by 22,000.[3] Census Bureau data highlighted the numbers by pointing to an increase in housing in the suburbs and a steep decline of home construction in Newark. Employment opportunities were shifting. The city that could claim 20 percent of all the jobs in New Jersey in 1910 by 1940 could claim only 11 percent. Of all wages earned in the state in 1909, 25 percent were earned in Newark; by 1939, the figure had plummeted to 10 percent. Wartime industries at its port and airport slowed but did not reverse the trend.

Industry was leaving the city for parts of the country where rents were lower, space more abundant, and labor cheaper.[4] An industrial exodus meant that less capital would be generated by companies and less taxes would be paid to the government. Repairs for housing and upgrades were postponed and then eliminated from the municipal budget, so that 31 percent of all dwelling units in Newark were below "the generally accepted standards of health and decency" by 1944.[5] That year, Dr. Charles Craster, in his thirtieth year as the city's health officer, wrote that like other large cities, Newark had a slum problem, with almost half the dwellings in the Central Ward in a state of deterioration and unfit for occupation. For Craster, the problem was a health issue that was responsible for the high morbidity rates from tuberculosis and other major diseases in these areas. The Newark city government had already received $14 million from the U.S. Housing Authority, via the Wagner-Stegall Act, to provide homes for 2,469 Newark families in six housing projects in the most blighted areas, and had been able to demolish houses on the Hill for their construction.[6] In the next decade, the Newark Housing Authority would utilize these funds to raze the old homes and three-story buildings in the north and central sections in the city and build public housing towers that sadly quickly deteriorated into new slums. Craster, who would retire in 1951 from his position, contended that the municipal government needed to create new public health prevention programs, but the shrinking tax base undercut Newark's ability to underwrite such initiatives.[7]

Weequahic in Transition

In 1950, Weequahic, the South Ward of Newark, was very much the center of the city's Jewish community. In the 1930s, the synagogues of the Hill had relocated to the Weequahic streets, following the relocation of their congregations and hospital. Rabbis removed the Torah scrolls from the old buildings and a parade of congregants from the Ahavas Achim and B'nai Jacob synagogues accompanied the scrolls to a new building on Avon Avenue.[8] Very few Jews lived in the deteriorating tenements of the Hill near High and Kinney streets. Some qualified to move into the newly constructed middle-class housing projects, and those who were too old to live alone and had no children to take them in were admitted to the Daughters of Israel Home for the Aged, which had once been Beth Israel Hospital. The borders of the Weequahic Jewish community ran from Clinton Avenue, where the old German community had lived, west to the Irvington city line, and south to the city border near Chancellor Avenue. To the east, Bergen Street and Elizabeth Avenue, both crowded with shoppers, ran parallel to the edge of Weequahic Park and the lake. A mile south, Newark Airport sprawled. Tucked into the southwest corner of the park was the Evergreen Cemetery, with two small parcels apportioned for the B'nai Jeshrun and Oheb Shalom burial grounds.

The World War II veterans who returned to the Weequahic section of Newark found the Beth little changed from its pre–World War II Depression years. Construction had been completed on a small addition that contained centralized ancillary services and a new auditorium, but the elevators were still slow and the ventilation still inadequate. In June 1951, with preparations under way for the jubilee anniversary of the Beth's founding, more than four hundred employees manned the hospital during a typical twenty-four-hour period, nearly three hundred patients filled the beds, and there were visitors at nearly every bedside, in the hallways, browsing the gift shop, and stopping for coffee in the expanded tearoom.

The Beth was a cacophony of care. The 1928 tower building, constructed before the industrial advances in acoustic bafflement, reverberated with the clacking wheels of gurneys, wheelchairs, and dietary carts, the clatter of typewriters, and the hum of electric equipment—all mingling with the voices of those providing care to those receiving it. On a summer day, the windows in every room were wide open; the hospital noises, among them the whir of a multitude of electric fans, reverberated through the neighborhood.[9]

Little had changed in the neighborhood since the early 1940s. Weequahic's frame homes, many built prior to the Beth, still lined the streets around the hospital. Some had been converted to two-family flats with a third apartment in the basement. Other houses on Lyons Avenue had become physicians' offices on the first floors and rooming houses on the upper floors rented to Beth graduate nurses, who paid rent from their hospital stipend for housing. The physicians and the nurses walked back and forth Lyons Avenue to Osborne Terrace to the hospital throughout the day and night. In the evening, the nurses, wearing their blue capes that billowed in the breeze and their caps pinned to their hair, strolled down to the Bergen Street to enjoy a snack at the local sweet shop.

In twenty-five years, the Beth tower building had become part of the Weequahic terrain. Its first-floor lobby served children as a shortcut home. Donna Marie Rey, who grew up on Lyons Avenue and would later receive a scholarship to attend the Beth Israel Nurses Training School, recalled that as a child she had figured out a shortcut from the Weequahic library to her home that included a surreptitious entry into the hospital from a side door and a quick dash across the front lobby—drawing the baleful eye of Gussie Cohen, the chief receptionist at the large central admitting desk—then down the front stairs and home on Lyons Avenue.[10] Every Sunday, Dr. Fred Cohen (no relation to Ms. Cohen) would leave his son to play under the watchful eye of Gussie; one day his son told him that he loved visiting the Beth because "they let you make as much noise as you want."[11] Even neighborhood pets came to the hospital building. One morning, Elmer, a black dog, appeared on the steps of Beth Israel Hospital and would not be budged from the front door. He settled down, apparently to wait for twelve-year-old Howard Kerdman, who lived nearby at Osborne Terrace and had been admitted to the hospital for tests. The *News* reported that Elmer patiently remained at the entrance to the hospital throughout the day and night, visibly relieved when Howard emerged from the hospital.[12]

The Weequahic neighborhood in which the Beth Israel hospital staff worked and lived, gradually changed in the 1950s as economic and demographic changes created an exodus of Newarkers to areas outside the city limits. By 1951, the population had been shifting outward from the Newark city line to land west and north in greater Essex County for nearly a decade. This outward shift encouraged the expansion of Newark's transportation arteries and construction of new roads. Newark, with its colonial origins, had several narrow avenues that extended west to its outskirts, literally evolving from dirt to wood planks, to asphalt, while streetcar and rail lines paralleled their routes. In 1951, the pockmarked pavements still supported rusting streetcar tracks. Roads such as Springfield Avenue extended out of the city and through the nearby suburb of Irvington, then west through

Maplewood and miles beyond to hamlets such as Pleasant Valley near Short Hills. The northern extension of the rail lines at Grove Street, Brick Church, and the Oranges had created the first suburbs of Newark even before World War I. From there, the Bambergers and the Lichtmans had commuted into the city for business.

Post–World War II suburbanization changed the patterns of traffic, increasing the demand for the new concept of high-speed multilane roads with clover-leaf exits onto a few streets in a city, first introduced to the public at the "Futurama" exhibit at the 1939 New York World's Fair. The 1944 Federal Highway Act initiated a joint federal-state effort to develop a system of highways, expanded in successive federal legislation, and culminating in the Federal Highway Act of 1956. The act provided more than 90 percent of the cost of constructing a network of limited-access roads to link cities with populations of more than 50,000. New Jersey had begun its highway construction at the end of World War II. In 1951, the first portion of the New Jersey Turnpike opened, and over the next years would open in sections, running northward from Bordentown to Newark's Raymond Boulevard.[13] The turnpike would pass east of Newark, cutting the city off from the Passaic River and destroying its meadowlands on its way north via bridges and tunnels to New York City.[14] The Garden State Parkway, which originated in the resort town of Cape May, stretched northward, a swath of asphalt through the western portion of Newark on its way to the New York State border. In 1957, the New Jersey State Highway Department proposed the creation of a fifty-nine-mile freeway, I-78, which would include portions of old Route 22 and connect Pennsylvania via Newark and the Holland Tunnel to New York City. There were plans for another highway routed through the Oranges to Morristown and for a third short freeway to replace Bergen Street that would connect the towns.[15] These highways gradually encircled and bypassed Newark.[16]

The construction of I-78 embroiled the Weequahic community in a bitter fight for its existence. In 1961, construction of I-78 had finally reached the western edge of the townships of Hillside, Elizabeth, and Union. The Hillside community residents fought the route of the highway foot by foot, especially the original plan to follow old Route 22 near the rail line, Lake Weequahic, and the airport. Hillside lobbied for a route that curved a half mile north of Route 22, bisecting the Weequahic community.[17] Although this route would cut through part of his city, Newark mayor Hugh Addonizio favored this path, declaring that the route was filled with slums and blighted housing. Even before construction began, Ralph Zinn, the chair of the Weequahic Community Council, warned that such plans would demoralize Weequahic and that many people were angry over the Newark city government's willingness to demolish almost eight hundred homes in the area and severely hurt the businesses on Chancellor Avenue and Bergen Street.[18] The battle for the final route resulted in twelve revisions of its alignment, the debate churning for almost three years while the state secured the right of way. The condemnation of houses and demolition began in 1964. The demolitions that destroyed synagogues, yeshivas, and many homes also brought the decelerating exit traffic to within one block of the Newark Beth Israel Hospital entrance.[19]

The battle over the construction of the I-78 freeway had created permanent physical and emotional divisions in the neighborhood. By 1967, the movement outward to the suburbs had greatly accelerated; the bustling Jewish community in which the Beth Israel hospital staff worked and lived was leaving, too.

A Jewish Community in Transition

In 1951, the bustling crowded streets in the south of Newark suggested a community permanence in the Jewish neighborhood that belied the truth: its institutions had sunk shallow roots in Weequahic. Only twenty-five years after leaving the Hill tenements, Jews were again in transit, from the Newark streets to homes in the new streets of the Essex County suburbs. They were moving into Cape Cods and split-level homes equipped with modern stoves, refrigerators, and washing machines, as well as squares of new grass sod on the front lawns. Each week, Jewish families could peruse the classified advertisement section of the weekly *Jewish News* called "Homes in the Suburbs," which described homes for sale that were adjacent to a country club that would accept Jews, as well as schools, shopping, and express commuting to Newark and New York. The suburbs were a magnet for families and for the businesses that provided services to them as readily seen in the *Jewish News* advertisements. Every February, Weequahic stores published special advertisements in the Friday issue of the *Jewish News* before their George Washington's Birthday sales. In the early 1950s, these advertisements filled several pages; by 1965 only four stores still advertised the sale.[20] Conversely, each week, more advertisements announced the relocation of kosher butcher shops, bakeries, and clothing stores to suburban shopping centers.

The growth of the suburban communities was spurred by the Serviceman's Readjustment Act, the "G.I. Bill," enacted in 1944, which offered to veterans low-interest loans from the federal government for home and business mortgages. Veterans, including many Beth Israel physicians, took advantage of this program. Dr. Eugene Parsonnet moved his family in 1951 from High Street in the Central Ward to a split-level house in Maplewood, four miles north and west of the hospital.[21] His son, Dr. Victor Parsonnet, a veteran of the Korean War, would move his family to the suburban town of Millburn in 1955. The Beth's physicians, such as Dr. Arthur Bernstein, who moved to Short Hills, embraced suburban life and continued their community activities in their new venue, rising to leadership positions in community centers and synagogues, and heading local United Jewish Appeal (UJA) drives.[22]

In 1951, the leaders of the YM-YWHA decided to relocate from the beautiful building across the street from the old hospital to a fourteen-room Weequahic home at 128 Chancellor Avenue with a soda bar, games, and meeting rooms for teenagers "right in the heart of this populous Jewish section."[23] However, there was some indication that this was a temporary relocation. The board of trustees of the Jewish Community Council suggested a very modest center for Weequahic because "the Center Board has felt it must provide where the bulk of the Jewish population still lives, which is Weequahic, but construction and planning should take into account possible population shifts."[24] Their information had indicated that the Jewish families who had moved to the suburbs had been replaced by Jewish families from other sections of Newark, but there was no telling how long Weequahic would continue to have a large Jewish population.

Synagogue leaders cautiously began to build satellite centers close to the new suburban communities. These new facilities offered Sunday-school classes, club activities, and Hebrew-school sessions. If the satellite thrived, the synagogue would close the city facility. Typical of these satellites was the Suburban House that B'nai Abraham Synagogue opened in time for the Jewish High Holidays in 1958. The same year, Congregation Oheb Shalom, founded in 1860 and opened in 1911 on High Street, moved out of the city altogether, establishing itself in South Orange in a new facility that would boast 1,500 seats; an overflow crowd of suburbanite Jews stood outside the building for its dedication.[25] Just after the High Holidays, on October 3, 1958, a banner headline in the *Jewish News*, the weekly successor to the *Jewish Chronicle*, gave notice that the community drive of the United Jewish Appeal's Red Cross would cover not just Newark, but "Newark and suburban areas."

The establishment of Israel in 1948 further complicated the financial pressures for older local Jewish institutions and new synagogues as contributions were diverted to the construction of the infrastructure for the new country. Zionists had found willing ears and open wallets in Newark as far back as the 1920s. Newark physicians had contributed to the establishment of a medical school at Hebrew University. In the aftermath of World War II and the Holocaust, the need for a Jewish homeland seemed more urgent than ever. After Israel pioneer-settler Golda Meir visited Newark in 1948, the Jewish Community Council borrowed $500,000 to donate to Palestinian Jewry, paying off the obligation with a vigorous fund-raising campaign in 1949. This pattern of borrowing and donating persisted until the mid-1950s, when Newark Jews were donating millions of dollars for Israel annually, much of it by purchasing Israel bonds.[26]

In Newark, the Children's Home of the Jewish Child Care Association (formerly the Hebrew Benevolent Orphan Asylum), which had functioned as a residential treatment center, closed its Clinton Avenue home in 1955.[27] The Theresa Grotta Convalescent Home, which had been built in a rural community of West Caldwell, found itself in the middle of a thriving suburb.[28] In 1957, the Daughters of Israel, once again displaying extraordinary finesse in real estate transactions, had negotiated with the City of Newark to acquire a Pleasant Valley property in exchange for the old Beth Israel Hospital property and renamed themselves the Daughters of Israel of Pleasant Valley. The *Jewish News* published a special supplement on March 2, 1962, regarding the relocation of the nursing home to its new facility on Pleasant Valley Way, adjacent to the Kessler Institute for Rehabilitation; the supplement was filled with advertisements for suburban shopping centers and synagogues, all welcoming the Daughters to their new home. A team of more than 250 persons, including thirty-two rescue squads, transported the men and women of Prince Street in a slow procession west on Orange Avenue, away from the Newark streets, to the new building, where the mayor of West Orange stood on the front steps to greet them.

"The current movement away from the city and into the suburbs was confronting every type of Jewish communal organization," declared an editorial in the September 5, 1958, *Jewish News*. The writer hoped that "the flight of the Jewish population from Newark does not become a flight from urban life into a fantasy land devoid of Jewish life while Newark's respected Jewish institutions were left to disintegrate. Some way must be found to avoid the tragic consequence of having Newark become a spiritually and culturally leaderless and poverty-stricken city." The editorial prompted pages and pages of responses from synagogues and association leaders, many denying that they were in flight and others denying that they had a responsibility to remain in Newark if their constituency chose to live in the suburbs' pleasant environs.[29]

A Jewish Hospital under Nonsectarian Auspices or a Nonsectarian Hospital under Jewish Auspices?

As the synagogue and association leaders debated whether the new suburban Jewish community would be devoid of Jewish spirituality and observance, a countermovement began by these same groups to enforce Jewish observance upon the older Jewish institutions in Newark, most notably the Jewish hospital. In 1949, the Synagogue Council of Essex County passed a resolution "that inasmuch as Beth Israel is regarded as a Jewish hospital that it be asked to observe Kashruth."[30] Such a commitment would require the hospital to serve only kosher meat, ritually slaughtered, and to refrain from serving milk and meat products in the same meal. Separate sets of dishes and utensils, one for milk dishes and the other for meat dishes, would be necessary.

Not surprisingly, Beth board members took immediate exception to this resolution. In 1949, the patient census demonstrated that fewer than half the patients admitted were Jewish, so there was little demand from patients for a kosher kitchen. Sophia Morris, the head of the Dietary Department since 1928, informed hospital superintendent I. E. Behrman that the general kitchen had a separate stove in a separate area, and glass dishes, for the preparation and serving of meals to patients who observed kashruth.[31] But, as she told Behrman, and he then informed the board, in the years 1939 through 1949, the department had received only one request for kosher food. Physicians' orders for special diets for their patients did not always follow the laws of kashruth. By the following spring, the board's Public Relations Committee unanimously agreed that the Beth was a "non-sectarian institution under Jewish auspices" and refused to go beyond accommodating observant patients.[32]

The Jewish Community Council went further than the protestations of the Synagogue Council over kashruth, making a broader set of demands: the elimination of Christian observances at the Beth, including events such as Christmas parties for staff and sale of Christmas gifts in the hospital shop. These proposed changes greatly angered the Beth's board. The hospital had welcomed non-Jewish employees and sought to ensure their comfort to promote workplace harmony and to retain employees. By 1949, nearly 85 percent of the staff was non-Jewish, as were more than half the patients.

The gift shop had stocked Christmas items in response to requests from the patients' visitors and hospital staff. For non-Jews, a hospital is a lonely place to be during the Christmas holidays; the red and green decorations on the wards and the exchange of gifts, especially for those children in the pediatric ward, were considered by the board to be appropriate and compassionate.

The JCC also asked for the regularization of Jewish ritual observances and the establishment of a permanent chaplaincy. The Beth had never employed a permanent chaplain because patients' ritual needs had long been satisfied by local rabbis, who came as needed to the hospital for services and holiday celebrations.[33] In addition, an ad hoc congregation including the Jewish staff and some community residents held services in the hospital auditorium. Attendance at the Beth auditorium services did not require the purchase of a ticket during the Rosh Hashanah High Holiday services as did the surrounding synagogues in Weequahic, which used the annual proceeds of their ticket sales for their year-long operation. The increase in attendance at the Beth services and at suburban synagogues was seriously affecting the finances of the synagogues remaining in Weequahic. The JCC sought to eliminate the ad hoc congregation, but did not understand that the attendees were Jewish staff members, who were on call for patients' care, and appreciated the opportunity to attend services within the hospital; and a dwindling and poorer Weequahic Jewish community unable to afford cost of the tickets.[34]

The controversy over whether the Beth embodied a Jewish identity was intertwined with the community funding issues, especially the allocations for the old Newark and new suburban Jewish institutions in Essex County from the funds raised by the annual United Jewish Appeal campaign. The choice of recipients and the amounts allocated became matters of intense debate in communities. Individuals wore different organizational hats at different times, including the Beth Israel physicians, who were hospital staff and active organizers for the UJA campaigns, further complicating the personal and institutional rivalries.

In 1951, the JCC pledged a flat sum of $100,000 to the hospital with an assurance of an additional 10 percent of all net funds raised over $2.3 million from the funds collected by the UJA.[35] The UJA fund drive was thus, in part, a drive for the hospital. What remained unresolved was what the contribution to the hospital meant in terms of policy. Did the JCC's generosity entitle it to shape hospital policy, especially with respect to the Jewish identity of the hospital? And to what extent would the council

endorse the Beth's independent efforts to raise the funds it needed beyond
the $100,000, especially if such efforts hampered those of other Jewish
agencies, including UJA, to raise funds?[36]

The rift between the JCC and the Beth proved too much for Beth board
president Abraham Lichtman. The JCC had pulled back its support during the
hospital's financial crisis in the 1930s, and now it was insisting that the hospital bylaws be modified to make anyone who made an annual contribution
eligible for membership on the hospital board, which would result in a membership whose loyalties were divided between the JCC and the hospital. On
June 25, 1951, a weary Lichtman announced that he was donating five thousand dollars to the Beth's Research Foundation and was resigning the presidency. "I wish to be relieved of a responsibility which I consider heavy. To
me, this hospital has been a labor of love . . . [but] in the last six months I have
suffered more with this hospital than the previous 16 years."[37] He continued
to chair the board while his brothers Harry and Fred served as board members. In the 1960s, Lichtman's son, Cecil, would join the board, keeping alive
and vital the family's strong connection to the hospital.

Simond T. Shifman, who succeeded Lichtman as president, spent
much of the years 1952–1954 locked in combat with the JCC over allocations
of UJA funds.[38] At the core of the controversy was the fund-raising campaign for a new laboratory building for the hospital. In 1949, Dr. William
Antopol, the director of the Laboratory Department, left his position for the
more modern laboratory and research facilities at the New York Beth Israel
Hospital. Dr. Lester Goldman, who succeeded him, pressed for the construction of a modern laboratory, justifying it with many of the same practical
arguments Dr. Danzis had made in 1921. The funds for the construction
would be raised through a campaign that would compete directly with JCC
plans for a campaign for its own new buildings in the suburbs, as well as
with the annual UJA drive for Israel. Undoubtedly aware that many in the
Jewish community had been born at the Beth or treated for illness there, the
JCC understood that many Jewish charitable dollars would be headed for
the hospital's coffers.[39] The acrimony escalated to a point at which the hospital nearly severed its relationship with the JCC.

In March 1954, an agreement resolved three issues: the hospital
would continue its own independent campaign for the laboratory; it would
hold in abeyance newspaper publicity or promotion until the end of the UJA
campaign; and it would be named a beneficiary agency in the 1954 UJA
campaign for maintenance purposes but receive no special funding for the
laboratory. After that, the hospital would be included in UJA campaigns as

a beneficiary agency, and every article about the hospital that appeared in the Jewish News would end with the statement that it was a member agency of the Jewish Community Council of Essex County, which receives funds from the United Jewish Appeal of Essex County.[40]

But the larger problem of the Beth and its relationship to the Essex County Jewish community remained unresolved. At issue was a change in demographics whose consequences reached far beyond those of objections to religious ritual. In 1959, Leo Yanoff, the new head of the JCC, assessed the Essex County Jewish community fund-raising commitments to the Daughters of Israel Home for the Aged, the Jewish Educational Association, the Jewish Community Center, and the Hebrew Academy. The impact of health-insurance carriers and the possibility of federal socialized health insurance was the impetus for his decision, made public in Yanoff's December 1959 address to the annual meeting of the JCC. The JCC would go "in the direction of devoting its energies and resources to the emotional, recreational and intellectual needs of individuals, not of medical care as in the case of Beth Israel and all other hospitals, [where] third party payments, such as Blue Cross, provide a larger part of fee income from patients."[41]

Increasingly transformation of the nonprofit voluntary hospital, as a delivery system for modern medicine and the thrust of the JCC efforts for the Essex Jewish community social services were diverging. The energies and resources devoted to the building, renovation, and expansion of suburban Jewish institutions was in stark contrast to the Newark Beth Israel Hospital, which received an increasingly smaller portion of allocations from the JCC and was ineligible to receive federal funds to make the changes necessary to modernize its facility.

The 360,000 Beds That Transformed American Hospitals

The Hospital Survey and Construction Act of 1946, sponsored by Senators Lister Hill of Alabama and Harold Burton of Ohio, provided funds to states to build sufficient hospitals to create a proportion of 4.5 hospital beds per 1,000 individuals. The act was praised by its supporters as a triumph of careful planning that would bring hospitals and health-care personnel to areas of rural America that had languished without adequate resources, while constructing new hospitals in advance to meet the demands of new suburbs that were replacing farmland in the outskirts of cities. Federal aid to states was authorized for surveying geographical areas, planning the construction, and authorizing grants to assist in the actual construction of both government and private facilities. Assistance was apportioned by a formula that gave preference to states deficient in rural hospitals. State, local, or private sources had to put up two dollars to every federal dollar, but states were not required to divert state tax revenues to these hospital projects; private fund-raising also could provide the funds. In the next twenty years, from 1946 to 1966, 4,678 projects would be funded, over 50 percent in communities with populations of under 10,000.[42]

The impact of the Hill-Burton Act was both measurable and immeasurable. Measurable was the hundreds of thousands of hospital beds created by the construction program and even more created with private endowments. The act had an immeasurable impact on the Jewish hospitals. A third wave of them emerged, located in new suburban areas. The first Jewish hospital of the third wave was the General Maurice Rose Hospital opening in 1946, in Denver, Colorado, named in honor of the state's "fighting general" and highest-ranking Jewish officer.[43] There would be a new Mount Sinai Hospital in Miami Beach, Florida, and a new Mount Sinai Hospital in Minneapolis, Minnesota—a seven-story nonsectarian 197-bed hospital dedicated to research and education, hailed as the most modern in the city.[44] In the suburb of Chicago, Illinois, the Louis A. Weiss Memorial Hospital opened as a nonsectarian facility in 1953.[45] In New York State, where Nassau and Queens Counties were among "the most under-hospitalized areas in the East," according to a survey by the Hospital Council of Greater New York, Long Island Jewish Hospital opened in 1954 with a $1.5 million grant-in-aid under the Hill-Burton Act.[46]

But, from 1946 to 1966, no Hill-Burton funds would flow to the urban hospitals built in the golden era of the 1920s and now in dire need of renovation. The hospitals, many operating under Jewish auspices, that were built in large industrial cities were considered high per-capita-income areas, even as they all suffered from an outflow of residents.[47]

One could indirectly measure the impact of the Hill-Burton funding that favored construction of new hospitals in less-populated areas in the hospital relocations and mergers of Jewish hospitals built prior to World War II. In Philadelphia, Pennsylvania, three Jewish hospitals consolidated as divisions of the newly named Albert Einstein Medical Center.[48] Similarly, in Brooklyn, New York, Beth Moses and United Israel Zion merged to become Maimonides Hospital. The Associated Jewish Charities of Baltimore, Maryland, chose relocation, replacing the Sinai Hospital in East Baltimore with a new medical center on a fifty-acre tract in the northwest section of the city.[49] The Cedars of Lebanon and Mount Sinai Hospital in separate sections of

Los Angeles, California, chose to relocate and merge at a new location, although the process extended over more than a decade.

In Newark, one voluntary hospital made the decision to close its city facility and relocate to the suburbs. In October 1954, the Saint Barnabas Hospital Executive Committee voted to close its facilities on Newark's High Street, and ten years later would open a $14-million Medical Center in Livingston, New Jersey.[50] Other Newark hospitals responded to the new economic realities by merging. As one hospital administrator observed: "The reasons for merger are many, but the common theme is change—change in economic factors, in medical practice, in demography, in travel time between doctor, patient, and hospital, and in such external factors as regional planning and third-party financing."[51] In January 1958, a joint agreement consolidated Newark's Presbyterian Hospital, Babies Hospital, Newark Eye and Ear Infirmary, and the Hospital for Crippled Children into one corporate structure, United Hospitals of Newark.[52] A year earlier, as the merger was being negotiated, the Beth had been approached to join the United Hospitals of Newark, but declined and remained an independent voluntary nonprofit hospital.

The Beth Israel Hospital Laboratory building was not built with federal or state funding. The Ladies Auxiliary spearheaded the fund-raising effort, raising money for a complete blood-bank wing, including a blood-donation area open six days a week, and then presenting Dr. Goldman with the keys to a new car for his commute from the suburbs.[53] The hospital medical staff provided nearly 35 percent of the funding (donations paid in full, not pledges), and Rippel Foundation and Ford Foundation grants supplemented the donations. On May 5, 1957, the five-story laboratory opened with a speech by Newark mayor Leo P. Carlin, the first mayor to be elected directly by the Newark voters, in accordance with the new municipal governing structure. It was an impressive glass-and-steel addition, spanning nearly 28,000 square feet, connected to the main building by a glass-enclosed bridge. The long laboratory tables stacked with state-of-the-art equipment were ready for the clinicians, technologists, and medical residents who would soon embark on a prodigious array of studies on hemophilia and sulfanimides. New advances in its hematology laboratory were made possible by an endowment from the Beth's board.[54]

The Beth Israel Hospital tower, once the embodiment of modernity, languished without federal and state funding. It was fast becoming the "nautilus shell," a still beautiful exterior that hid an ugly deteriorating infrastructure, derided by Dr. Joseph Doane in his 1945 AHA report on voluntary hospitals. Board member Alan Sagner in December 1956 sounded the first call for consideration of the Beth's future, expressing his conviction that "some thought should be given to long-range planning of this hospital." Sagner, born in Baltimore in 1920 and a graduate of the University of Maryland, moved to New Jersey in 1945 to join his brother-in-law in the construction business. He quickly became involved in the politics of the suburbs and the city and its Jewish community. His experience in construction placed him on the Plant and Facilities Committee of Newark Beth Israel Hospital; like his predecessors, he became more and more involved in "something both important and rewarding."[55] Sagner's call in 1956 for a study of the "population and transportation trends" in conjunction with "contemplated engineering plans before spending huge sums of money" was consistent with the postwar recognition that planning must precede construction and be responsive to community needs. He recognized that part of the Newark community the hospital was created to serve—the Jewish community—was departing Newark at the very time that costly hospital repairs and upgrading could not be postponed.[56]

To assess costs, the board engaged "independent engineers to conduct a survey of the entire hospital."[57] In 1958 and 1959, engineering firms estimated the total cost of repairs at $2,202,000, an amount almost equal to the cost of the entire hospital complex in 1928. The cost of repairing the aging plumbing alone would be $600,000.

In 1965, the question arose once again of whether Newark Beth Israel should leave Newark or, at the very least, establish a satellite hospital in suburbia closer to its traditional patient base. After all, the new, modern Saint Barnabas Hospital in Livingston was attracting patients to its air-conditioned facility and ample parking lot, and dramatic demographic changes, along with the new realities of reimbursement for hospital services by prepaid insurance plans or federal funds, left little alternative to bold planning.

In September, Alan Sagner, now heading the Administrative Committee, presented a plan that would strengthen the hospital as a center of advanced medical care while keeping it in its present location in Newark; his proposal would set the Beth's course for the next quarter century.

Familiar with the planning required to successfully complete construction projects, Sagner explained that his analysis indicated that in previous hospital construction, "present and future needs were viewed from a fragmented approach," which were periodically completed as needed. He observed that "with the passage of time, the present plan covering our projected needs will not be adequate to carry the increased loads in specific areas and when the buildings are finally completed the Hospital would still have the same image." He "favored a new approach, encompassing an entirely new concept—a total plan that allows for the integration of all previous plans into one large building complex." The architectural drawings reflected not the renovation of buildings but a new set of pavilions next to the existing hospital structure, including a garage capable of accommodating 410 cars. Sagner proposed that the hospital double its facility in anticipation of admitting more patients, not fewer. These patients would travel from the surrounding suburbs, even from other New Jersey counties, able via the newly constructed highways, to seek renowned medical specialists and therapies they could get at few places other than the Beth, with parking facilities to accommodate these patients and their families.[58]

Sagner explained that his plan "would require a greater sum of money and a more dynamic approach to raising the amounts needed" than past fundraising had involved. He estimated the building costs at $8.5 million, of which $3 million would come from a joint fund-raising endeavor into which the Beth had entered with four other hospitals (Columbus, Saint James, Saint Michael's, and United), the Greater Newark Hospital Development Fund. The Development Fund was in the midst of a $15 million campaign to modernize all five hospitals by spring 1967.[59] Another $6 million would have to be borrowed. Sagner thought that the annual budget must be increased by $400,000 per year to cover interest and amortization of the loans over a twenty-five-year period. Some of that might be offset by fees from the parking garage; another $100,000 might be saved by centralizing the dietary service rather than preserving the multiple kitchens that had served the Beth's patients since 1928; finally, the interest on the $6 million would be chargeable as an expense to Blue Cross and recovered in the hospital's per diem allowance. The plan presented the future of the hospital as thriving and expanding, attracting patients from the entire region.

The board approved Sagner's plan a month later.[60] The following January, Sagner was elected president of the board, succeeding Gil Augenblick, who had served for four years. Few knew that at the time, Sagner was motivated less by the expansive, long-term plan for the future of the Beth than by the sense that there was no alternative in 1965. He did not voice to colleagues the Hebrew phrase that echoed in his mind: "*Ain brera*," no other choice.[61]

The Transformation of the Hospital Workforce

During the post–World War II period, Vannevar Bush's agenda for medical research had been embodied in a series of federal laws whose main intent was to support research and programs addressing the public's demand for improved and affordable health care. The National Heart Act, passed in June 1948, was the first act to provide grants for the training, diagnosis, and treatment of heart diseases. It was quickly followed by the National Dental Research Act, providing funds to states for the training and treatment of dental diseases. The Omnibus Medical Research Act of 1950 expanded the mechanisms of support for research and training, followed by the Health Amendments Act of 1956, which authorized support for increasing the number of trained nurses and other professional public health staff.

While federal legislation was promoting research and improving health-care facilities and training, it offered little direct benefit to those involved in providing the supportive and ancillary services for patient care. In a classic case of demand versus supply, the advancement in new life-saving medical technologies created the demand for professionally trained technicians who could operate new equipment and render diagnoses. The numbers of formally trained technicians lagged behind the demand to hire them and hospitals escalated their wage offers to recruit them. But the wages of food service, housekeeping, custodial, and laundry employees, as well as of clerks in the offices and the wards, continued to be among the lowest, in part, because there was a ready supply of untrained newcomers, many Puerto Rican and African American, who were standing at the entrance doors each morning, ready to take unskilled jobs.

Beth hospital chef James Hopkins recalled the dawn when he stood waiting near the entrance to the Beth's kitchen, hoping for a job interview. His sister told him to be there at 5:00 A.M. because that was when the elderly woman who might hire him began her workday. And right on time, Sophia Morris did indeed walk briskly up the path from the nurses' residence, wearing an old hospital uniform and a smile for the young man. Learning that his sister already worked at the hospital, Morris beckoned Hopkins inside. For the next forty years, he, too would begin his day at the Beth.[62]

Positions classified as nonprofessional and unskilled, such as the dietary positions that reported to Morris, were exempt from the minimum-wage provisions of the federal Fair Labor Standards Act.[63] In 1962, it was estimated that at least 750,000 hospital unskilled positions in dietary, housekeeping, and supportive positions in the ancillary and administrative areas were outside of the federal minimum-wage law.[64]

The issues that the Beth Israel Hospital staff faced divided the professionally trained from the nonprofessional employees. Each group would attempt to redress its concerns by organizing in opposition to the hospital management, but with different outcomes.

Professionals— the Beth Nurses

In 1950, the Beth Israel Hospital nurses were increasingly dissatisfied with a wage-and-benefit package that was falling far below those of other city hospitals and the newly opened Veterans Administration hospital in the suburbs. Nearly half the Beth's nurses left their workstations on November 15, 1950, to demonstrate that negotiations between their representatives and the hospital's executive director, I. E. Behrman, had reached an impasse; the walk-out forced the shutdown of the fifth floor of the hospital and the postponement of elective surgeries. That year, the federal government had extended the Social Security Act to cover its nearly 10 million hospital employees, requiring that their paychecks be adjusted for the deduction. Behrman had proposed to the staff nurses a new salary-and-benefit package that increased their vacation days, but reduced the hourly wage for part-time nurses and raised it for full-time nurses, while eliminating their monthly twenty-five-dollar stipend for housing—a package far less generous than those offered by other hospitals in Essex County, including other voluntary hospitals.[65] It was not the salary but the elimination of the stipend that stymied the negotiations. As nurses began to voice their concerns, they also asked for the right to select duty in the services that most interested them. Behrman refused their requests, and they walked out. The nurses returned to work the next day, declaring that they did not want to do anything to hurt the nursing school or the hospital.[66] An agreement was reached between George Furst, the chair of the Beth's Nursing Committee since 1939, and Vice President Simond Shifman; but Behrman was barred from all further negotiation meetings.

The resolution of the 1950 salary crisis did not solve the broader problem: the inability of the Beth Israel Nurses Training School to meet the increasing demand for student and graduate nurses to staff the hospital. During World War II, the school had briefly affiliated with the University of Newark for a program that secured federal funding for training the U.S. Cadet Nurse Corps and finally achieved national accreditation.[67] Peacetime brought an end to the cadet program, a drop in the number of students from the Red Cross, and mass resignations of graduate nurses.[68] The school found itself competing for applicants with the City Hospital Nursing School, which offered its students a wide variety of clinical experiences, a nurse faculty possessing graduate degrees, low tuition with an annual stipend, and a diploma curriculum that could be transferred as two years of college credits toward a bachelor of science degree.[69] Increasingly, those who opted for careers in nursing wanted to earn a BS degree from an accredited university.[70]

Fannie Katz, who became the director of the Beth Israel Nursing Department and Training School in 1952, pursued another source of nurses for the hospital through the Foreign Nurses Training Act, supported by the American Nursing Association. The program offered educational and practical experience to foreign-trained nurses, who were given a two-year exchange visa to come to U.S. hospitals and provided room, board, and a stipend for living expenses.[71] In November 1954, the Nursing Department launched an exchange program to provide on-the-job training to foreign nurses.[72]

The exchange nurses brought a high level of skill to bedside care at the Beth and an appreciation for U.S. physicians, whose camaraderie they found refreshing. Many remarked that they were not used to physicians talking to them directly and including them in the discussions of the management and assessment of patients.[73]

Over the next two decades more than five hundred professional graduate nurses from other countries arrived in Newark to work at the Beth. Katz's assistant, Cecile Champagne, worked tirelessly to prepare the paperwork that enabled their entry to the United States, and Beth staff and volunteers met them at the airport and took them directly to the hospital. One exchange nurse remembered a blur of papers and waiting lines and then being escorted to meet Katz, who shook her hand and simultaneously shouted to her assistant, "Champagne!" The nurse thought to herself, "What a hospital! They're serving champagne for my arrival."[74]

During the Cold War, immigration restrictions had limited the supply of immigrant nurses from Europe. By 1965, the Beth and many other U.S. hospitals found a ready supply of nurses in the Philippines, where nursing schools were equivalent in quality to many U.S. diploma schools. The program was so successful that in 1966, the Beth dedicated a new residence hall for foreign-exchange nurses. The opening ceremony displayed the flags of sixteen nations and was attended by diplomats who were addressed by Dr. Rodolphe Coigney, director of the World Health Organization.[75] By the time the building opened, the Nurse Training Act of 1964 was providing funds for construction of new nurse-training facilities, including a grant to the Beth Israel Hospital. By the mid-1960s, the American Nurses Association had taken the position that all licensed nurses should be trained in institutions of higher education. The era of diploma schools such as the Beth Israel Nurses Training School was drawing to a close.[76]

Nonprofessionals—the Unionization of Beth Israel Hospital

In 1959, Martin Cherkasky, the director of Montefiore Hospital in the Bronx, presented a changing profile of the unskilled labor force in his Jewish hospital and other voluntary nonprofit hospitals, like Newark Beth Israel:

> The low pay scale attracted primarily two groups of workers: untrained people and newcomers to New York, mainly Puerto Ricans and Negroes [who had recently migrated from the South]. These recent arrivals in the community take these jobs as a first foothold in the city. As soon as basic wage-earning skills are acquired and enough phrases in English are mastered, they leave for better paying jobs. At Montefiore Hospital, this influx resulted in an annual turnover rate as high as 300 percent, particularly in the dietary and housekeeping departments which absorb the major number of the low-paid employees.[77]

The Hospital Workers Union emerged to become the champion of these lowest-paid employees. Local 1199 of the Retail Drug Employees Union, which had existed since 1932, began to gain strength in the 1950s when the dynamic Leon Davis, a former pharmacy student and committed member of the Communist Party, took over its leadership. In 1954, he was joined by Moe Foner, a bold organizer from District 65 of the Wholesale and Warehouse Workers, a committed radical, and the son of Polish-Jewish immigrants.

The Hospital Workers Union's first big victory came at Montefiore Hospital when 628 employees out of 900 eligible to vote chose Local 1199 as their bargaining agent in late 1958. The hospital and the union negotiated a contract with a modest increase, time-and-a-half pay for work beyond a forty-hour week, a grievance procedure, and minimum provision for sick leave and annual vacation time.[78]

But the Labor Management Relations Act of 1947 (the Taft-Hartley Act), which gave unionized employees the right to bargain for benefits in their contracts and recognized the right of employees to seek health plans as a component of their salaries, specifically excluded nonprofit voluntary hospitals from its provisions—based on the contention of the American Hospital Association that hospitals should be exempt from legislative acts that require compulsory bargaining of hospitals with employees. Hospital workers could organize a union but had no federal protection for collective bargaining efforts. Nevertheless, by 1960, there was still a patchwork of unions in Jewish hospitals; for example, Mount Sinai of Milwaukee signed a contract with local 1572 of the AFL-CIO, and Mount Zion hospital in San Francisco signed a contract with the Building Service Employees International Union. The Teamsters Union, United Auto Workers, and even the Tavern Employees Union all had members who were hospital employees.[79] The Hospital Workers Union gained dominance among the other hospital unions by associating their cause with the civil rights movement.[80] The union raised funds in support of the 1955 Montgomery bus boycott and participated in the 1960 picketing of Woolworth's in New York City to protest lunch-counter segregation at Woolworth stores in the South. Dr. Martin Luther King Jr. considered himself an ally of Local 1199 and vice versa. When Local 1199 launched a strike at six New York hospitals, King, the civil rights movement's most charismatic leader, described the struggle as "more than a fight for union rights . . . it is a fight for human rights and human dignity."[81] In early September 1964, a New Jersey court ruled that hospital workers in the state should be allowed collective-bargaining rights, a decision upheld on appeal. By now, Local 1199 organizers had unionized sixty hospitals in New York City and recruited 20,000 members. Within a month of the court decision, Local 1199 targeted twenty-two hospitals in New Jersey for organization efforts.

By the end of September, the organizers' first target, Clara Maas Memorial Hospital (formerly German Hospital) in northern Belleville, had voted in favor of union recognition, shortly followed by Saint Barnabas Hospital. The following month, Moe Foner told *Modern Hospital* that the drive in New Jersey was "the most dramatic organizing campaign in recent years, not only in the hospital field but in any field."[82] Leaflets included endorsements by King of the Southern Christian Leadership Conference, Roy Wilkins of the NAACP, James Farmer of the Congress of Racial Equality, and A. Philip Randolph of the Brotherhood of Sleeping Car Porters. Union leader Leon Davis did not hesitate to cite racial issues in his attacks on the hospitals, characterizing them as denying hospital workers, most of them African Americans, the most elementary right of representation in the workplace, and the hospitals as surgical sweatshops that made up hospital deficits through substandard wages.[83]

How then could the Beth be most effectively organized by 1199? The union organizers spotted two vulnerabilities in its management. In February 1959, Behrman, in poor health and recognizing the onset of a new era of hospital administration, resigned after twenty-three years of service, join-ing Lichtman as a consultant to the board for the next ten years. He was suc-ceeded by Dr. Jacob Rosenkrantz, a graduate of the College of Physicians and Surgeons at Columbia University, who had served in the U.S. Army Medical Corps during World War II. From assistant director of professional services at the Veterans Administration Hospital in the Bronx, he had advanced to director of professional services at the newly opened East Orange Veterans Hospital, a position he held for four years. From 1956 to 1959, Rosenkrantz had served as the administrator of the Southern Division, formerly Mount Sinai, of the Albert Einstein Medical Center hospital system in Philadelphia.[84]

By 1960, when Rosenkrantz assumed the position, the Beth staff had grown to 850; almost one-third (258) had between five and thirty-five years of service, and of these nearly 45 had more than fifteen years of service.[85] An entire level of hospital management staff, almost all women, had supervised the ancillary departments of the hospital for a quarter of a century, practicing the hands-on management style that nurtured community spirit among those within the hospital walls. Rosenkrantz did not seek to dissuade the women from seeking retirement. Many nonsupervisory older employees also retired, and turnover steadily increased. Some of the women managers had lived in the nurses' residence, and their vacant rooms created a visible and emotional void for the student nurses, lowering morale and increasing resentment. From 1962 to 1964, almost all of the women managers had retired, producing an uneasy transition and turnover.[86]

The second vulnerability was the anti-union sentiment expressed by Rosenkrantz, who asserted that he was "unalterably opposed to a union in a hospital," declaring to colleagues that unions "destroyed the normal hospital administration triad: Board of Trustees, Medical Staff, and Administrator, by imposing an outside party to determine what is proper for the hospital in terms of employee practices."[87] He particularly opposed Local 1199's tactics, stating that the union had "made a race question of it and are calling it freedom."[88]

Local 1199 organizers selected a Beth female employee to actively campaign for unionization on the hospital premises, during working hours, correctly predicting that Rosenkrantz would first confront and then summarily fire her. He did and at seven o'clock the next morning, a group of employees gathered in front of the hospital, threatening a mass walkout in her support.[89] The Administrative Committee recommended that two attorneys for the board negotiate with the union to set terms for a general election.

The attorneys, Harold Grotta (the grandson of Theresa Grotta) and Alan V. Lowenstein, both well known in Newark's Jewish community, had the board's complete confidence and assumed responsibility for negotiations. They reassured board members that they would not encourage agreement to

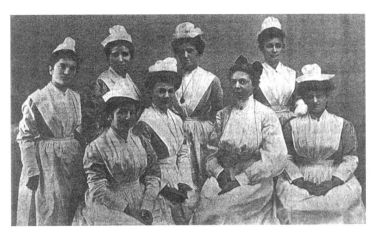

FIGURE 1. The first nurse staff of the hospital (the converted Pennington mansion), from *Report of the Newark Beth Israel Hospital and Dispensary, January 1, 1901 to January 1, 1906. Back row*, R. Gleicher, K. Sinis, L. McGill, B. Levy; *front row*, D. Gleicher; S. Kaufer; C. Feitzinger, director of the nurse training school and superintendent; B. Hunkele. *Courtesy of the Jewish Historical Society of MetroWest and featured in the exhibition "Born at the Beth: Newark's Jewish Hospital since 1901."*

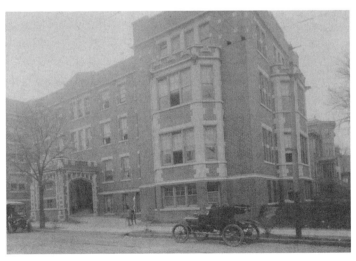

FIGURE 2. The Newark Beth Israel Hospital, corner West Kinney and High Streets, circa 1921. The frame building adjacent to the hospital in the background is the old Weston mansion that briefly served as the nurses' residence and then as the hospital laboratory, 1910–1928. *Courtesy of the Jewish Historical Society of MetroWest and featured in the exhibition.*

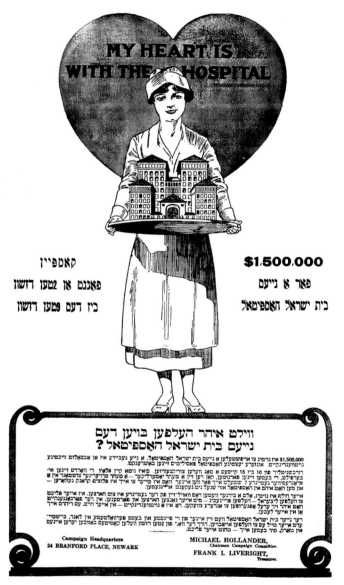

FIGURE 3. "Miss Beth," who epitomized the modern hospital in the 1924 campaign for a new Newark Beth Israel Hospital building; this full-page advertisement appeared in the June 1, 1924, *Der Tog*.

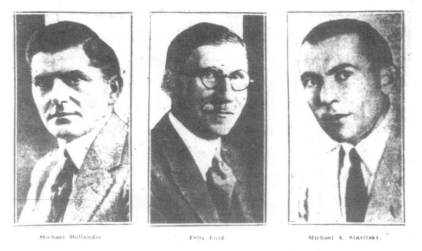

Michael Hollander   Felix Fuld   Michael A. Stavitsky.

FIGURE 4. Michael Hollander, Felix Fuld, and Michael Stavitsky, *left to right,* who headed the 1924 and 1928 Newark Beth Israel Hospital campaign drives for the new hospital. *Library of Congress.*

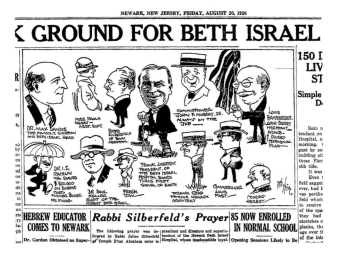

FIGURE 5. "150 Defy Rain to See Liveright Symbolize Start on Institution," a *Newark Jewish Chronicle* cartoon that gently satirized the August 18, 1926, ground-breaking ceremony for the new Beth Israel Hospital on Lyons Avenue near Osborne Terrace. Just before the ceremony, a brief rainstorm had transformed the construction site into a soggy mud bog.

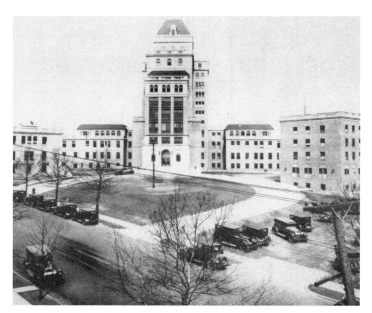

FIGURE 6. Newark Beth Israel Hospital on Lyons Avenue, circa 1930, its front lawn transformed into a parking lot. *Courtesy of the Jewish Historical Society of MetroWest and featured in the exhibition "Born at the Beth: Newark's Jewish Hospital since 1901."*

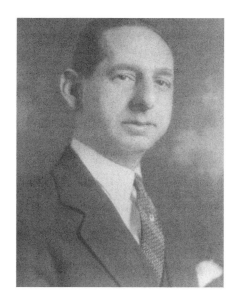

FIGURE 7. Abraham Lichtman, chair of the hospital board, 1935–1951, credited with saving the hospital from bankruptcy and closing during the Great Depression. *Courtesy of the Jewish Historical Society of MetroWest and featured in the exhibition.*

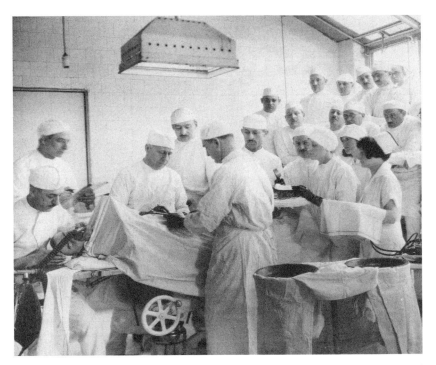

FIGURE 8. Dr. Max Danzis, *third from left*, performing surgery in Newark Beth Israel Hospital operating pavilion, circa 1930. One of the founders of the hospital, Danzis was chief of medical staff, 1920-1940. *Courtesy of the Jewish Historical Society of MetroWest and featured in the exhibition.*

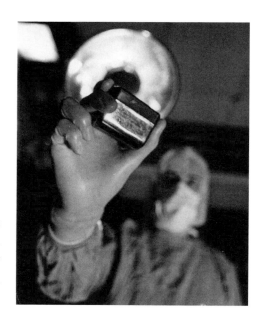

FIGURE 9. Dr. Victor Parsonnet holding an implantable pacemaker. *Courtesy of the Jewish Historical Society of MetroWest and featured in the exhibition "Born at the Beth: Newark's Jewish Hospital since 1901."*

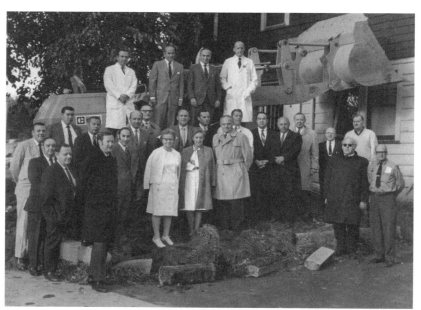

FIGURE 10. Poised to demolish the last remaining house on Osborne Terrace in preparation for phase 3, the construction of the pavilion complex. *Top row*, Alan Sagner, *second from left;* Dr. Victor Parsonnet, *far right*. Chair of the board, 1966–1973, Sagner implemented the phased-construction plan and renamed the hospital the Newark Beth Israel Medical Center in 1968. *Courtesy of the Jewish Historical Society of MetroWest and featured in the exhibition.*

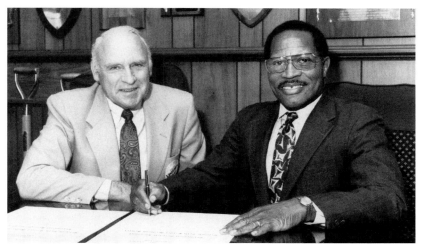

FIGURE 11. Lester Bornstein, who joined the hospital in 1957 and served as executive director, 1968–1995, with Sharpe James, South Ward councilman and Newark mayor since 1986. *Courtesy of the Jewish Historical Society of MetroWest and featured in the exhibition.*

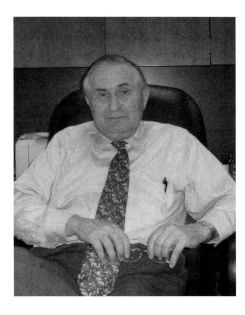

FIGURE 12. Lester Lieberman, chair of the Beth Israel Hospital Corporation, including the Newark Beth Israel Medical Center, 1980–1996, who oversaw construction phases 4–9 and founded the Healthcare Foundation of New Jersey. *Courtesy of the Jewish Historical Society of MetroWest and featured in the exhibition.*

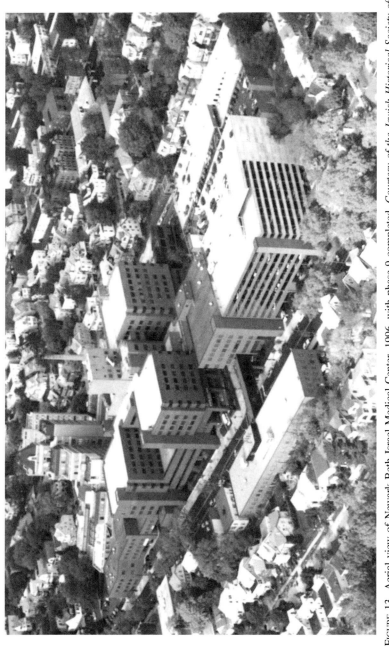

Figure 13. Aerial view of Newark Beth Israel Medical Center, 1996, with phase 9 completed. *Courtesy of the Jewish Historical Society of MetroWest and featured in the exhibition "Born at the Beth: Newark's Jewish Hospital since 1901."*

any contract not in the best interests of the hospital, no matter how great the pressure. On October 9, 1964, the Beth employees gathered in the auditorium and voted to have Local 1199 act as the bargaining agent for the hospital's 300 nonprofessionals. Afterward, Lowenstein said the representatives of 1199 "conducted themselves as ladies and gentlemen. . . . The union conducted itself through its representatives, including its counsel, with dignity, intelligence, and cooperation. This showed their confidence they would succeed."[90]

By the end of October 1964, every major hospital in Newark was unionized. The Beth's board members extended their unanimous thanks to Grotta and Lowenstein, and the latter advised them how to behave in future labor relations: "The hospital is embarking on a new development which industry has faced for the past 30 or 40 years. We must learn to deal with the problems of personnel on the same level as industry has learned." Lowenstein understood that fair and equitable treatment could be realized only if the hospital's financial existence was secure. Therefore, he added that with the prospect of hospital technicians unionizing, the Beth must study its personnel administration carefully and try to "hold to the economic adjustments we would normally make if the union were not here."[91] The following year, when Local 68 signed up five boiler-room engineers at the Beth, Grotta worked directly with union organizers to negotiate a contract.

Paying for Hospitalization

As the Newark Jewish community grappled with the shift in its geographical distribution and ethnic identity, the Beth Israel Hospital administration was grappling with the transformation taking place as their patients presented the requirements of their insurance carriers to the staff of the hospital billing, accounting, and social work departments.

The first to identify the transformation in payment for hospitalization was Minnie Edelshick, the director of the Social Services Department. In 1949, Edelshick, whose staff conducted pre-admission interviews to assess the patients' ability to pay for hospitalization, identified that the Beth "all-inclusive rate plan" was incompatible with the itemized services reimbursement plan of the Blue Cross New Jersey Hospital Plan. Effective April 15, 1949, the Beth and a number of other Newark hospitals adopted the reimbursable cost formula, compatible with the Blue Cross plan. When Behrman explained to the Beth board that the reimbursable cost for the hospital per ward patient rate was slightly higher than the all-inclusive rate, the change was approved unanimously.[92]

In 1950, Edelshick presented statistics demonstrating that almost 43 percent of patients admitted to the hospital were covered by the Blue Cross third-party payment plan. The Jewish philanthropic mechanisms of support for the hospitalization of Jewish patients had greatly diminished. To Behrman, these numbers bore out the idea that Newark Beth Israel was no longer a charitable hospital surviving on the largesse of Jewish philanthropy, but a non-profit voluntary hospital engaged in balancing the expenses per inpatient day with the reimbursements from insurance carriers.

In the 1950s, competition among prepayment plans and an increasing demand for coverage resulted in a marked increase in the number of Americans with health insurance, from 77 to 132 million. The number with surgical coverage grew from 54 to 121 million; with medical coverage, from 22 to 87 million. Blue Cross enrollment escalated from 30 to 52 million between 1948 and 1958, with Blue Shield members across the nation in that period jumping from 8 to 40 million and paying nearly $3 billion in premiums.[93]

The increase in the number of insured patients meant an increase in hospital utilization; hospitals and insurance administrators feared that physicians were ordering unnecessary tests and extra days in the hospital for well-insured private patients because it was so convenient to see them in the hospital. Increased use heightened hospitals' reimbursement demands and pressured the "Blues" to seek rate increases. However, controlling use was never easy; it raised the "spectre of bureaucratic intrusion into the sacrosanct relationship between patient and physician."[94] Still, the data were unmistakable: hospital expenses per patient per day more than doubled between the mid-1940s and the mid-1950s. As Rosemary Stevens observed: "Expense per inpatient day was a crude measure—not allowing, in particular, for the increasing amount of outpatient care being given in these years, nor for the changes in hospital productivity," but there could be no mistaking the national trend, as "average expenses per patient day rose from less than $10 in 1946 to over $44 in 1965."[95]

In May 1952, Behrman negotiated a 5 percent increase in payments from the Hospital Service Plan and the next year reported that the number of Beth patients covered by Blue Cross had increased astoundingly to almost 70 percent. The fifty-year-old policy of the hospital to request payment at the time of admission no longer made sense. Very few patients paid any amount to the cashier in advance of their hospitalization. At the time of discharge, when patients received a hospital bill, they submitted a claim to their insurance carrier for reimbursement, and the processing of this claim extended the delay for the hospital to receive payment. Hospital insurance rates for reimbursement of services were often less than the amount charged by the hospital, further complicating receiving full payment. Behrman solved this problem by quietly discontinuing the pre-admission policy and instituting a hospital cash-indemnity plan whereby the hospital would submit charges directly to the insurance carrier and the patient would be billed for only the difference between the insurance carrier rates and the hospital charges.

Blue Cross and other insurance carriers reimbursed their subscribers for the cost of semi-private rooms and allowed patients to upgrade to private rooms; it was in the best interest of the hospital to encourage patients to choose these accommodations rather than a bed on the ward. By 1956, the number of ward patients, at that time, the source of "clinical material" for medical training, had dwindled to such a low number that the hospital's accreditation for residency in surgery was in jeopardy. The board agreed to pay for two ward beds at a cost of $12,000 per year in order to provide the opportunity for residents to enhance their medical education via the treatment of patients who consented to be studied.[96]

The escalating reimbursement schedules helped offset the ever-increasing costs of technology and improved patient care. In 1957, an adjustment resulted in Blue Cross sending the Beth $140,000, the anticipated increased cost of operation. The latest news about the hospital's negotiations with Blue Cross on one matter or another topped almost every meeting agenda.

Medicare

In 1959, the health care sector in the United States was bracing for the advent of federal health-insurance legislation, which had not passed during the Truman and Eisenhower administrations but would certainly be part of the both Democrat and Republican political party platforms in the 1960s. The goals and constituencies of the AHA and AMA had diverged in the early 1950s as the AHA assumed the accreditation of hospitals in the formation of the Joint Commission of Accredited Hospital Organizations (JCAHO). The AMA constituency contended that the central point of medical care was between the physician and patient and the AHA institutions contended that the central point for provision of medical care was the hospital. Hospitals were bearing the burden of increasing costs not fully covered by private insurance carriers, the need for new equipment and renovation of their facilities, and the shift to an older patient population that did not have the financial means to pay their bills. The AHA began to favor the concept of social security legislation.

In 1963, the passage of the Kerr-Mills Act created a medical assistance program for the aged, a boon for voluntary hospitals. The next year, hospitals and medical professionals readied themselves for the passage of the supplement to the Social Security Act that would create Medicare. In New Jersey physicians talked of refusing to serve patients who would receive hospital care paid by Social Security, fearing that this new federal program was the vanguard of socialized medicine. Rosenkrantz denounced such reactions: "Beth Israel Hospital will always serve persons in need of medical care regardless of the method involvement in payment of bills. If federal legislation is passed concerning medical care for the aged, we will obey the law."[97] The plans for a boycott of Medicare patients faded, but fears remained that socialized medicine would overwhelm the hospitals.[98]

Medicare was established as part of Lyndon Johnson's Great Society program to revolutionize health-care distribution to the elderly and the poor. Its major provisions, which went into effect (under PL 89–97) in 1966, offered a compulsory hospital-insurance-benefit program to persons sixty-five and over, a voluntary supplementary plan to finance physicians' care, and an expanded medical assistance program for the medically needy.[99] Basic benefits in the original law included up to ninety days of inpatient hospital care per illness, outpatient care, post-hospital care in a qualified nursing home for up to one hundred days per illness, home-health services, and physician services, with various deductibles and coinsurance required of patients. Hospitals were now guaranteed payment by the federal government on a schedule of "reasonable costs."[100]

The Department of Health, Education, and Welfare charged the Social Security Administration with administering the new programs. Hospital reimbursement for Medicare patients was organized through fiscal intermediaries, buffers between the federal government and the voluntary, for-profit, and local-government hospitals. The AHA favored intermediaries to protect hospitals from government bureaucrats. Hospitals could select their intermediaries, and over 90 percent in the nation chose Blue Cross.

Stevens states: "Medicare represented the art of the possible—familiar patterns—in terms of program implementation, too. Compulsory hospital insurance for the elderly under Social Security was designed as if it were an extended Blue Cross program. Medicare . . . assumed a basic division between hospital and medical insurance, Part A was to cover hospitals, Part B, physicians."[101] As with Blue Cross, the emphasis was on acute inpatient hospital care. Medicare was never meant to offer comprehensive medical coverage but reimbursement for services rendered, with beneficiaries covered for a specific number of days for each diagnosis. Hospitals were to be paid on a per diem basis.

Hospital administrators had to prepare their institutions for the strain that the new federal system would place on existing hospital services and resources. The process of bringing hospitals into the program began with a January 1966 mailing to nearly 10,000 institutions that met the statutory definition of a hospital, followed by a second mailing in February to 8,000 inviting them to participate, and an evaluation of more than 7,000 utilization plans submitted by these hospitals for certification as Medicare eligible. Medicare went into effect on July 1, 1966, in more than 6,200 hospitals. Six months later, the coverage for extended care services to nursing homes and rehabilitation facilities needed to be ready, so more than 13,000 facilities were undergoing certification concurrently.[102]

The hospitals' preparations .were fraught with apprehension. Many hospital administrators feared that aged patients would defer their care, and all would seek admission on July 1. They anticipated an increased demand for outpatient, extended care, and home-care facilities. Those eligible for Medicare benefits might give up their Blue Cross or other third-party insurance and shift to supplementary insurance to cover coinsurance and deductibles. Physicians feared that Medicare patients, who would be able to enjoy semi-private hospital accommodations and the benefit of being treated as private patients by their own physicians, might not be amenable to serving as "teaching material." If that were the case, then private patients would have to be asked whether they would consent to be seen by interns and residents so that the hospital could sustain its training program.

Supervisors of the administrative departments feared that the new system would unleash an onslaught of paperwork that would overwhelm their staff. In 1967, after the first year of the program, Rosenkrantz reported: "There has been a definite increase in the number of admissions and hospital stays caused by the plan's beneficiaries, but the load has been absorbed with only moderate strain." The experience at the Beth paralleled that reported by hospitals nationally, according to Rosenkrantz, who explained that the hospital was "not flooded by patients over age sixty-five. Despite many problems, our utilization committee functioned efficiently. This does not mean that there were and are no problems, but they were not insurmountable. The introduction of Medicare went along smoothly, the result perhaps of the careful pre-planning."[103]

The statistics bore him out: "The first year of Medicare saw the admission of less than 4 percent more aged patients compared with a like period during the previous year." Indeed, the Beth "experienced an 11.8% increase" in the years prior to Medicare. What changed was the number of total days of care, Rosenkrantz observed: "Our Medicare patients were responsible for 26.9% of the total days of care, even though the group represented 14.2% of the total admissions." Between 1966 and 1967, "3,380 Medicare patients were responsible for 35,181 hospital days." Rosenkrantz believed that Medicare's biggest advantage for the elderly was that it allowed them to consult private physicians rather than remain unattended because they could not afford adequate care.[104]

Certainly there were problems occasioned by the new system. The onslaught of forms affected outpatient Physical Therapy, Pharmacy, and Medical Records Departments the most. The Beth's billing system, admissions, and medical record keeping had to be automated, as the utilization reviews would require quick access to medical records and bill statements. In the first years, payments to physicians were not prompt and federal payment schedules for particular procedures were below those of Blue Cross. Still, physicians and hospitals, not federal bureaucrats, were in charge. Rosenkrantz concluded: "The Medicare program is excellent social medicine, providing for the health of millions of older individuals."[105]

Transition Converges to Turmoil, Newark, 1966–1968

Newark's 300th anniversary, commemorating Puritan Robert Treat's arrival, began on May 18, 1966, with a parade complete with marching bands and banners praising the contributions of the many ethnic groups that across time had contributed to Newark's accomplishments. Newark's mayor and other leaders welcomed the mayor of Newark-on-Trent, England, and predicted a bright century to come. The celebration did not focus on the transformation of the city since its 250th anniversary celebration: Newark was now officially designated an economically depressed city.

The tricentennial celebration launched two campaigns: one that promised Newark its own medical school and a second that sought to persuade Newarkers that the area where the medical school might be located was sufficiently blighted to justify razing the buildings and relocating residents to public housing in other locations of the city. In 1954, Newark had lost a campaign to Jersey City for a medical school. But Jersey City's victory had been Pyrrhic—from 1954 to 1961, the private medical college had incurred massive operating expenses that the city could no longer afford. New Jersey governor Richard J. Hughes and the state's legislative leaders appointed a fact-finding committee that on July 28, 1964, endorsed a purchase of the school's assets from Seton Hall University for $4 million; in 1965, the New Jersey State educational system purchased the medical college, and plans were set in motion to move it to Newark.

There was one major obstacle: the medical college wanted to relocate to another part of the state. Its president, Dr. Stanley Bergen Jr., and the college trustees were eyeing the 138-acre Dodge estate in Madison, New Jersey, which they considered a "beautiful bucolic setting available to the State of New Jersey at reasonable cost—versus an inner city site in Newark."[106] However, Mayor Addonizio, determined to bring the medical college to Newark, offered land next to the City Hospital, which had been renamed the Harrison S. Martland Medical Center. The trustees, hoping to quash the negotiations, made a demand that they thought would cause Newark to withdraw from the negotiations: 150 acres of downtown Newark must be razed for the medical school's new structure and campus. The mayor's staff later admitted that they had never expected to deliver more than 30 acres, believing that the medical college was less interested in the land than in scotching a move to Newark.

Much to the chagrin of the medical school administration, Newark officials met their demand to raze an area that encompassed not only the most decaying blocks, but also neighborhoods of working- and lower-middle-class residents. The area would be declared an "urban blight" so that Newark would be eligible to receive federal assistance for the destruction of the housing. African American residents of the so-called blighted area noted that at least some of the area included middle-class housing. Hughes Allison, the author of the Joe Hill detective novels and whose father had been the president of the Newark NAACP, showed a reporter his Wallace Street home and others that had been renovated by their owners and now even had central air-conditioning.[107]

On January 4, 1967, title searches, a prelude to condemnation of buildings, began with the goal of razing the blocks in the central city by March 1, 1968. News articles about the swirling controversy appeared almost daily. The Weequahic community opposed the medical college, contending that the city, which had already lost the tax base of thousands of urban families and businesses displaced by the construction of I-78, seemed destined to lose even more by destroying more housing in the city. The North and Ironbound Wards said little, but Central Ward residents began to organize. Members of the Committee against Negro Removal marched on city hall, the first organized protest. But, a survey commissioned by the United Community Corporation of Newark (UCC) lowered the estimate of the number of families likely to be affected to 727 and reported that most Newarkers polled were in favor of a medical school someplace in Newark; those faced with displacement wanted only to be given sufficient reimbursement to move to equivalent private housing, not public housing.[108]

What then caused the opposition to coalesce and to escalate? At least one reason was the equation of urban removal with other acts of discrimination against African Americans. Tensions in Newark were boiling over between different ethnic groups. Two incidents raised the tension between African American and Jewish residents. In 1966, an arson fire at Ahavath Zion destroyed its Torah scrolls and prompted its rabbi, who was also the Beth Israel Hospital chaplain, to relocate the congregation outside the city. In downtown Newark, elderly Jewish business owners struggled daily against robberies and the atmosphere of fear. In April 1967, picketers marched against a Jewish meat market on Clinton Hill, complaining of mistreatment, and forced the owner to close.[109]

That month, a new anti–medical school protest began. In downtown Newark a group of picketers held signs saying "Damn the Med School" or "There's No Place for Black People to Go." Charging the NAACP with inaction, picketers urged passing African Americans to burn their NAACP cards.

The protesters, many of whom were not Newark residents, were sufficiently savvy to penetrate the UCC, which had been created as an antipoverty agency by Rabbi Jonathan Prinz, the son of Rabbi Joachim Prinz of the B'nai Abraham synagogue. In May 1967, the young Rabbi Prinz's resignation from the UCC was quickly followed by the president's and a change in UCC leadership. New leaders who opposed the medical school's construction did not hesitate to tell the City Council that the medical school was a "gross example of racism and denial of the rights of the people." One longtime Central Ward resident commenting about the municipal and UCC leadership said: "The people who are the backbone of the community feel they are not at the moment being given consideration or being effectively consulted on policies or programs that affect them."[110]

In June 1967, the *News* headlines trumpeted that President Lyndon Johnson had nominated Thurgood Marshall to the Supreme Court, but Newarkers also read two other stories on page one more critical to the community. There was an article about the thirty hours of testimony against the Medical School during which the new associate director of the UCC threatened that if the medical school were built before new housing was completed, "the blood will run down the streets of Newark."[111] There was a third article on page one describing what would come to be called the Six Day War in Israel. The controversy over the medical school festered.

Toward the end of June, the Newark City Council announced that the medical school would be built, but would not carry out the plan to destroy 150 acres that had stirred so much controversy in the community. The $5 million pre-engineered facility would rise on an 11.5-acre tract in an area already set aside for the construction of a state health center; the proposed site was already 80 percent cleared. However, the news was too little, too late. The tensions between African Americans and the city that seemed willing to bulldoze their streets for a highway and their homes for a medical school had transformed Newark into a tinderbox. All that was needed for a bonfire was a spark.

On the evening of Thursday, July 13, 1967, physicians in Newark Beth Israel's emergency room were treating the usual complement of sick children, elderly suffering from heat exhaustion, and women in labor. The peak load of patients was at noon, and the busiest days were Saturday and Sunday, when many patients came in on the way home from church. The lacerations and orthopedic cases were mainly the products of pediatric accidents. The emergency room staff rarely saw the products of urban violence.[112] That was about to change.

Two policemen entered, between them a man in handcuffs—John W. Smith, a driver for the Safety Cab Company, who an hour earlier was tailgating a patrol car. When the police stopped him, there was an exchange of profanities, followed by an altercation and an arrest. Smith was taken to a holding cell at the Central Ward precinct, where by 10:40 P.M. a crowd of 250 had gathered. At the request of some in the crowd, Smith was taken to Beth Israel Hospital for a checkup. Although the doctors thought he might have a broken rib, he was returned to police headquarters to scotch the rumor that had spread through the Central Ward neighborhood that the police had killed him.[113]

Early Friday morning, a brick shattered a store window at Montgomery and Belmont Avenues; a full-scale riot ensued. High Street and Springfield Avenues were the center of the looting and burning. As injured riot victims jammed Martland Medical Center, nurses on duty said that it reminded them of the Korean War. "Even the reporters who were counting persons with gunshot wounds had to stop tallying" as ambulances arrived with bullet holes in their windshields.[114]

Victims with lacerations from flying glass and bullet wounds streamed into the Beth, overflowing the emergency-treatment rooms; new incoming patients had to be treated in the entrance hall. Beth Israel had become a "casualty station."[115] Arrivals in need of surgery were being moved into surgical suites around the clock. The house staff and nurses worked double shifts, catching sleep on hastily assembled cots. Hundreds of people were camped out in hallways, many exhibiting signs of shock. Others seeking sanctuary from the rioters crowded into Temple B'nai Abraham. Members of the Beth Israel staff recall going up on the roof of the hospital and watching rioters race up and down nearby streets, pursued by the police. Staff who lived outside the area remained within the hospital's walls, fearing that if they left in their cars, they would be stoned and beaten.[116]

The aftermath of the riot was eerie. A citywide curfew enforced by police cleared the streets. For the first time in more than a century, the Hill was silent. On the heels of the state troopers and police came the reporters and photographers, who found Prince Street stores in ruin. So many houses were destroyed or burned that demolition proved more practical than reconstruction. In the weeks and months to come, the houses of the central city that had served generations of newcomers were bulldozed and scooped away.

The assassination of Dr. Martin Luther King Jr. the next year did not cause a second riot in the city. Rather, on April 8, 1968, some 25,000 "white suburbanites and Negro ghetto dwellers," in a column more than a mile and a half long that filled High Street from curb to curb, marched "side-by-side . . . in a display of racial understanding that was torn by riots last July." The "solemn procession . . . silently passed the remnants of violence, boarded up store fronts, charred shells of houses and stores, in hopes of creating a dialogue of peace between white and black."[117] From High Street, which would be renamed Martin Luther King Boulevard, they marched through Lincoln Street and Quitman Place and past the Abyssinian Baptist Church at 225 West Kinney, where King had spoken just eight days earlier.

Ladies Auxiliary members volunteered to provide coverage at the Beth Israel Hospital so that as many employees as possible could join the march that day. Sagner marched, as did many of the board. It was not a parade, but a movement of hope through the streets.[118]

The Ladies Auxiliary, manning the desks and workstations that day, carried out their tradition of supporting the hospital staff begun nearly forty years earlier, but they clearly realized that they were performing tasks in a hospital and a city markedly different than their predecessors had known. Mrs. Samuel Einhorn, had become president of the Ladies Auxiliary in June 1967 and a year later, in June 1968, delivered a speech that reflected the concerns of many. Recalling for her listeners the events of the previous summer, Einhorn observed that "Newark Beth Israel Hospital is staffed by many who are not Jewish, serves many who are not Jewish, and is located in an area no longer predominantly Jewish supported by mostly non-Jewish funds. . . . This then is our hospital, one located deep in the city, away from the descendants of its founders, serving amid the disadvantaged and close to areas of tension. This is what history in 1968 asks us to accept and support."[119]

Einhorn was emphatic in urging her colleagues and members of the Jewish community to support the hospital and its core mission to be a non-sectarian institution with "the obligation to make medical care available to all who need it." But it was time for the old image of the Jewish hospital as part of the history of the Hill and Weequahic Jewish communities to change. "The image of Beth Israel . . . needs redefinition. It is a medical center engaged in highly sophisticated and original medical research, utilizing specialized and highly complex medical equipment and techniques and providing extended and rehabilitative care. It is no longer an ethnic institution but rather a serving center, an integral part of the community and dedicated to it."[120]

In 1965, Sagner had conjured the Hebrew phrase *"Ain brera,"* no other choice, when he proposed keeping Beth Israel Hospital in Newark and making it a regional medical center.[121] In 1968, Einhorn may have had that phrase in mind as well.

CHAPTER 7

Medical Research at Midcentury

❦

By mid-century, Newark Beth Israel's buff-colored Spanish style tower building had been a part of Newark's skyline for nearly a quarter century. Those who had worked through the night in the tower could sip their morning coffee looking out across the city. Dr. Rita Finkler, who spent many such nights at the Beth, recalled how she enjoyed greeting the dawn from the tower's top floor: "I often saw the beautiful sight of the sunrise which I watched from the tenth floor of the maternity suite. Ah how good it was to have an early breakfast and feel that you really earned it."[1]

The institutional culture of the Beth at midcentury combined warmth, encouragement, and opportunity in a way that produced institutional loyalty among staff and physicians alike. In 1964, Kenneth L. Tyson, an undergraduate chemistry major, walked up the Lyons Avenue hill from Bergen Street to interview for an internship with laboratory director Dr. Lester Goldman, well known in Newark for riding herd on his medical technology students. The towering building seemed to loom higher as Tyson approached, and inside, he stood awestruck. For nearly forty years, the imposing lobby with its walls carved of rosy Tavernelle marble, well-proportioned arches, decorative spiral columnettes, and terrazzo floor had momentarily stunned first-time visitors. But amidst the cool marble, Tyson was warmed by the friendliness of the staff members who guided him to Goldman's office. The laboratory director greeted him with a combination of kindness and interest that made the young non-Jewish man feel very much at home. And indeed for the next thirty years the Beth was home for Tyson, who became a manager and ultimately the Beth's senior vice president.[2]

The warmth and high spirits that impressed Tyson also characterized the Beth's medical staff, perhaps in part because by then many of its members were the relatives of an earlier generation of Beth physicians. The hospital's 1964 annual report listed the family of Dr. Louis Reich, brother-in-law of Dr. Max Danzis, which included Drs. Mortimer, Abraham, and Henry Reich. Drs. Lustig, Goodman, and Schotland were all related by marriage to Dr. Henry Reich. Dr. Walter Rados was carrying on the work of his parents, Drs. Andrew and Berta Rados; Dr. Edward Comando, the work of his father, Dr. Harry Comando. Dr. Rita Finkler's daughter, Dr. Sylvia Becker, was in practice with her husband, Dr. Marvin Becker. Drs. Robert, Saul, and Herbert Lieb, all cousins, worked in the wards. The Kern family contingent included Dr. Meyer Kern, whose son and grandson were in practice, as well as his nephew and two cousins. Dr. Virginia Drobner, daughter of Dr. Louis Brodkin, was in service at the Beth, and brothers Samuel and Harvey Einhorn practiced together.

What Tyson felt on his first visit was more than a family atmosphere. The warmth was expressed in the Beth's creed, adopted in 1928. Perhaps inspired by a 1924 American Hospital Association pledge, it was composed by a Beth Israel employee whose identity remains unknown:

> Personal attention, notable for its warmth and sincerity, and inspired by a sympathetic recognition of the human element, is the powerful but gentle handmaiden of science employed by doctors, nurses, and attendants at Beth Israel Hospital. Patients are people—not cases—at this hospital. The sick and convalescent here are not laboratory specimens to be examined, treated, re-examined, and catalogued. Rather they are men, women, and children—human beings—and are treated as such. The value of the human touch as a power for healing is never lost sight of at Beth Israel.[3]

The words struck a responsive chord in altruists who chose health care. Looking back at his career as the head of the Department of Surgery, Dr. Samuel Diener recalled: "I was the happiest person in the world to be a doctor. I couldn't wait to get to work. I loved it so much."[4]

As the identity of Newark Beth Israel Hospital was transformed during the tumultuous midcentury years, physicians, surgeons, nurses, and the professional, technical, and ancillary staff who worked in the aging ornate tower managed to transform the hospital into a distinguished research and regional medical center.

The Beth at Fifty

In 1950, board members struggled to fix a date for a jubilee celebration. Should they count fifty years from the date that the Daughters of Israel incorporated, from the date that the Daughters of Israel and the Hebrew Dispensary Association agreed to merge in 1901, or from the date that the first Beth Hospital, on High and West Kinney streets opened its doors?[5]

Few physicians who had begun their careers at the "Old Beth" on High Street still practiced at the hospital on Lyons Avenue. A new generation of medical staff, including many veterans, served at the hospital, where physicians seeking postgraduate training competed for one of three residencies—medicine, surgery, or gynecology—some using the G.I. Bill to defray the cost of their three-year appointments.[6] While these younger physicians could probably not have cited Vannevar Bush's report concerning the future of science, they were increasingly familiar with the funding mechanisms being created by both private industry and the federal government to support research, and aware of the need to combine teaching and research in the practice of progressive medicine.

Medical progress often seemed especially swift in the postwar era. At the Beth, as at other hospitals, penicillin and other antibiotics were being dispensed in the pharmacy. New Jersey had selected the Beth Israel Hospital as the site of the first radioisotope center, where all isotopes for clinical use would be available.[7] The most recent accreditation approval report of the American College of Surgeons (ACS) had commended the hospital on the excellence of its cancer clinic; a tissue pathologist had been appointed; and the Schering Corporation, which manufactured the state-of-the-art technology in the field, supplied equipment to Dr. Leff and the Radiology Department to test in the new field of angiocardiography.[8] The opening of the new hospital auditorium enabled the hospital to host a meeting of the New Jersey OB/Gyn Society, advancing its reputation as a venue for scholarly and professional discourse.[9] The auditorium was also put to good use for the annual ceremonies and open house for Hospital Day, the birthday of Florence Nightingale that became the occasion to honor hospital volunteers.

The *Journal*: A Chronicle of Achievement, 1950–1976

In 1949, President Abraham Lichtman had marked the beginning of jubilee planning by endowing an in-house medical journal, in honor of his late wife, Dorothy. To unanimous board and medical staff approval, the *Journal of the Newark Beth Israel Hospital* was launched in January 1950. Its inaugural blue cover featured a hospital emblem designed by Dr. Aaron Parsonnet, and its end pages included advertisements for the Newark insurance firm of Rachlin and Hollander and offers for institutional and individual subscriptions.[10]

The *Journal* was one of many in-house journals published by Jewish hospitals unaffiliated with medical schools. Mount Sinai Hospital in New York and Michael Reese Hospital in Chicago had both initiated journals in the 1930s, Brooklyn Hospital in 1939, and, in the 1950s—along with the Beth—Sinai Hospital in Baltimore, Sinai Hospital in Detroit, Mount Sinai Hospital in Chicago, and Mount Sinai Hospital in Minneapolis. Others, published medical-staff newsletters such as Mount Zion in San Francisco and in Los Angeles, the Cedars of Lebanon and Sinai hospitals.[11]

The purpose of the Beth *Journal* was to establish in the national medical community the hospital's identity as a modern teaching and research institution:

> The *Journal* exists as the sounding board and recording device for the work of the medical staff of the hospital. We strive to report the enormous amount of clinical and investigative experience of the people working at the hospital. We print whatever is worthy of reporting and recording of the many interesting cases and problems occurring at our very active hospital. We have always planned our pages for their educational value and as a stimulant towards better medicine. The material presented is a true cross section of the hospital work, clinical and laboratory; and is representative of the work in medicine, surgery, obstetrics, gynecology, anesthesiology, pediatrics and radiology.[12]

From 1950 to 1976, the *Journal* chronicled the achievements of the hospital's medical staff as the nonprofit voluntary hospital became a regional medical center for New Jersey. The *Journal* offers a distinctive perspective on the hospital post–World War II in research articles by a new generation of residents, descriptions of new departments, and accounts of new technologies and new surgical procedures.[13]

The first editorial advisory board represented the "Old Beth." Dr. Abram Abrams, the first chief editor, joined the hospital as an intern in 1916 and also served on staff at Newark's Presbyterian Hospital. Dr. Henry Davidson, who also was a Beth intern, had become the chief of neuropsychiatry for the New Jersey Veterans Administration and was editor of the state medical journal. Dr. Max Danzis had received the Edward J. Ill award from the Academy of Medicine of Northern New Jersey. Dr. Aaron Parsonnet, one of the founders of the American College of Cardiology, had coauthored two books and fifty papers in his field. They were joined by two men whose names would become synonymous with New Jersey medicine: Dr. Henry H. Kessler, formerly an attending orthopedic surgeon at the Beth, director of the New Jersey Rehabilitation Commission before World War II, and the founder of the Kessler Institute for Rehabilitation; and Dr. Harrison S. Martland, the medical examiner of Essex County, famous for his study of radiation poisoning among female workers who had dipped their brushes into pots of radium-infused paint, licked them to sharpen the points, and painted the watch faces that glowed in the dark.

As soon as the *Journal* began publication, it became the editor's sad task to include obituaries, beginning with a tribute to Aaron Parsonnet. For many years, Dr. Arthur Bernstein had been expected to respond to a summons even in the middle of the night from Parsonnet, his brilliant, quirky mentor, to discuss an idea or to serve as the sounding board for a nocturnal insight into some medical mystery. One Sunday afternoon, responding to a frantic call, Bernstein arrived at the Parsonnet home to find the distinguished sixty-year-old physician, who had written so extensively about heart disease, sitting upright in his favorite dining chair, dead of a sudden massive heart attack.[14]

Dr. Max Danzis by midcentury was the grand old man of the Beth, one of two surviving physicians who had practiced in both the Pennington and Old Beth on High Street.[15] In the ten years since his retirement from practice, he had become a skilled orator whose speeches marked every significant hospital milestone.[16] The *Journal*'s October 1951 editorial announced that he would be in charge of the jubilee anniversary celebration November 5–10, 1951; the date chosen to commemorate the incorporation of the merged two associations. Danzis presented to the hospital and the public a veritable cavalcade of thirty motion-picture documentary shorts, one shown every afternoon and every evening, often accompanied by a formal address by a guest professor from a medical school. The final jubilee event was a dinner dance at Newark's Essex House.[17]

Two years later, Danzis died from natural causes, not from the influenza he feared.[18] *Journal* editorials lauded Danzis's life and the causes he championed, especially the training and education of medical students. The self-made man was memorialized by an annual lecture in his name and a medical education scholarship fund to subsidize the training of medical students.[19] The grand old man was succeeded on the *Journal* editorial board by Dr. Rita Finkler, by now the grand old lady of the Beth, an emeritus consultant.[20] Finkler, in her jubilee year of practice and research, ever dynamic, had refocused her research to the study of the endocrinology of menopause.

The jubilee program had been conspicuous for the absence of attention given to the research studies performed by Beth medical and laboratory staff, such as the ongoing work on hemophilia funded by the hospital research foundation.[21] The *New York Times* noted that Beth physicians had developed a new human blood-plasma product designed to be injected into hemophiliacs to replace the protein factor missing in their blood, and that the results of their research were presented before a meeting of the Genetics Section of the Carnegie Institute.[22]

Subsequently, the *Journal* announced the creation of an annual issue devoted to a specific field of medicine so that the medical staff could present their original research and clinical reviews of hospital cases. The first of these, which detailed the theoretical and practical aspects of the basis of radium in medicine, generated "a deep sense of pride in the medical staff of this institution, pride in the administration that made this department possible, and pride in the staff of the department . . . to be able to present so fine a scientific analysis."[23] The annual issues covered a wide variety of fields. The 1956 *Journal* symposium issue was devoted to surveying and analyzing the Beth's clinical cases of gastric cancer. A review by the resident staff included 671 gastrectomies, including 116 cases of gastric carcinoma, 95 cases of diverticulitis, 115 cases of colon carcinoma, and an eight-year survey of intussusception, the infolding of one part of the intestines into the other. Subsequent symposeal issues addressed obstetrics and gynecology, pediatrics, surgical specialties, laboratory, cancer, radiology, emergencies, special procedures, the thyroid, and the urinary system.

The Beth medical staff did not initially pursue federal funding for their work. In 1958, a resident independently applied for and received a $4,000 fellowship grant from the U.S. Department of Health to study the effect of tobacco on the vascular system.[24] It was a prestigious award, but the hospital received only $500 for overhead costs, which seemed to some Beth board members insignificant compared to the funding the hospital had received from the Rippel and Ford Foundations for construction of the new laboratory.

Medical research was often encouraged by gifts from the Ladies Auxiliary. In 1956, Bernstein recruited Dr. Seymour Ribot, an attending physician at the Veterans' Hospital in East Orange, whom he had met through their collaboration on United Jewish Appeal activities. Ribot was transfixed when he entered a room adjacent to the Emergency Room and saw the latest gift to the Department of Medicine from the Ladies Auxiliary: a twin-coil artificial-kidney dialyzer.[25] He remembered staring at the amazing machine and thinking that the gift was the equivalent of receiving a supersonic airplane. Fascinated, he was inspired to retrain himself in the new field of renal dialysis.[26] By 1958, he and Gerald Weiss performed the first successful renal dialysis procedure in New Jersey. The April 1963 *Journal*, devoted to the outcome of his initial work, included original articles by Ribot and his colleagues concerning their experiments on dogs, the role of the artificial kidney in acute nephritis, and related research on exchange transfusions and the venous system.[27] Throughout the next decade a steady influx of new electronic equipment appeared in the Beth, including a hypothermia machine for open-heart surgery and an artificial-kidney unit.[28]

Research activities at the hospital reached a peak in 1961, as fifty staff members engaged in thirty separate projects, with an additional twenty proposals at the preliminary planning stage. While one group was focusing on the study of heart arrhythmias, another studied whether hardening of the arteries was linked to an inflammation of the lining of the arteries. Still others were studying leukemia, with the goal of effecting a therapeutic treatment with transplanted bone marrow.[29] And the *Journal* was listed in the *Index Medicus*, taking its place among the foremost medical publications in the world for reference and study.[30]

If the grants came gradually, the research progressed rapidly. By 1955, the Department of Cardiodynamics was engaged in some of the most innovative work. An observer wrote: "It was fascinating—the magic thread of the catheter tube, directed by skilled hands, slowly inched its way through the throbbing veins of the boy to the various chambers of the heart, telling a revealing tale to doctors who were watching it on the fluoroscope—a tale that would be minutely analyzed later before a conference of physicians." Two teams of Beth doctors were actively exploring catheterization studies of "blue babies" to assess whether the infants were candidates for the new heart-surgery procedures.[31]

When President Dwight David Eisenhower suffered a serious heart attack in September 1955, the medical crisis captured the attention of Americans—to the benefit of cardiology research already being vigorously pursued at the Beth.[32] The October 1955 *Journal* symposeal issue, dedicated to myocardial infarctions, began with a clinical review of 888 cardiac cases treated at the hospital, authored by eighteen doctors on the medical service. An article coauthored by Dr. Victor Parsonnet, named for his grandfather, described a post-mortem study of myocardial infarction using a new injection technique; Parsonnet had a personal interest in the etiology of sudden myocardial infarctions.[33] His *Journal* article signaled the beginning of the Beth's ascendance as a cardiovascular center. Cardiovascular research work at the Beth progressed under the sponsorship of the Beth Israel Research Foundation, which provided some funding and assisted researchers in obtaining external grants, including funds for basic research on the development of a heart pacemaker.[34]

Throughout the late 1950s and early 1960s, the Beth continued to build its medical reputation in cardiac surgery. Drs. Templeton and Gibbon laid out an in-depth evaluation of the progress of cardiac surgical procedures and the use of heart-lung bypass to save the cardiac patient in a 1958 *Journal* article.[35] In 1962, the medical and technical staffs were sufficiently prepared and trained in perfusion protocols so that the artificial heart-lung machine was used successfully.[36]

The Beth Pacemaker Program

In 1959, Parsonnet proposed the creation of a separate hospital institute for research on cardiac, pulmonary, renal, vascular, cerebral, and cancer diseases, an ambitious program that would place the hospital in the vanguard of medical institutions in New Jersey.[37]

Parsonnet had long mused about the possibility of artificially affecting the heart rhythm; by the late 1950s, technology finally made this doable. The first implantation of an impulse generator, performed in Sweden in 1958, set off a reaction in the medical community equivalent to the nation's response to the Sputnik launch; it marked the start of a new era in cardiac surgery. The "pace race" took off in 1960 with the first successful U.S. surgery, performed by doctors in the Buffalo Veterans Administration Hospital, followed in a few weeks by a similar procedure performed at the Boston Beth Israel Hospital. At first, pacemakers were external, with wires connecting the heart through an incision in the skin to a battery at the patient's side. According to cardiologist and historian of medicine W. Bruce Fye, the demand for implants "skyrocketed" across the nation when a "fully implantable system" was invented. Fye estimates that in the United States, more than 150,000 pacemakers were implanted within fifteen years.[38] Parsonnet and electronic engineer Dr. George H. Myers described this new specialty, biomedical engineering, in part inspired by work in the nation's space program, in a January 1964 *Journal* article.[39]

The work of the Newark Beth Israel Cardiopulmonary Laboratory doctors and engineers concentrated on tackling the toughest problem: pacemaker longevity. The first generation of pacemakers lasted only two years;

the key to extending their work life was a continuous power source. In the years 1961–1966, Newark Beth Israel doctors performed twenty-two complete reoperations and numerous minor operations on their first ninety-three patients (fifty-four had required nothing beyond the original implant). They experimented with sources of bioenergy in the body, studying the motion of the diaphragm and then attaching ceramic plates to the descending aorta so that its expansion and contraction could generate electricity.[40]

By 1968, Beth surgeons had performed 250 pacemaker implantations, had established a fully functioning critical cardiac care unit and a thirty-two-bed nursing unit, and were running an outpatient clinic to monitor their patients. The cardiodynamics section had achieved international renown under the leadership of Parsonnet, Gilbert, and Zucker. Parsonnet and Myers had led a Beth team to the forefront of clinical research in the first decade of pacemaker surgery.[41] More clinical research and the increasing demand for pacemaker implantation heightened the popularity of cardiology as a field in continuing medical and graduate medical education. In 1960, there were 72 cardiology training programs and 142 cardiology trainees nationally; by 1972, 280 programs and 1,260 trainees.[42]

Parsonnet had earlier proposed to the Atomic Energy Commission that a pacemaker could be powered by nuclear energy—a microsized plutonium machine whose radioactivity would produce heat, converted to an electrical current. The Newark pacemaker received the go-ahead from the commission in early 1969, and the first atomic pacemaker was implanted in a dog at the National Heart Institute of the National Institutes of Health on March 26, 1969, with Parsonnet participating in the surgery. The first U.S.-made atomic pacemaker human implant was performed at the Beth in March 1973.[43] Over the 1970s, the lithium pulse replaced atomic pacemakers, but the work of the researchers had positioned the Beth as the leading hospital in New Jersey for advanced heart surgery. The Beth's cardiac researchers continued with work on non-invasively programmed pacemakers that transformed them from electromechanical devices to microcomputers that could be reprogrammed remotely.[44]

Progressive Care of Patients

When Dr. Jacob Rosenkrantz succeeded Behrman as executive director of the hospital in 1959, he used the *Journal* to circulate his initial ideas and goals for transforming the care and treatment of patients from their admission to discharge. In his first article, "The Hospital Administration and Medical

Staff Responsibilities," Rosenkrantz wrote that a modern progressive hospital needed to respond to patients' differing needs for care in different facilities within the hospital. Patients who required the most constant nursing would be treated during the acute phase of their illness in an intensive-care ward unit (ICU) for three to five days. As their recovery progressed, these patients would be moved to the area of the hospital dedicated to intermediate care, ideally either in the same building or in a separate building on the grounds of an acute general hospital. Patient care would include actively managed convalescence—new modalities of rehabilitation.[45]

Rosenkrantz noted that increasingly, patients admitted to a hospital expected to return to full activity; achieving such a goal required not just convalescence, but active rehabilitation. There must be separate facilities for rehabilitation on the hospital campus or at another site where rehabilitation goals could be met, while staff provided a compassionate environment of palliative, long-term care for patients with chronic and incurable conditions. The hospital staff as a team of "health care providers" must engage in "an active comprehensive medical care program designed to focus the resources of the whole team—physician, nurse, dietitian, social worker, psychologist, psychiatrist, physical therapist, chaplain—. . . in the treatment of the whole patient."[46]

Rosenkrantz's proposal for an ICU within the hospital was supported by the medical staff who urged its creation to maintain the accreditation status. The board approved the proposal, and by 1964, construction was under way for a new kitchen and cafeteria, converting the old interns' wing and old cafeteria into a twenty-six-bed ICU.[47]

The construction of specialized units, such as the ICU, transformed the modalities of patient diagnosis and treatment. Traditionally, medical school students were trained to go to the bedside and focus a "clinical gaze" upon patients to acquire basic information about their condition. Now, the patient was transported to a special area, each area equipped with specialized machinery for diagnosis and treatment, performed by nursing and technical staff who specialized in the specific phase of medical care. The physician still came to the bedside, but reached for new electronic and automated devices to assist in diagnosis and scanned the printed results of the automated analysis of blood counts, pap smears, and blood-chemistry determinations to assess the progress of a protocol. Drs. Parsonnet and Hossein Eslami (the first recipient of the Danzis Medical Education fellowship) coauthored an article about extending the "clinical gaze" even further with the use of telemetric monitoring of artificial aortic prostheses for observing arrhythmias.

The Lack of a Medical School

From its first issue in 1950, the Beth's *Journal* editors had periodically expressed concern about the lack of a medical school in Newark, arguing that "although our hospital has many excellent teachers on its staff, it is not affiliated with any teaching institution and the need for the staff to express themselves in Medicine has been keenly felt." The *Journal* would, in part, meet this need by affording an opportunity [for Beth physicians] to train themselves in the scientific evaluation of their cases and in the correct method of presenting these for the formal use of medicine as a whole.[48]

A committee appointed by New Jersey governor Alfred Driscoll had in May 1950 begun to consider a 500-bed medical center in Newark that could be "a base on which to establish a medical school in New Jersey by furnishing extensive and modern facilities as well as a wide variety of cases for study by physicians in training."[49] Driscoll's committee narrowed the possible sites to two cities. Newark anticipated that it would be chosen, but, in 1954, Jersey City was selected instead.

By 1962, the American Medical Association Council on Medical Education indicated that twelve new medical schools were being planned across the country, five at universities.[50] In 1962, twelve years after Yeshiva University's School of Medicine and Dentistry received its charter, New York's Mount Sinai Hospital initiated a plan to establish its own medical school. The $30 million medical school would transform Mount Sinai Hospital into a Biomedical Center, the school built on the city blocks adjacent to the hospital.[51] The Mount Sinai Medical College affiliated with the newly formed Graduate Center of City University of New York, "creating a total biomedical and health-sciences complex of high quality to help New York City meet its pressing needs for the education of many more physicians and related scientific and technical personnel."[52]

"Medical Education in the Community Hospital," a 1963 *Journal* editorial, made explicit the problem that the Beth shared with many other Jewish voluntary nonprofit hospitals. It defined three types of hospitals in terms of their relationship to medical education: (1) institutions affiliated with a medical school, (2) nonaffiliated hospitals with meager facilities and a questionable teaching program, and (3) nonaffiliated hospitals with fine facilities and medical staff and an extensive program of residents and interns. The ability of the Beth to establish and maintain its own *Journal*, its editors contended, demonstrated that the Beth Israel Hospital was a category 3 community hospital, capable of providing the same level of training and research as medical school teaching hospitals. But the Beth interns wrote a response to the *Journal* that articulated the gnawing concern of the medical staff. They contended that every institution could benefit from exposure to outside viewpoints, and "possibly the development of a formal or informal affiliation with an outstanding nearby medical college could lend new strength in this direction, particularly in the area of basic sciences, so vitally important in expanding our clinical acumen."[53]

Furthermore, residency programs were increasingly granted to teaching hospitals. Residents preferred institutions with a clear commitment to education and the facilities to support it. So did the board that certified specialists and would be the final arbiter of which physicians with graduate training in a specialty could be certified in that area. According to medical sociologist William G. Rothstein, "In 1962–1963, only 24.5 percent of the 1,464 hospitals with approved graduate programs were affiliated with medical schools. They trained 49.1 percent of the 12,024 interns and 61.9 percent of the 36,162 residents. In 1974–75, 67.5 percent of the 1,683 hospitals with approved residency programs were affiliated with medical schools and they trained 92.9 percent of the 33,509 residents."[54] No wonder, then, that physicians at the Beth, and especially its interns, were anxious for affiliation with a medical school.

The pressure increased when the Federation of Jewish Philanthropies of New York accepted a recommendation that ten Jewish voluntary hospitals consolidate into hospital centers, in affiliation with medical schools, to provide improved care and to expand teaching and research. In 1965, the Beth Israel Hospital had offered its facilities to the newly formed University of Medicine and Dentistry of New Jersey (UMDNJ) so that its program could continue after the college gave up its quarters in Jersey City. Bernstein obtained from the Beth's board unanimous approval to actively pursue an affiliation between UMDNJ and the hospital.[55] But, as the February 1966 issue of *Modern Hospital* reported, the medical college decided to relocate its third-year students to the East Orange Veterans Administration Hospital Department of Medicine and fourth-year students to the new Saint Barnabas Medical Center in Livingston, while providing some externship programs for medical students in the Newark City Hospital because of its ample "medical material."[56]

Trends in Internships and Residencies

The post–World War II trend toward specialization had been nourished by the 1944 Servicemen's Readjustment Act (G.I. Bill of Rights). In

1945, the Veterans Administration (VA) issued a regulation that payments to physicians pursuing residency training would be made to cover tuition and living stipends and could be made to hospitals that met acceptable standards, whether or not they were affiliated with medical schools. The stipend greatly increased the number of residencies offered—in general surgery, the number rose from 808 in 1940 to 4,000 in 1950.[57]

In 1952 there were more than 22,000 residencies; five years later, more than 30,000; and by 1970, more than 45,000. The AMA Council on Medical Education, inundated with applications from hospitals, simply did not have the staff to conduct site visits to all new programs in hospitals. Paper applications alone were sometimes enough to earn accreditation; teaching programs were sometimes less than adequate.[58]

Internships were a separate but related issue. In 1951, to regulate competition for interns among hospitals and order the process whereby interns could apply to hospital internship programs, the AMA's Council on Medical Education, the Association of American Medical Colleges, and hospital organizations established the National Intern Matching Program. Now there would be rules by which hospitals and prospective interns could select each other, including a time each year when hospitals had to offer their appointments. The matching plan brought order out of chaos.[59]

In 1953, it was still a buyers' market for interns, who could choose between "the university hospital where traditionally good teaching and supervision are expected, or the non-university hospital which has effected a carefully planned program of medical education under the supervision of qualified physicians."[60] The Beth Israel brochure for internships and residencies in 1953–1954 describes the Newark hospital as "a general, non-sectarian Hospital approved by the American Medical Association and the American College of Surgeons . . . with ready access to the New Jersey Academy of Medicine . . . and within ten miles of New York City and its many medical centers."[61] Patterns of discrimination that persisted until the 1960s meant that applicants to the Beth's programs were disproportionately Jewish, and much of the competition for the best students for postgraduate training was from other Jewish hospitals. If Jewish students could often find positions only in Jewish hospitals, the Beth made clear in its publicity that it did not discriminate and that its programs met the highest medical standards. The Beth offered twelve one-year internships, a four-year residency program in the Division of Surgery, and a three-year program in the Division of the Hospital. Residents received an extensive coordinated program that included practical experience, didactic lectures, regular clinical-pathological conferences, training in the use of the hospital medical library and the special pathology library, and a formal basic medical science program conducted by the departments of Laboratories and Radiology.

In 1961, Rosenkrantz appointed Dr. Irving L. Applebaum to serve as the first full-time medical education director for the hospital. A Newarker, Applebaum had completed his initial training at Saint Michael's and the old Essex County Isolation Hospital, had come to the Beth in the postwar period, and had served as an editor of the *Journal*.[62] As medical education director, he was in charge of the teaching program for the residents, postgraduate courses, and the comprehensive training programs that must be designed to meet the requirements of specialty boards. He was also responsible for the recruitment of interns and residents. In 1962 and 1963 the Beth was the only hospital in New Jersey to be assigned its full quota of thirteen general rotating interns for its 1963–1964 internship program by the AMA's intern-matching program.[63] In fact, the Beth was one of the few nonaffiliated hospitals that filled all its intern and resident slots, thanks to aggressive marketing, competitive salaries, and stipends comparable to those of New York's Beth Israel and Mount Sinai Hospital programs.

The Millis Commission's 1966 report on the issue, *The Graduate Education of Physicians*, produced as dramatic an effect on physician medical education as had the 1914 AMA Council on Medical Education requirement for hospital internships. Dr. John S. Millis's eleven-person Citizens Commission on Graduate Medical Education issued a final report critical of the value of medical internships in educating physicians. At the time, mixed internships provided training in medicine, surgery, and often one other specialty. Some medical practitioners, who felt this was too narrow, preferred the rotating internship, which provided training in a number of different specialties. As a result of the Millis Commission's recommendations, the rotating internship with no major focus on a specialty soon declined. By the end of the 1960s, 80 percent of internship programs in the nation either focused upon one specialty intensively or, like the Beth's, "rotated" with an emphasis on a specialty, usually leading to graduate training in that field. Thus, the Beth positioned itself on the cutting edge of medical education.

Medicare and the Challenge of Federal Intervention

By the mid-1960s, the Beth was consumed with planning for the avalanche of paperwork and surge in admissions anticipated with the passage of Medicare legislation. Rosenkrantz had been making changes since 1961;

revamping the lobby to accommodate a family room for consultations and removing Gussie Cohen and her central reception desk and the old switch-board.[64] The hospital automated its clerical work, installing a mainframe data-processing computer to reduce the time to produce weekly reports. The production of the hospital payroll, a biweekly project that had once taken four employees four days to perform, became a ninety-minute task completed by a single employee.[65]

Medicare requirements altered the work of the administrative sections of the hospital: admissions, accounting, and medical records. Until World War II, the Social Service Department would have been a key component of the administrative sections for this change, but, in 1964, after the retirement of Minnie Edelshick, the new department head stated that its staff was "getting away from financial screening of patients for hospital admission and focusing more attention on the emotional components of illness." The social workers continued to contact the community agencies for direct services or assistance, including orthopedic appliances from the Crippled Children's Commission and the Flo Okin Society, and layettes from the Infants Welfare League.[66]

The Admitting Office assumed the duties formerly performed by social workers; its director, Etta Greenwald, described the impact of the Medicare Act upon her office:

> The year 1966 brought us MEDICARE, a boon to the eligible patient, but to the admitting office: more requests for semi-private beds, more signatures, more explanations, more confusion, longer stays (particularly the elderly patient who has no one to care for him at home and no room in the nursing home) and not enough beds in the hospital. These patients are entitled to semi-private rooms and they insist on our better semi-private accommodations, and rightfully so, creating increased pressures.[67]

The Medical Records Department became responsible for providing information to insurance carriers, Social Security offices, and regional Medicare entities; and for responding to the numerous private requests from patients and their representatives. The Accounting Department had the most challenging task in the hospital: the massive transformation of patient billing to a fee-for-service system compatible with Medicare categories. By January 1, 1968, they had to establish a code for every diagnosis, service, procedure, and supply item. If the Beth's coding system and its new forms for coding did not meet legislative requirements, there would be a lag in cash flow, making it difficult to meet bills and payroll from the federal agency reimbursements.

The Beth also was required to create a utilization committee composed of physicians, social workers, and administrative staff that could study patients' medical charts to ensure that the facilities were not "overused." The inception of a utilization program entailed a careful assessment of a patient's age, previous hospitalizations, and plan for rehabilitation, including transfer to long-term facilities certified by Medicare. The Social Service Department presented a troubling finding to the Beth Utilization Committee that Medicare patients remained in the hospital an average of 2.5 times longer than non-Medicare patients.[68] Committee member Greenwald identified the cause of this discrepancy in an inefficient procedure for patient discharges, resolved by revising the discharge policy to enforce an earlier discharge time.

Beth Israel Hospital's Self-Assessment in 1967

In the summer of 1967, when the four days of riots disrupted the entire city, the medical and administrative staffs were still learning to cope with Medicare paperwork. Tanks and checkpoints for entering the city on Lyons Avenue made travel almost impossible for the physicians attempting to enter the Weequahic streets, yet Ribot recalled not having missed a day of work during that period.[69]

Hospital communities live in the present. The medical staff's attention moves from diagnosis, to treatment, to recovery with each patient. There is little or no time for reflection or reminiscences. Strong emotions are of necessity kept in check and sublimated in protocols for patient care. The rhythm of the hospital is always grounded in the present and oriented toward the future. And yet, the human drama of the Newark riots was not easily transcended. There was a need to examine and assess all that had gone on and what it meant. In December 1967, board president Alan Sagner encouraged everyone at the Beth to assess the recent past. He set the tone in his president's report: "The physical, emotional, and financial damage caused by the disastrous riots may give one pause and force him to ask himself, 'Was there any good done during the past year?' "[70]

Every department responded with a positive accomplishment that reflected the staff's mission of providing care to the community. On behalf of the physicians, Bernstein explained that the Physicians Committee had agreed to make the Beth the health center for the community. Their first action to promote preventive healthcare would be to administer to all admitted routine chest X-rays, and perform pap smears as part of routine gynecological examinations for all women. The Outpatient Department Committee was to address emergent medical problems: clinic services were to be offered during the evening and on weekends, including special clinics for adolescents at the Endocrine Clinic, where all important hormonal problems could be addressed. Gilbert, heading Thoracic and Cardiac Surgery, stressed the importance of adjusting emergency-room procedures and preparation to the nature of the injuries most frequently seen, citing "a perceptible increase in the amount of chest trauma, accidents, knifings, and gunshot wounds" and noting that "these chest traumatic wounds have reached a level never before seen in this hospital."

Dr. Irving K. Perlmutter announced that the Maternity Department and its newborn nursery were finally consolidated and separated from the rest of the hospital population, nearly thirty-seven years after the request was made by Ruth Schindel of the Jewish Maternity Hospital. These youngest hospital patients were benefiting from new protocols for intravenous feeding and blood tests that had resulted in a drop in mortality. Dr. Mervin E. Fischman, the department head, reported that the seventh floor was now an adolescent unit for children

The Radiology Department under the direction of Dr. Spindell had begun a two-year in-house program to prepare applicants for the certification examination administered by the American Society for X-ray Technologists. Dr. Edward Fram was training technicians to perform a new procedure, called mammography. The Otolaryngology Department was shifting its focus from tonsillectomies to neck and head malignancies. Dr. Gilbert Sugarman, director of the Tumor Registry, reported that cases of malignancies presented by patients had increased and accounted for 3 percent of all hospital admissions. Goldman reported that the Laboratory Department was increasing the automated aspects of testing procedures for chemistry and blood work screening, making possible rapid and prompt analysis that would enable the cytology service to increase its capacity and better support the department charged with analysis of tumors.

The newly established Institute for the Study of Cardiodynamics, Heart Disease, Pulmonary Disorders, Vascular and Cerebral Vascular Surgery, Cardiac Surgery, and Renal Diseases had begun operation with funding from the Beth Research Foundation as well as National Institutes of Health, the Atomic Energy Commission, and the state and county heart associations. It had initiated an inhalation-therapy program and an outpatient clinic for follow-up of pacemaker patients.

Dr. Sol Parent reported that, after nearly thirty years, the Medical Education Department had replaced the mixed-internship schedule with eleven different combinations of rotating internships. Dr. Hossein Eslami had been appointed the new director of surgical education.

For Ellen Blidsoe, the executive housekeeper, 1967 was the year that the housekeeping staff received new equipment and new uniforms, and she had joined the Hospital Infections Committee, redefining her department as being on the front line of the hospital infection-control program. Other ancillary services departments reported that if they had not been able to make improvements, they had at least been able to maintain the same level of service.[71]

Director of Nursing Fannie Katz reported that in the past year, the Nursing Department had shifted to the use of licensed practical nurses, alleviating the heavy workload that fell to registered nurses at the Beth. A new policy of encouraging continuing education for the nursing staff had resulted in a 60 percent increase in the continuing education hours for which staff applied. But, Katz also acknowledged that the future of professional nurse education would be at the college and graduate level, although the Beth was one of thirteen Jewish hospitals still offering diploma schools.[72] The Beth Israel Nurses Training School would soon close in 1968, and its new school building would be sold to Essex County Community College, which would conduct courses for student nurses on the hospital campus.

Rosenkrantz's report as executive director was, in his own words, "but a summary sketch of some of the departments and their activities." A few months later, in May 1968, *Modern Hospital* noted that he had become assistant dean of the New York Medical College and director of the Flower Hospital. He would be succeeded at the Beth by Lester Bornstein, who had joined the hospital in 1957.

The Newark Beth Israel Medical Center

In 1968, the hospital board approved the renaming of the hospital as the Newark Beth Israel Medical Center (NBIMC). The following year, the NBIMC affiliated with the newly named University of Medicine and Dentistry of New Jersey (UMDNJ).

For the first time, the Beth created full-time positions for physicians on its staff in conjunction with faculty appointments at the medical college. When the Beth recruited Dr. M. A. Kirschner to be its first full-time director in the Department of Medicine, the offer also included a tenured position at the UMDNJ. Similarly, Dr. Jules Titelbaum became a tenured faculty member when he was recruited for the Pediatrics Department. Later such full-time department directors as Dr. Kamil Gal in pathology and Dr. Paul Pedowitz in ob/gyn joined the faculty, as did Drs. Parsonnet, Bernstein, Cohen, Ribot, and Donald Brief of the Beth.[73]

The appointment agreements were typical of Jewish hospital affiliations. In 1969, the Miriam Hospital in Providence, Rhode Island, became a Brown University–affiliated institution, with its clinical facilities used for teaching and its faculty members receiving joint appointments.[74] The trend of affiliations continued as the 375-bed teaching hospital of the Albert Einstein College of Medicine at Yeshiva University amalgamated with the 773-bed Montefiore Hospital and Medical Center; Montefiore assumed full responsibility for both hospitals.[75]

Between 1969 and 1972, the Beth played an increasing role in the undergraduate teaching program of the UMDNJ as plans went forward for integrated postgraduate-training programs in medicine, surgery, and pathology. The Beth's Department of Medicine integrated its house-staff training program with those of Martland Medical Center (later University Hospital) and East Orange Veterans Administration Hospital to form a single core program in internal medicine. Not long afterward the Beth's Department of Surgery engaged in a similar core program.

The Beth's identity as a medical institution was enhanced by not only the increasing role of its medical staff in research and medical education but also the plethora of health services it offered patients. In succeeding years, the hospital sought partnerships with other institutions, gradually developing its muscle as a regional center that offered tertiary care in a variety of specializations. In 1973, the NBIMC affiliated with Saint Elizabeth General Hospital, which designated Beth staff to head its Department of Pediatrics and to train its residents.

Constructing the Future

On September 9, 1974, the first patient-care floor of a new pavilion, the result of the Beth's ambitious multiphase construction program, quickly filled its thirty-four beds. For the first time in the history of the tower building, its patients barely noticed the September heat, resting comfortably cool in air-conditioned rooms with Venetian blinds sealed between the thermopane windows. Television equipment at the nurses' station helped nurses monitor patients. Smoothly functioning modern elevators transported dietary carts, linens, gurneys, and medical staff from one floor to another. Patients and their families entered the Abraham Lichtman Lobby and were treated in the Alan Sagner Department of Medicine and Patient Care.[76]

On September 30, 1974, the surgical team scrubbed in their new operating room on the new pavilion's third floor. Many had to modify their scrub preparations, as they no longer had to duck the condensing water that had trickled from the ceiling of the old 1928 facility. Nearly a half century earlier, the first surgical procedure in the tower building had been performed by two generations of the Parsonnet family: Drs. Max Danzis and his son-in-law Eugene Parsonnet. That Beth tradition was continued in 1974, by Dr. Eugene Parsonnet and his son, Victor, who together performed the first surgery.[77]

Other hopes for modernization expressed in the 1967 annual report were realized within the next decade. By 1975 a newly expanded Radiology Department had ultrasound and computerized tomography equipment. The new admitting pavilion included an automated telephone system and an adjacent laboratory for the battery of blood tests required for every admitted patient. With two X-ray rooms and facilities to perform full surgery, the Emergency Department could now treat the high volume of patients presenting acute problems; the department added two social workers and had handled nearly 40,667 patients, of which 3,264 were admitted in 1974.[78] The Laboratory Department passed accreditation by the American Association of Blood Banks and finally phased out the use of freshly drawn blood in favor of plasma. The Accounting Department finally transferred its entire system to a main-frame computer and boasted that it had reduced its costs by $200,000 every year since 1969.

Two important changes were evident in the medical posture of the Beth by 1975. The first was the emergence of the NBIMC as a regional center for particular specialties, consistent with the 1973 Social Security Act amendments that had transformed the provision of health care from municipalities to various geographic areas and created the Professional Standards Review Organization (PSRO), a federal regulatory agency charged with the review of hospitals' quality of care. The Beth became a regional center for heart surgery and was also the designated tissue bank for kidneys. The Ob/Gyn Department transformed itself into a regional perinatal center to handle high-risk pregnancies and support a neonatal intensive care unit. The Dental Health Center had become a regional center for the treatment of handicapped dental patients. The good work of the Beth hospital staff in the 1960s was rewarded when the NBIMC became the first hospital in Essex

County to be given the authority by the PSRO to perform its own quality reviews.[79]

The second change evident by 1975 was the number and variety of department lectures, publications, and grants. Several Department of Medicine staff served on the editorial board of *Abstracts and Facts*, the monthly publication that cited the works published by the University of Medicine and Dentistry of New Jersey and the Beth Medical Center. The medical staff publications appeared in the most prestigious peer-reviewed journals.

The Twentieth-Century Transformation of Hospital Care

The period between the 1960s and the 1970s saw startling changes in how medicine was practiced in the United States and in the kind of facilities required. Increasingly, hospitals were transformed into places where patients came for treatment but did not stay. Many diagnostic and surgical techniques once requiring the aseptic environment and postoperative care available only in a hospital could be safely performed in a physician's office suite, the patient returning home after the procedure for rest and recuperation without the risk of nosocomial infection. The intensive use of an ever-increasing variety of antibiotics meant that fewer and fewer patients died of infections; in consequence, as one analyst explained, "more of the hospital's resources could be used for the diagnosis and treatment of the chronic degenerative diseases of old age: cancer, heart disease and stroke, arthritis and emphysema." As antibiotics also reduced the need for pediatric and infectious disease facilities, "outpatient visits increased from 65 million in 1954 to more than 180 million in 1970."[80]

New techniques—sonography, electrocardiography, and later magnetic resonance imaging—revolutionized the diagnostic process; test results could be processed faster and with greater accuracy and consistency by computer. The clinical gaze of the physician was brought inside the body as never before.

Ambulatory surgery was made increasingly possible by new anesthesia combinations and computer-assisted visualization technology enabling the tiny incisions and insertion of micro-instruments for microsurgeries. Prosthetic devices such as artificial heart valves, artificial blood vessels, and ultimately, artificial hearts made "spare parts" surgery a reality. The hospital became a "highly technical, high-cost, acute curative institution in which perhaps as much as seventy percent of the facilities and personnel are . . . related to the care of surgical patients." Further, "intensive-care units for patients with heart attacks, strokes, severe injuries, neonatal disease, infections resistant to antibiotics, and burns" revolutionized staffing, concentrating "specialists and their technology to specific areas of the hospital."[81] The process of recuperation was no longer under their purview; patients recovered at home with supportive services provided by outpatient services in the ancillary departments of physical therapy and occupational therapy.[82] At the same time, community needs transformed outpatient care; the dispensaries and clinics of the early twentieth century were reborn in the 1970s as health-care centers. The Beth, like other inner-city hospitals, created an entirely new health-care center at the hospital staffed by physicians. Routine health care could now be provided without impeding the emergency room's ability to treat acute cases and emergencies.

New peer-reviewed journals proliferated to serve specialists' needs for the latest from laboratories and research centers; other publications redefined their purpose. In April 1974, *Modern Hospital* re-created itself as *Modern Healthcare*.

The editors, using the same editorial format and space as the inaugural editorial in September 1913, commented that the traditional compartmentalized segments in health care were "uncoupling and recoupling into combinations of extended care facilities, consortiums of hospitals, and multi-hospital chains, due in part to . . . external forces [such] as government regulation and inflation, and further, because the delivery system is demanding closer working relationships, the traditional barriers between the various stages of care—acute care, chronic care, rehabilitation care, and so on—were falling."[83]

In 1970, Menorah Hospital and Medical Center in Kansas became the last Jewish hospital to initiate an in-house journal, which ceased publication in 1973. In 1969, the *New York Mount Sinai Hospital Journal* became the *Mount Sinai Journal of Medicine* for its medical school. Many other Jewish hospital journals had ceased publication, unable to similarly transform themselves. If the editors of the Beth's *Journal* had hoped that their in-house publication would be the precursor of a medical journal for the UMDNJ, that was not to be. In June 1975, the editorial staff informed the board that it was considering terminating the *Journal* because the medical staff was no longer using its pages for publication of their work. The board voted to continue publication, perhaps sensing that its termination one year before the seventy-fifth anniversary of the hospital would come as a sad ending.

The hopes of the founders of the *Journal of the Beth Israel Hospital* had been realized in one generation: to become a research hospital affiliated with a medical school. At the Beth, research and education had become as much a part of the daily routine as patient care. As for the blue-jacketed first issue of the *Journal,* it took its place in the anniversary display cases as a fond memory of the Beth's rich past.

CHAPTER 8

Redefining the
Beth's Community

*B*y 1969, scarcely twenty years had elapsed since World War II veterans, including physicians and nurses from Newark Beth Israel Hospital, had returned to the bustling, noisy neighborhood surrounding the Beth. Much had changed. There were different sights, smells, and sounds in the neighborhood around the Newark Beth Israel Medical Center. Construction crews were converting Lyons Avenue, three blocks north of the hospital, to an overpass for the six-lane I-78. The noise of the construction crews for the freeway would be replaced with the low rumble of automobiles and trucks, their exhaust fumes tinging the air with the faint odor of gasoline. Jet traffic at the Newark airport, three miles south of the hospital, filled Weequahic's sky. And then there was the hum of idling engines from the moving vans ever more frequently parked along Weequahic's streets as an exodus of shopkeepers and residents that had begun before the 1967 riot accelerated in response to the violence.

Bergen Street, once the commercial hub of the Jewish community, lined with shops that advertised in the *Jewish News*, had become a silent street of vacant stores. The Weequahic Jewish Community Center that had opened in 1954 closed in 1969. Those who could were departing and resettling in areas outside the city limits; the poor remained, suffering the consequences of a city in decline.

By 1969, Newark was characterized by *d*'s. There was *devastation*. Only a narrow ribbon of asphalt remained to remind passersby that Prince Street had once flourished, its poultry shops and bakeries replaced by weeds, swaying in the breezes. There was the *detritus* of highway construction that littered blocks near I-78: more than sixty abandoned and boarded-up single homes and apartment houses surrounded by piles of sharp rocks, garbage, abandoned cars, and rats—all potential traps for neighborhood children.[1] The highway had widened streets to be service roads for the highway exits that were unsafe to cross. Reporters chose Schley Street to symbolize the impact of the 1967 riot, not realizing that its abandoned buildings and garbage were the products not of the rioting, but of the old street, which had once connected the Old Clinton Hill neighborhood with the eastern edge of Weequahic, having become a dead-end into the freeway.[2]

There was now ever present *danger*. Pedestrians were not robbed, but beaten and robbed. Vandals set fire to the pews at B'nai Abraham, forcing the congregation to finally close its doors in 1969. In 1971, one year after Kenneth Gibson was elected the first African American mayor of Newark (the first African American mayor of a major U.S. city), his father was lying in a hospital bed at the Beth recovering from a violent robbery.[3] Violent muggings occurred in the Beth's parking lots and even in the hospital lavatories. On one New Year's Eve, medical staff were horrified to find the chief resident lying unconscious and bleeding on the front steps to the entrance.[4]

A *New York Times Magazine* article described Newark as "a study in the evils, tensions, and frustrations that best describe the central cities of America."[5]

A Test of Leadership: Lester Bornstein

The escalating urban crisis in Newark tested leadership in every institution that served the city, including Newark Beth Israel. In early 1968, after Dr. Jacob Rosenkrantz resigned, the Beth's board appointed Assistant Director Lester Bornstein to succeed him. Superintendent I. E. Behrman, who was impressed with the World War II veteran's extensive credentials, had hired him in 1957.[6] Bornstein, much decorated for his bravery at the Battle of the Bulge, had learned hospital administration as a commissioned military officer at Walter Reed Hospital. During the Korean conflict, he helped establish an army hospital on Kyushu, Japan. By the time Behrman interviewed him, Bornstein had earned a master's degree in hospital administration and had served as an administrator of Barnhart Hospital, a Jewish hospital in Paterson, New Jersey.

Despite Bornstein's years of experience at the Beth, board president Alan Sagner insisted on a six-month trial period, arranging for Bornstein and him to share an office. The two worked at desks pushed together so that they could more easily discuss every decision, especially those bearing on the future of the hospital. During that period they mulled over many of the issues lucidly advanced in a somber 1967 *Modern Hospital* article in which Richard Johnson contended that urban hospitals "located in deteriorating neighborhoods, have three basic courses open to them: to flee to the suburbs, stay in the city and adapt to changing conditions, or to change from a community to a regional hospital."[7] Like many other Jewish voluntary hospitals, the Beth met all the "community criteria" described in the article as contributing to crisis: an exodus of a socioeconomic group formerly served, an increase in the average age of the group that remained, a surrounding neighborhood whose single-family dwellings had become multifamily units, a decline in family income, and an increasing crime rate. The Beth also met Johnson's "hospital criteria": an obsolete physical plant, the buildings' worth almost fully depreciated, crowded departments, inadequate parking, rapid increases in emergency visits, and insufficient real estate in the hospital's possession to support expansion.

During Bornstein's trial period he wrote an article for the May 1968 issue of *The Reporter,* the Beth's in-house newsletter, responding to the position expressed by many that when the Jewish community had moved out of Newark, the hospital should have chosen to follow:

> My friends, I want to set the record straight. This hospital was built to fill a need, that need has changed, but a new need exists and it exists in Newark. And this is where we are going to stay because our services are vital to this community. . . . If Newark has become a slum area, if Newark has become a pocket of poverty, if Newark has degenerated from the city it once was, then now more than ever before is not the time to desert it. . . . Now is the time to look beyond the present—not at what it was—but at what Newark can become and our Hospital has the opportunity to be a forerunner in giving this city a hopeful tomorrow.

By October, Sagner was convinced that Bornstein was the right man for the job and the board appointed Bornstein executive director of the newly named Newark Beth Israel Medical Center. Together, he and Sagner would pursue a dual strategy: to adapt as a community hospital to Newark's changing demography, while evolving into a strong regional presence in New Jersey, a magnet for patients from the mid-Atlantic region.

Rebuilding Hospital Community from the Inside

Bornstein brought to the job his buoyant enthusiasm for the hospital's work and some concrete measures to improve working conditions. In his newsletter article, Bornstein had told the Beth community: "Our pride must be injected and protected and it must start with the employees . . . from the orderlies who wheel the stretchers, the porters who mop the halls, the volunteers. . . . And then it must be inevitably transferred to the patient." Simultaneously, Bornstein would work to shore up the hospital's internal sense of community and morale, which had been tested both by the changes in Newark and the broader changes in how hospitals functioned in the rapidly evolving health-care environment of the late 1960s. It was a tall order. The 1967 Annual Report had soberly noted that the accomplishments of the hospital staff had been carried out while it had suffered a 100 percent turnover in almost every department.

Bornstein recognized that in order for the NBIMC to attract employees, his task was to make the hospital campus safe, while trying not to create a walled compound similar to the Martland Medical Center, which had put barbed wire atop its walls after the 1967 riot. For the first time, a security force patrolled the perimeter of the hospital around the clock and monitored the security cameras positioned at every doorway. Bornstein hired personnel specialists experienced both in recruitment and employee relations in order to build and retain the new workforce.

Bornstein also recognized that the new staff for a regional medical center would have to be responsive to the changes in hospital position descriptions. From 1969 to 1970, the number of employees needed to care for a hundred patients in a modern hospital jumped from 280 to 292.[8] In the 1928 inpatient wards, nurses and the women's auxiliary volunteers had filled all the supportive positions; auxiliary volunteers on a 1970 modern nursing unit would assist tiers of caregivers, from ward clerks to nurses' assistants, licensed practical nurses, registered nurses, and head nurses. The 1928 patient wards had been served by social workers, dietitians, and diet aides; now the support staff to the bedside expanded to include phlebotomists, respiratory therapists, and occupational therapists. Administrative, technical, ancillary, and maintenance hospital departments were all changing as the scope of their work was altered by the transformations in technology and advances in medicine.

Now, specialties in nursing required graduate degrees and continuing medical education; a nurse practitioner, for example, possessed an undergraduate and a master's degree. The Beth's Nurses Training School had been absorbed into the Essex County Community College. There were new job descriptions for older occupations: social workers were providing therapeutic counseling to patients, as their assessments for the ability to pay were no longer a part of the admissions or billing process. X-ray technicians needed the knowledge, skills, and ability to operate sonography transducers in the new field of diagnostic medical imaging. Laboratory technologists were

required to perform an expanded array of laboratory tests. Pathology technologists were being retrained in the use of the electron microscope. Nurses
specialized in new hospital areas: neonatal intensive care units, dialysis centers, and chemotherapy units.

The care of patients was shared by those who provided direct care and
those who worked indirectly to promote patient recovery. No longer would
several skilled operating engineers manage the entire physical plant; now
there were specialists for all the equipment. A new cadre of staff monitored
the mainframe computers and programmed the systems. Rows of clerks at
keyboards entered patient data; others processed forms for reimbursements
for inpatient and, in increasing numbers, for outpatient services.

The key to recruitment and retention of personnel was identifying the
new skills and special training employees would need. For example, an
operating-room instrument technician might have brought a single tray to
the operating suite in the 1950s; by the 1970s, the technician needed to
assemble nearly a hundred instruments in rows that paralleled the stages of
complex operating procedures, as well as respond to the requests of the surgeons as they worked. What would the instrument technician need to know
by 1980?

Bornstein found in Kenneth Tyson an individual who could help him
develop the workforce that the hospital needed. Tyson had worked in the
Beth's laboratory for Dr. Lester Goldman and his successor, Dr. Kamil Gal,
but had recently taken a job at another hospital to move into administration.
Bornstein invited him back to the Beth for an afternoon talk and, during its
course, learned that the former Beth medical technologist was a Newarker,
that he had recently met and married a Filipino laboratory technologist, and
that he possessed an enthusiasm both for the changes in medical technology
and for the camaraderie of physicians and nurses. Bornstein told Tyson that
the NBIMC would pay his tuition for an MBA degree. Then, he constructed
a series of supervisory positions in the technical and ancillary sections to
give Tyson managerial experience; finally Tyson became an assistant director reporting to Bornstein. Tyson's command of the technical issues in medical advances, coupled with his formal financial training and his loyalty to
the institution, complemented Bornstein's experience and enabled them to
transform the hospital staff.[9]

While some areas of the hospital required more specializations and
staff, others were undergoing a reduction in need. In 1951, the Beth Israel
Hospital in Boston estimated that 125 different kinds of items needed to be
mended and maintained, from towels to white coats to sterile covers.[10]

In 1967, Newark Beth Israel still had special rooms for the mending and seamstress staff who made caps for the nurses, mended thousands of patient gowns, and tailored coats and jackets for physicians, interns, residents, and laboratory staff. The laundry-room staff still used the mangles and equipment brought from the old High Street hospital. However, the manufacturing of disposable linens of the 1960s brought revolutionary change; there would be no more mending of bed sheets, towels, and surgical materials. Bornstein initiated a policy of attrition as these staff members retired. When the Prudential and Mutual Life Insurance Companies gave Newark hospitals a $6 million grant to create a central laundry on Freylinghuysen Avenue, Bornstein outsourced the Beth laundry and made sure that the new facility hired Beth laundry staff not eligible for retirement.

Bornstein studied the patterns of nurse turnover carefully and learned that the nurses were still overburdened with clerical work, insufficient assistance in the evening, and frustrating linen shortages, especially in the evenings. A new recruitment package that offered flexible and compressed workweek schedules, and a hefty salary increase enabled him to stop hiring extra nurses from agencies for the medical and surgical wards. Dr. Arthur Bernstein, now an elder member of the Beth medical staff, secured a $500,000 grant to train nurses to work in coronary-care units and both physicians and nurses in the field of renal dialysis.[11] The recruitment incentives of specialized training and flex-time reduced the need for importing foreign nurses, as well as the contracts with agencies whose rates were nearly double the salaries of the staff nurses.[12] By 1990, for the first time, Beth Israel's nursing staff levels reached 100 percent.

Rebuilding the Surrounding Community

Restoring trust and a spirit of cooperation between the Beth and the communities it served required Lester Bornstein and members of his staff to mount new outreach efforts that served the needs of Newark's changing population. The South and Central Wards still were home to a substantial group of elderly and poor Jews, and Jewish High Holidays services were held in the hospital tower auditorium for those who lived nearby. Bornstein and his staff obtained an agreement with the Essex County Jewish agencies to set up a special clinic for the elderly Jewish residents and a transportation fund so they could afford visits for preventive care.

The Essex County Welfare Federation collaborated with the NBIMC to provide direct medical and dental services to hundreds of families of a new wave of Russian Jewish immigrants, as well as a comprehensive program of ambulatory preventive care and counseling services with interpreters who could speak both Yiddish and Russian. The Beth provided free immunizations and examinations to children for school admissions and summer camp, reminiscent of the Maternity Auxiliary campaigns. Beth physicians also offered a special service for these immigrants: a circumcision program for children and adults who had been prohibited in the Soviet Union from practicing this ancient Jewish ritual.[13]

Federal and state grants awarded to Newark enabled the city to establish a network of seven Community Health Service Centers to provide health education, early diagnosis and treatment, and a sliding-fee schedule based on ability to pay.[14] The NBIMC Outpatient Department ultimately became one of these health centers, harking back to an era when hospital dispensaries had served poor immigrant communities.

The most dramatic demographic change continued to be the growth of Newark's African American population. The city's political machine, which had long reflected the Irish, Italian, and Jewish immigrant populations, was superseded by the African American residents and their control of the Central and South Wards. The 1966 Newark mayoral race first pitted former mayor Leo P. Carlin, an Irish American, against the incumbent, Hugh Addonizio, an Italian American. They were challenged by Kenneth Gibson, a young black American and civil engineer, who with no political experience was resoundingly defeated by Addonizio. Native Newarkers liked to say that "whatever is going to happen in a city, happens first in Newark," perhaps remembering that in 1936, the Newark councilmen had chosen Meyer "Doc" Ellenstein as their first Jewish mayor. In June 1970, Kenneth Gibson became the first black mayor of a major Northeastern city, winning close to 43 percent of the vote.

Bornstein reached out to the South Ward by creating a Community Health and Planning Committee that included members of the local associations. The committee identified ways to tackle immediate public health hazards in the neighborhood, including rodent and vermin control, the cleanup of empty lots, and the removal of dead trees. Beth medical personnel offered community health information seminars at local community centers. The NBIMC formed a first-aid squad among residents to shore up the inadequate municipal ambulance service in the city's South Ward. The National Council of Jewish Women, like Jewish women's associations nearly seventy years earlier, opened a daycare center on the hospital site for children of employees. By 1970, nearly ninety Weequahic high school students were part of the

Beth's Medical Explorer Scout Post and Future Physicians Club, which offered programs to guide students toward careers in medicine.[15]

In September 1968, the Prudential Life Insurance Company stated that it would provide $97 million in loans to Newark institutions and companies for the rebuilding of the city. The Pru, long a mainstay of the city, had erected Newark's first skyscraper office building on Broad Street in 1901. During the 1918 epidemic, its employees had stayed in the office building day and night to process the thousands of insurance claims generated by the deaths; it was said that some employees, sick themselves, died at their desks. The company had offered jobs to Newarkers during the Great Depression and in 1954, when suburban flight began in earnest, had committed to staying downtown. Now the company was once again coming to the city's rescue, committing $47 million to the construction of a massive downtown office and hotel complex, the Gateway Center, near the old Morris Canal that had become Raymond Boulevard.

A *New York Times* article cautioned that there was a growing divergence between two Newarks as a result of this bold initiative. The first Newark remained the commercial and financial center, with a need for more office space. There would be the construction of the new Gateway Center to meet the office needs as well as a new $200 million airport complex. As the article noted, Newark was becoming the first U.S. city to have a workforce made up of suburban commuters. But there also would be a second Newark, in the streets near the downtown, notably the Central and South Wards, existing in parallel, whose recovery would progress far more slowly, its residents enduring a high unemployment rate, few job opportunities in the downtown high-rises, and deteriorating housing.[16]

As construction got under way downtown to create the Gateway Center, bulldozers and pile drivers razed old homes that had stood on Osborne Terrace adjacent to the Beth's tower building, in preparation for the biggest addition in the history of the hospital. Pursuing its dual strategy, the Beth was physically recasting itself as a regional medical center whose strength and services would benefit the poor living in the houses on the blocks adjacent to the hospital. However, to its neighbors, the construction looked like part of the first Newark, even though the hospital stood in the midst of the second.

Building a Regional Medical Center

The operation of a hospital and the functions performed in its physical facilities are constantly changing with advances in the diagnosis and treatment of its patients, in turn propelling giant leaps forward in the surgical suites, laboratories, and wards. These changes require the acquisition of new equipment, even the redesign of rooms, all while the existing hospital infrastructure is undergoing tremendous wear and tear. These necessary and constant changes could render the new facilities and equipment outdated by the time they were completed and obsolete within a decade.

Beth board president Alan Sagner understood the complexities of hospital construction when in 1965 he proposed that the board approve a phased series of construction projects that would transform the Beth's physical image and vastly increase its breadth of services.

Sagner and the Beth's board agreed that projects already completed be redefined as phase I and the ongoing projects as phase II. In phase II, new elevators, ducts for air conditioning, and upgraded electrical capacity had extended the 1928 tower building to its limit. As President Frank Liveright and Dr. Paul Keller had understood in 1922, when the renovation of an aging facility is not feasible, the only choice is to build a new structure. Phase III, scheduled to begin in 1968, would be the most ambitious component of the new plan, transforming the very look and character of the hospital. The new pavilion building would replace the large lawn and circular driveway in front of the tower entrance. A new entrance would extend the hospital south toward the city street, Osborne Terrace. Phase IV would focus on work across the street and would include a parking garage and the renovation of several adjacent buildings. Together, phases III and IV would comprise the core of a modern, regional medical center, attracting patients from surrounding New Jersey counties.

In the aftermath of the Newark riots in July 1967, board members were worried about pursuing an ambitious and expensive construction program, suspending construction projects for nearly a year. In September 1968, the Prudential Insurance Company sent word that it would commit a $10 million loan, payable in twenty years, for the hospital's expansion and renovation, as part of the Pru's program to help all Newark hospitals better serve the community.[17]

The loan was insufficient to dispel the doubts of many board members. Sagner commissioned a report by Eugene D. Rosenfeld Associates that would revisit the institution's options, especially the possibility of establishing a suburban presence. The report confirmed that the NBIMC did not have the resources to build a satellite hospital.[18] The consultants recommended that the plan to make the medical center a regional tertiary care institution go forward, concentrating on developing those areas of medical specialization in which the NBIMC already excelled or could excel: "The medical staff should be training, teaching and doing research in this area (inner Newark) and we can continue and develop in that way."[19]

In early 1969, as board members continued to debate the future of the medical center, Albert Rachlin raised his hand and rose to address them. His father had been clerk-of-the-works for the 1928 hospital construction, with the advice and guidance of his grandfather who had built many of Newark's neighborhoods. For the past few years, he had been acquiring parcels of land, house-by-house on Bungalow Court, adjacent to the hospital, in preparation for phase III. Rachlin began his remarks by proposing that a plaque be prepared to honor Abraham Lichtman, who had died a few months earlier. Then he warned them that time was running out: "We are already at the point where the same money we now have available will build far less than it would have when first planned. . . . And if we do nothing, we will make no mistakes and also will get nothing done."[20]

The board heeded Rachlin's admonition and proceeded with phase III. But, an important component of phase III had to be eliminated. Plans called for incorporating the Theresa Grotta Restorative Center, a Jewish convalescent facility, into the new Pavilion, so that Medicare patients could progress from the acute care wards to a rehabilitation facility on the same site. In 1968, changes in the architectural plan could not incorporate the convalescent facility. The delay in phase III had created a greater problem. The Beth was transforming itself into a regional medical center just as the federal government was enacting regulatory legislation that would seriously entangle the expansion of voluntary nonprofit hospitals.

Regionalization and Regulation

As the federal government increased its funding for the provision of health care to millions of Americans, policymakers sought ways to avoid spending excesses, especially those resulting from the duplication of services. In 1966, Congress passed the Comprehensive Health Planning Act (PL 89–49), which provided $125 million in grants to states to assist them in establishing their health programs and required all states receiving funds allocated by the Hill-Burton Act, other public health acts, and the Social Security programs such as Medicare and Medicaid to establish state and local health-planning agencies. The act specified that each state must submit a comprehensive plan that established a single state agency engaged in health planning, with a state planning council composed of representatives of federal, state, and local agencies, and of groups concerned with health planning. Effective July 1, 1968, each state council would implement a statewide program for capital expenditures for replacement, modernization, and expansion without duplication of services and in an efficient and economical manner.

By 1972, twenty-three states, including New Jersey, had adopted legislation requiring hospitals to obtain certification or permission from state councils prior to beginning any new construction exceeding a specified sum. All public and private voluntary hospitals were required to comply with their state certificate-of-need (CON) regulations. The decision of a state council to grant a hospital a CON would be based upon existing state or regional plans for the provision of medical care. CONs and regional planning were important innovations in the ever-increasing number of state comprehensive health-planning programs.[21] Federal amendments to the Social Security Act also enacted the same year gave a state health-planning council more teeth by granting states the authority to deny Medicare, Medicaid, and Title V (the Maternal and Child Health Program) reimbursement to hospitals and other facilities whose capital expenditures it did not approve.[22]

The New Jersey state agency created the Hospital and Health Planning Council of Metropolitan New Jersey, which divided the state into regions: Region II included the counties of Essex (Newark), Morris, Union, and Warren. The state planning councils were redefined as health planning agencies in 1975, with the right to approve or disapprove capital expenditures and a hospital's applications for a federal loan or grant.

All public and private hospitals within a region were required to justify every addition or major expenditure, describing how the changes fit into a long-range plan for the geographical area, and, if necessary, why a particular hospital was the best site for a new service or new equipment. Every change that NBIMC was planning for its phased construction would now have to be reconciled with a regional plan covering four counties. These plans included a demographic profile of the local, city, and regional communities being served, as well a description of other health services and providers in the region and their interrelationship; patient-origin services; utilization patterns; fiscal data; and a forecast of future needs. Each change in each component of an NBIMC construction phase would require a separate written justification that filled a minimum of twenty single-spaced pages.[23]

At times, the construction specifications in different phases contradicted one another, resulting in maddening problems and added expense. Dietary carts already purchased were too wide to be wheeled into elevators that had just been installed in the new Pavilion. Similarly, the Pavilion lobby had been designed with automatic doors in the drawings, but then deleted as a cost-saving measure and replaced with hinges whose "hold open" devices affected the heating and air conditioning sensors.[24]

When Sagner was selected to head the New York Port Authority in November 1973, Leonard Lieberman succeeded him as NBIMC president. An executive president of the Pathmark supermarket chain, intelligent and innovative, he had pioneered the concept of supermarket generic brands. At the Beth, Lieberman made phases III and IV construction the focus of his tenure, defining his job in terms of three basic construction questions crucial to the hospital's future as a regional medical center: (1) when to build more floors and what should be on them, (2) when to build a garage and a materials handling center, and (3) what to do with the center tower.[25]

Construction was progressing, thanks to an increase in the Prudential loan to $11 million in 1970. Lieberman's first action was to renegotiate the Prudential loan to $15 million in order to cover the increasing costs.[26] The construction coincided with the decision of the Federal Hospital Council to address the issue of urban hospital obsolescence by expanding the scope of the 1946 Hill-Burton Act; the Beth finally obtained a federal matching grant. Originally intended to support only phase IV, the grant, to the board's relief, was allowed to apply to completing phase III construction as well.[27]

Leonard Lieberman found that one of the most frustrating challenges he faced was the ambiguity that often pervaded the regulatory environment. The Beth's master phase-construction plan included a staged series of construction projects that erected six-story shells designed to be expanded inside and vertically, adding new floors as funds became available. When a hospital department moved into the new Pavilion building, its former rooms were renovated for another department. Preparing the required justifications became more difficult because different sections of the old hospital building and the new buildings fit into different categories as defined by different New Jersey State agencies. What had seemed to be an economical and logical approach was stymied by the myriad regulations from various federal and state agencies.

The Department of Housing and Urban Development (HUD) implemented the fast-track National Housing Act, which guaranteed that a hospital project with a HUD mortgage could start construction before the sequence of plan preparation, permit approvals, and mortgage endorsement got under way—accelerating construction by as much as a year.[28] Unfortunately, at the same time, the NBIMC phase IV CON application was frozen because the construction coincided with the University of Medicine and Dentistry of New

Jersey Hospital construction. New Jersey placed a ninety-day moratorium on all Newark hospital projects to determine whether the two hospital plans were redundant—a virtual paperwork log-jam—while the respective construction crews continued to bill both hospitals.[29]

At the November 10, 1974, dedication ceremonies that marked the opening of the new NBIMC Pavilion, the hospital community and Newark celebrated a milestone in Newark's rebuilding. Unlike previous hospital openings with their parades and week of tours and speeches, the Pavilion opened and went into full operation immediately, pausing only for a ribbon-cutting ceremony and photographs with hospital doctors, officials, and staff and city dignitaries.[30] The Pavilion housed twelve operating rooms, sixty-eight additional hospital beds, a radiology suite, and a new emergency ward. In his remarks at the ribbon-cutting ceremony, Newark mayor Kenneth Gibson declared the Beth one of the finest institutions of its kind and added: "I pledge to you, that it will continue to have all the help my administration can give it."[31]

But the health care environment of 1969, when the Pavilion was designed, had changed by 1974. Some parts of the Pavilion were outdated by the time the ceremonial photographs were being taken. Although the gap between planning and construction steadily decreased as the phased construction continued, astounding advances in medical technology threatened in many areas to make planned equipment and layouts obsolete. The 1968 plans for the Departments of Radiology and Radiation Therapy were out of date by 1971; a complete redesign of the electrical distribution and outlets was required.[32] Only a few years later, while still in the midst of construction, the Radiation Therapy Department plans had to revamped again to accommodate linear accelerators and computer automated technological (CAT) scanning machines not even on the horizon five years earlier.[33] Advances in surgical protocols for kidney transplantation meant the organ-preservation laboratory had to be redesigned to incorporate machinery to perform the perfusion process for kidneys and other organs, with added safety and security precautions for a staff that worked around the clock in twenty-four-hour shifts.[34]

Plans immediately began to convert one floor of its inpatient rooms to an ambulatory or "in-out" surgery unit for the surgical procedures that no longer required hospital admission. The advent of ambulatory surgery created new procedures for preadmissions laboratory work, new specialties in anesthesiology, and a new configuration of surgi-centers, reequipping the operating room for the new field of arthroscopic surgery. Another change seemed to hark back to the early twentieth century: a new generation of women demanded at-home births with the aid of nurse-midwives. The Beth inpatient maternity department had to construct neonatal intensive care units, step-down nurseries, and birthing rooms that simulated the at-home experience, while providing fully trained nurse-midwives to assist in uncomplicated deliveries. All of these renovations would require CON applications and approval prior to beginning construction.

As phase IV began, Alan Sagner's phased construction planning finally delivered dividends. Items deleted or curtailed in phase III could be reviewed and restored in the phase IV master plan. For example, to cut costs, the phase III construction committee deleted plans to locate a sink in each patient room in addition to the one in the patient's bathroom. When Dr. Jules Titelbaum requested that the sinks be put back into the specifications to encourage the hand washing necessary to hospital-staff hygiene, so important in protecting patients from infections, his request could be accommodated only in phase IV plans.[35]

Regionalism versus Localism

The Beth was literally crafting in concrete its dual strategy: creating a regional medical center while at the same time adapting the hospital in ways that would best serve the surrounding community. Even as the Beth's leadership was persuaded that it had selected the best strategy for the institution's future, members of the local community were offended by the very phase of the hospital's plan that could not be sacrificed if it was to become a regional care facility: parking.

Insufficient automobile parking had always been an issue for the Beth. By 1930, the front lawn of the hospital was being used as a parking lot. In the 1950s and 1960s, every plot acquired by the hospital was covered with asphalt and converted to parking spaces. It was apparent by 1965 when the phased-construction concept was accepted that the parking problem could be solved only with multilevel construction. In fact, the proposed parking garage was the linchpin of the written justifications filed with the planning council that the Beth deserved designation as a regional medical center, capable of receiving patients who traveled from the outlying counties in Region II of New Jersey.

The initial plans were to construct an underground garage, but the uneven terrain and drainage eliminated that option; a multilevel structure would have to be above ground. Plans also called for the garage to be jointly financed and shared with Essex County Community College, however, in 1970, the college sold back the building and withdrew from the garage agreement—which meant the garage could no longer be justified as a "city facility." Community residents soon noticed that there were cars with New York plates parked on their streets. The hospital was not using local labor, but a New York City construction firm. The project was not helping reduce local unemployment in the least. Perhaps the most critical issue was the sheer size of the structure, which straddled Lyons and Lehigh Avenues. The garage was in danger of becoming a symbol of the two Newarks, built for the suburbanites working or seeking care at an institution in a neighborhood whose residents often could not afford to own a car.

Bornstein met with the Lehigh Avenue Block Association, which requested an affirmative action plan for the hiring of employees who would construct the garage. Further, board member Lester Z. Lieberman (no relation to Leonard Lieberman), drawing upon his extensive engineering experience, worked with the architects to design the garage to look like an extension of the phase III pavilion, so that the imposing boxlike structure would aesthetically blend in with the patient centers and be less offensive to the community who had to live with it as a physical presence.[36]

Among the most vociferous of the hospital's critics was Newark city councilman Sharpe James, who had grown up in the South Ward and now was its representative. Could the Beth persuade James that it wanted to serve his community? Bornstein, an avid tennis player, was unaware that nearly a half century earlier, Dr. Paul Keller had envisioned a recreation area complete with tennis court for the rooftop of the nurses' residence. Learning that the councilman also liked the sport and cared deeply about the lack of adequate recreation space for community residents, Bornstein proposed to James that the NBIMC erect a tennis court on the roof of the new garage for the neighborhood children. It was an offer greatly appreciated and began an ongoing alliance and personal friendship between James and Bornstein.[37]

By 1976, when phase IV was under way, the sources of funding included a Hill-Burton matching grant, a Title X of the EDA Mental Health grant, and an FHA-GNMA loan, for a staggering total of almost $38 million. The regulations and deadlines for applications for each of these grants required the full-time attention of attorneys and hospital executives.

Phase IV construction was scheduled for completion in 1978 to coincide with the fiftieth anniversary of the opening of the tower building. And, indeed, by September, the phase IV project was ready for public use, save only for the punch-list items that require attention at the very end of all construction projects. Lester Z. Lieberman's reward for a job well done was more responsibility. In December 1978, labor attorney Harold Grotta became the NBIMC president and Lieberman became vice president.[38]

The completion of phases III and IV enabled the NBIMC to be designated as a New Jersey Region II acute care regional medical center. The pavilions also markedly changed the physical appearance of the hospital. However, few in Newark could look at the aerial photographs of the two pavilions buildings, constructed side by side on Osborne Terrace in an orderly square, and recognize that the it bore a striking resemblance to Frank Grad's 1922 preliminary architectural plans for a pavilion of buildings designed for the High and West Kinney Streets location and the design that he had envisioned for the new site if all the parcels of land had been acquired.[39]

Building the Late Twentieth-Century Beth

In 1980, engineer Lester Z. Lieberman succeeded attorney Harold Grotta as president of the board. Like so many others of his generation on the board, Lieberman was a Newark product, born at the Beth and with a degree from the Newark College of Engineering. The experience of watching the Beth hospital staff care for his daughter during a life-threatening illness galvanized him to become involved in the administration of the hospital. Lieberman had the skills and experience to finish what others had begun: to complete the transformation of the medical center to serve the region and its neighborhood.[40]

Lieberman pressed forward to phase V, the renovation and expansion of four treatment areas in both the center tower building, now called the East Pavilion, and the new Pavilion, supported by government grants and loans and an array of local philanthropic Jewish organizations. A multi-disciplinary Flo Okin Oncology Center was dedicated by the women's cancer-relief organization to those who had founded the organization in 1932. The Ruth Gottscho Kidney Foundation supported renovation of the fourth floor of the tower building with its inpatient and outpatient dialysis and kidney-transplant units. The Nuclear Medicine Center was expanded and placed near the new Radiation Therapy Center, which received a linear accelerator from the Beth Israel Women's Auxiliary.

Construction would continue in phases V through IX from 1980 through 1995. As plans were readied for each phase, Lester Lieberman had to identify design flaws of buildings constructed in an earlier phase that had to be corrected for proper completion of the next structures. Sometimes the correction came with great cost and aggravation. In 1986, for example,

Lieberman learned that the six-story phase III Pavilion could not sustain the crosswinds that would threaten its doubled height in a later construction phase. After a long and positive relationship with the architectural firm that had built the structure, the hospital now sued the architects for the $1 million needed to correct the design flaw. Although the court agreed that the firm had not performed adequately, the architects did not pay for the correction of the design as twelve years had passed from the date the Pavilion had opened to the start of the new expansion and the statute of limitations had expired.[41]

Despite such setbacks, Lieberman pressed onward. The final complex, connected by pedestrian bridges, would span three streets. By phase VIII, a building for hospital offices that had been needed since the early 1960s finally went up; nested within the parking-garage structure, its offices were built along an extension to a building on the west side of Lyons Avenue. A 1993 $54 million CON from the State Health Planning Council for phase IX construction financed a modernized laboratory, expanded emergency-room services, and a new state-of-the art ambulatory care center in place of the 1928 three-story outpatient-clinic building on the south side of Osborne Terrace, adjacent to a second expanded 1,000-space parking garage. This center complemented the Pavilion brick for brick, creating a continuous complex connected by a pedestrian bridge over Osborne Terrace. The street below was a pleasant thoroughfare open to both pedestrian and local car traffic.[42] By 1995, the NBIMC campus was finally an integrated structure, and the board named the new ambulatory care center for Lester Lieberman in honor of his work.[43]

The interns and residents who came to the "Pavilion Beth" began their postgraduate training in an acute care regional medical center affiliated with the UMDNJ. No longer merely a community hospital, the NBIMC offered programs judged as best in the state. These women and men completing their medical training each received a *Staff House Manual* reminding them that they were coming to a Jewish hospital that had been long committed to postgraduate education since its founding, had begun training interns in the first decade of the twentieth century, and had run a fully accredited residency program since 1947. The section "House Staff Philosophy" reinforced the nature of medical training in a voluntary hospital:

> We believe that both the attending staff and the house staff have a
> mutual responsibility for the care of each patient. . . . This can only
> be done when there is a full exchange of ideas between the bright

minds of the young interns and residents, leavened by the experience of the attending physician. . . . It is true that not every attending is an outstanding teacher, similarly not every house staff officer is another Osler, and . . . not every case is "interesting," but every case is a human being with a problem that must be treated.[44]

But some still recalled the earlier era, among them Dr. Eugene Parsonnet, whom many nurses called "Dr. Gene," who walked the halls of the Beth's new Pavilion to visit elderly patients whom he had treated and who remained his friends. Until his death in 1986, Dr. Gene made the rounds of the patient floors, "kibitzing" gently with the young nurses and stopping by the bedsides of patients to practice "the healing touch" as he had done for nearly a half century. The central air-conditioning and acoustically sound-proofed construction kept the rooms cool and silent, punctuated by the chatter of daytime television programs and the continuous beeps of the myriad of monitoring equipment and intravenous trees that tethered the patients to wires and tubes. The doctor and his patient could look out of sealed picture windows high above Weequahic on a vista of Newark and beyond, to the east, the faint outlines of the New York City skyline.

Hospital Medicine in the Era of Cost Containment

The physicians who practiced in the Beth Pavilion would reap the benefits and liabilities of practicing in a medical system that bore little resemblance to the one that Dr. Eugene Parsonnet knew. By the 1980s, the federal government had escalated its expenditures for health-care services from $12 billion in 1950 to $139.3 billion in 1976. Most of these funds were allocated for research, training, and facility construction.[45] An increasing component of federal government funds came from the agencies of the Department of Health and Human Services, including the National Institutes of Health, the Social Security Administration, and the Health Care Finance Administration.

More than 70 percent of U.S. expenditures for health care went to the elderly and the poor through Medicare and Medicaid. Containment of costs in these programs became an important federal priority by the early 1980s. As part of its effort at "scientific management" grounded in standardization, the federal government developed a scheme of "prospective payment," whereby it would pay hospitals predetermined amounts for particular medical procedures. A bill signed by President Ronald Reagan in 1982 provided for a new modus operandi: instead of reimbursing hospitals for costs tallied after treatment, a set fee per case would be determined in advance of treatment by the diagnosis. Diagnoses were categorized into one of 467 diagnosis-related groups (DRGs). For example, among the cardiovascular diagnoses, DRG 103 was the designation for a heart transplant, DRG 129 for cardiac arrest.

Critics of the DRG system, such as the historian Rosemary Stevens, observed that the DRGs "challenged variety in medicine." Underlying the system was the flawed assumption that "cases falling into each group are relatively homogeneous, in terms of medical technology, use of hospital labor, and length of stay," suggesting that "medical practice can be standardized into defined expectations and procedures." The new system posed "a direct threat to the clinical autonomy of physicians and to the traditional division between medical and administrative responsibilities in the hospital" in the name of standardization. The incentive for each hospital would be to cut costs so that they would not spend more than the amount available from the federal government.[46]

In preparation for full implementation of the DRG system, NBIMC hospital unit chiefs indeed began to cut costs. However, at times they miscalculated because they did not fully understand the terminology and process of cost reimbursement, as an exchange of memoranda between Bornstein and Dr. Victor Parsonnet amply illustrates. Parsonnet's memo described the changes that were made in the interest of cost containment in the preoperative, intraoperative, and postoperative procedures in heart surgery: discontinuing urine and sputum cultures and pulmonary function studies "except when specifically indicated," changing the oxygenization system, and reducing the drugs used postoperatively where possible. His estimate of savings was nearly $800 per case, and as his department performed four to five hundred procedures each year, he estimated that these measures would save the NBIMC almost $1 million annually. Bornstein's carefully worded reply thanked him for his efforts but explained that the terms "costs" and "charges" were defined differently by federal regulations and private insurance carriers. The department's cost-containment plan would save the hospital close to $300,000, not $1 million.[47] The DRG system clearly applied an unwelcome pressure to cut costs that was felt even by physicians and surgeons who wished their institutions to remain competitive.

Together, DRG and CON regulations could strangle urban voluntary hospitals trying to comply with both. An urban regional medical center granted a CON for a particular specialty was also expected to admit the sickest patients, those most in need of its specialized care. Statistics for these patients, measured by DRG and related regulations, never took into account that, for patients suffering from the particular condition in which a hospital specialized, such institutions might have higher mortality figures than other institutions. This combination created problems for the Beth in the 1980s. The hospital had received a CON and designation as an acute coronary facility in New Jersey and by 1987 also obtained a CON for a two-year demonstration project in heart transplants. The designation necessitated admitting the most acutely ill coronary patients, potential recipients of a transplant. The Beth did not screen out the sickest with an eye to the potential impact on its mortality data. Not surprisingly, many such patients did not survive. When the mortality data were reported, the Beth temporarily lost its permission to conduct transplant surgery.

The impact of the DRG system was most keenly felt in small municipal and voluntary nonprofit hospitals that offered good care but could not compete in efficiency with larger for-profit hospitals. Thousands of 100-bed hospitals, most built with Hill-Burton funds, now blanketed the health-care landscape in areas that had once been rural and were engulfed by expanding suburbs. Municipalities and county governments operated these hospitals, providing emergency services and care to the indigent while struggling with their own budgets. These small outmoded hospitals had to compete with Veterans Administration facilities, teaching hospitals, and larger voluntary nonprofits to offer attractive salaries to the best medical personnel.

The Rise of the For-Profit Health-Care Corporations

What kind of hospital could compete in an arena of CONS and DRGs? The 1980s saw a surge in the formation of for-profit hospital-network chains, which expanded by carefully identifying areas whose residents could afford medical care but were currently served by the small aging 100-bed public hospitals. The chain would offer to take over such a hospital from a municipality and finance the improvement of care and services by charging fees for services; many communities found these offers attractive and accepted the bids. Small voluntary nonprofit hospitals were also vulnerable to these attractive bids and were bought by the financially robust hospital chains. Between 1980 and 1982, one-fourth of the phenomenal growth of the for-profit chains came from the purchase of public and voluntary nonprofit hospitals. Following the purchase, the aging hospital was renovated or razed for a new facility, new physicians were given short-term incentives, and the new hospital raised its fees and reduced services for those unable to pay them.[48]

University-affiliated teaching hospitals were among the few entities that could successfully counter the for-profit bids. In 1983, the Baltimore City Hospital was an aging three-building complex—a tuberculosis sanitarium, an acute care building, and a nursing home, all built in 1925 and located in the depressed East Baltimore neighborhood. When a for-profit network approached the Baltimore city government, the Johns Hopkins University Medical Center, a formidable university teaching hospital, counterbid and transformed the municipal into a satellite, Bayview Center. The action strengthened the viability of Baltimore's voluntary nonprofit hospitals, including the local Jewish Sinai Hospital, which had relocated to the northern suburbs in the early 1950s.

Not every teaching hospital was financially strong enough to counter the for-profit bids. The University of Chicago hospital staff was issued pocket manuals listing the cost of each laboratory test, to enforce cost consciousness.[49] In cities where the for-profit network hospitals were able to establish themselves successfully, the indigent and the uninsured poured into the few voluntary nonprofit hospitals, sharply reducing their ability to survive.

The Beth Healthcare Services Corporation

The NBIMC, like many other voluntary hospitals, countered the for-profit hospitals by restructuring its organization. As early as 1971, board member Alan Lowenstein had proposed that the NBIMC be restructured to possess the diversity of both nonprofit and for-profit entities. In 1973, the NBIMC created a nonprofit corporation to acquire the land, building, and other assets of the Columbus Redwood Nursing Home, which was then leased to the Theresa Grotta Center for Restorative Services.[50] The corporation then lent Theresa Grotta $300,000 to pay the mortgage for the property and facility, enabling a strong affiliation with a suburban health-care facility, but without a formal amalgamation.[51]

By 1985, the Beth Healthcare Services Corporation was organized into taxable and nontaxable corporations. The nontaxable corporations included the Newark Beth Israel Medical Center and the Newark Medical Research, Education, and Development Foundation, which held a sublease linking the medical center to the research firm of Hoffmann-LaRoche for research conducted in the tower building. The Beth Medical Services Corporation owned 80 percent of the Morris Avenue Association, an off-site facility providing immediate care and medical services. The associates managed Doctors on Duty, nicknamed doc-in-the-box, that provided immediate

care and dispensary services to employees whose employers signed agreements with the physicians' practice. In the 1920s, local businesses like the
Hollander Fur Company had hired doctors for the care of their employees; in
the 1980s, local businesses signed contracts with Doctors on Duty to perform pre-employment physicals and assess workers' compensation claims
and to discount medical services for their employees.[52] Parkside Urban
Renewal Associates was a partnership between Beth Israel Medical Services
Corporation and Newark Kidney Center Associates that in turn served as
landlord to the Parkside Dialysis Center, an outpatient facility. The Beth
countered the financial power of the for-profit hospitals, then, with the diversity and flexibility permitted by its Healthcare Services Corporation.

The DRG system only heightened the disadvantage in the medical
marketplace of the smaller municipal institutions and the voluntary nonprofits. By 1985, even as their revenues began to flatten, four for-profit hospital chains owned or managed nearly 12 percent of U.S. hospitals: Hospital
Corporation of America, American Medical International, Humana, Inc.,
and National Medical Enterprises, Inc.[53] Would economic necessity compel
the Beth to join such a chain? What would be the effect of such chains
on those who depended most on voluntary not-for-profit hospitals such as
the Beth?

By the mid-1980s, some Jewish hospitals began to show marked
problems. In 1985, Los Angeles's Cedars-Sinai Medical Center laid off 250
staff members.[54] In Chicago, Michael Reese Hospital's cuts were even
harsher: eliminating 1,000 of its 4,880 full-time jobs, for example, cutting
two of every three cashiers and eliminating weekend hours, and cutting the
number of meal entrees from seven to three.[55] The number of closures of
community hospitals accelerated. The American Hospital Association
established the Ad Hoc Committee on Hospital Closures after two successive years (1988 and 1989) that each recorded a closure or conversion of
eighty-one hospitals. The committee issued guidelines on managing hospital closures and noted that conversion of services should be a goal, but that
when closure was the only option for a hospital in an "overbedded area," the
overall outcome might improve the health-care system.[56]

This industrialization of U.S. medicine produced cut-throat competition. What should voluntary nonprofit hospitals do to survive? This question not only faced Jewish hospitals but also represented a crossroads in the
nation's medical care. As it had so many times before, the Beth looked to
its history of survival to cope with the new economics of hospital care.
Dr. Lee K. Frankel, in a foreword written for the 1930 Newark Beth Israel

Annual Report, described the response of the voluntary hospitals to the Great Depression; his words now seemed chillingly prescient:

> The hospital is a changing institution. Its surroundings are chang-
> ing. . . . I think it may be accepted as a fact that in the past the hospi-
> tal has been largely an isolated independent unit. Has the time come
> for us to think in terms of the community instead of the individual
> institutions? I am wondering whether the time has not come when
> we shall have to think in this city and other cities as well, of a public
> coordination of the activities of incorporated hospitals; . . . another
> questions arises, which I approach with even more temerity. That is
> the question whether the time has come to consider limiting the
> activities of incorporated hospitals to definite zones or areas. . . . Is it
> preferable to continue the present policy of hospitals receiving their
> patients from any section of the city, or from outside of the city, or to
> divide the city geographically so that each hospital shall be the cen-
> ter for the care required within a limited area. . . . Changes are taking
> place. Those of you have watched have seen [that] there is a ten-
> dency toward consolidation or merger of hospitals.[57]

Frankel's words defined the outlook and options that U.S. hospitals, including the NBIMC, would confront at the close of the twentieth century.

CHAPTER 9

The Changing Shape of Health Care

*T*hose who fully comprehended that late twentieth-century medicine was increasingly organized according to an industrial model understood that hospitals must chart their courses for the future accordingly. Gaining strength in the world of industry often required consolidation to control costs and maximize profits. Confronting similar economic problems, hospitals adopted a similar solution.

Forces in the Trend toward Merger

In 1974, when *Modern Hospital* changed its name to *Modern Healthcare*, journal publisher David McKelly explained that he made the change because "the shape of health care is changing." Turning to hospitals, specifically, he observed:

> Around the country, some hospitals are building extended care facilities or associating themselves with existing units. In several cities, notably Detroit and Hartford, hospitals are organizing themselves into consortia which will allow each institution to concentrate on specific parts of the health care whole, thus maximizing the institutions' resources and eliminating the duplication of effort and service. Multi hospital chains both non-profit and investor-owned, are sprouting and growing, indicating that the corporate form of management in health care is demonstrating its efficiency and effectiveness.

If the charitable voluntary hospital institutions that had served their local communities were receding into the past, it was because of broader changes in society, the economy, and medicine, according to McKelly:

> In part because of such external forces and government regulation and inflation, and further because the delivery system is

demanding closer relationships, the traditional barriers between the various stages of care—acute care, chronic care, rehabilitation care and so on—are falling. While there are and will continue to be differences in methods and techniques, the trend is toward the formation of a common interest—providing health care to the people.[1]

Modern Healthcare signaled to its readership that the inpatient hospital facility was increasingly only one piece of a much broader health-care network. By the 1980s, the U.S. hospital system, a mosaic of thousands of small municipal and voluntary nonprofit hospitals fostered by the Hill-Burton Act, was reassembling into a far less variegated image as they were acquired by the mega-health-care network chains and transformed into franchises. Many urban voluntary nonprofit hospitals pursued a two-pronged response to this onslaught, establishing affiliations with other hospitals to expand their geographical presence while restructuring their own organizations to accommodate nonprofit and for-profit components. It was a risk. Such reconfigurations could weaken their identity as nonprofit institutions and dilute their commitment to their original missions to serve vulnerable populations most in need of quality low-cost medical care.

In 1986, a study by the prestigious Institute of Medicine (IOM) presented the problems of this competition between for-profit and nonprofit medical institutions. An article in the widely read *New England Journal of Medicine* discussed the implications of the IOM study, observing that "the challenge to not-for-profit institutions is not only how to deal with new and difficult economic realities but how to do it so that the community functions that many hospitals have performed over many years are preserved." IOM data, which revealed that "the activities of some not-for-profit hospitals can hardly be distinguished these days from those of their investor-owned competitors, may be true in some ways (e.g., the growth of multi-institutional systems and for-profit subsidiaries) but not true in others." The increasing similarity of not-for-profits and for-profits had serious implications for the former because they would "have a more difficult struggle to maintain their credibility, support, and tax exemptions."[2]

Others predicted the demise of voluntary nonprofit hospitals altogether. A *Wall Street Journal* business bulletin quoted a hospital administrator who proclaimed: "By the mid-1990s . . . we'll see 1,000 hospitals belly up."[3] The article reassured readers that the loss of the voluntary nonprofit hospitals would not adversely affect the U.S. health-care system—of seven thousand hospitals in the United States, the loss of a thousand hospitals would still leave sufficient beds for the population.

A historical perspective provided by the historian Rosemary Stevens in the 1980s suggested a less apocalyptic outcome. Stevens compared the burgeoning of the for-profit networks to the brief resurgence of proprietary hospitals in the 1920s. Describing U.S. hospitals as "diverse and multipurpose institutions" with a "tradition of serving specific communities of interest, providing opportunities and hierarchy in medical and health-care professions, and providing sites for training, employment, and voluntary work," she was not prepared to write off voluntary nonprofits; such hospitals had in the past managed to retain their traditions while "adapting very rapidly to external incentives" no less effectively than did their for-profit rivals.[4]

Although Stevens did not single out Jewish voluntary nonprofit hospitals, she might have used them to bolster her argument. Pessimists characterized Jewish hospitals as among the most vulnerable of the voluntary nonprofit institutions. Many that continued to serve their communities were now venerable names functioning in aging facilities in large impoverished inner-city neighborhoods, true nonprofit entities with profit margins of less than 1 percent.[5]

However, by the 1980s, many U.S. Jewish hospitals, both the general and the specialized, were also the resilient survivors of twentieth-century crises, including cycles of economic depression, recession, and wartime inflation. These hospitals had changed as the state of medicine had changed, often razing and rebuilding entire units—laboratories, radiology, surgery, and ancillary services and expanding to become regional medical centers like the Newark Beth Israel Medical Center (NBIMC). These hospitals that had depended on philanthropic legacies and community donations, survived the Depression, restructured their accounting and record systems to the reimbursable cost systems of third-party insurance carriers, and restructured again for the myriad of Medicare, Medicaid, and federal grant program regulations, now readied themselves for the next cycle of adaptation.

Mergers

A period that witnessed the proliferation of hospitals and specialty institutions was always followed by a period of their collapse and merging that responded to the unsettled economic environment. The 1920s—the golden age of skyscraper and specialty hospital construction—foundered amid the economic pressures of the Great Depression. By 1930, the New

York City municipal government merged twenty-two municipal and charity hospitals with a total of 14,138 beds. This giant merger encouraged the consolidation of other voluntary hospitals in New York City such as Columbia Presbyterian, which absorbed Babies Hospital, Sloane Hospital for Women, New York Neurology, Herman Knapp Eye, and New York Orthopedic.[6]

The 1930 *American Jewish Yearbook* listed sixty-two U.S. Jewish hospitals, sanatoria, and convalescent homes in twenty-five communities. There were specialized hospitals for the care of incurables and the chronically ill, and sanitariums for those who had tuberculosis.[7] This list omitted the numerous local Jewish associations that maintained orphan homes, homes for the aged, and day nurseries, all providing medical care. The list appeared extensive, but did not reflect two mergers that had already occurred within the Jewish institutions that provided health care.

By 1930, the Jewish or Hebrew dispensaries had completely melded into the Jewish hospitals. In the first decade of the twentieth century, the doctors' storefront offices in Jewish immigrant neighborhoods had become merged with the fledgling Jewish hospitals. The concept of the dispensary was retained in the outpatient clinics on the hospitals' premises, dispensing care for nonacute cases. Indeed, the Beth's dispensary continued to operate on Charleton Street from 1900 through 1908, when the second Newark Beth Israel Hospital opened. In the 1970s, the ambulatory clinics and neighborhood health centers could be described as the newest versions of such facilities.

By 1930, the Jewish maternity specialty hospitals were being actively merged or amalgamated into the newer general Jewish hospitals, exemplified by the Beth's amalgamation with the Newark Jewish Maternity Hospital. Many aspects of the care they provided were retained in the general hospitals: the separation of maternity patients from those with communicable diseases, limited visiting hours to permit hospital routine to continue unencumbered by outsiders roaming through halls or sitting at patient bedsides and interfering with caregivers, and the provision of counseling services as a component of antenatal treatment. The independent birthing centers and antenatal clinics that were created in the late 1970s and early 1980s resembled, in their separation and services, the maternity hospitals that had existed fifty years earlier.

How many Jewish hospitals existed prior to the Great Depression? The answer has always been problematic when consulting Jewish publications such as the *American Jewish Yearbook*. In 1940, the Beth's Dr. Max Danzis, writing an article on graduate medical training, turned away from these Jewish sources. Instead, he counted hospitals, nonsectarian and sectarian, operating under Jewish auspices, which met the standards set by the American Hospital Association (AHA), the American Medical Association (AMA) Council on Medical Education for internships, and the American College of Surgeons (ACS). His approach identified thirty-six general Jewish hospitals. A review of earlier ACS lists identifies three Jewish hospitals that had previously received accreditation and had closed during the 1930s: in Omaha, the Isaac M. Wise Memorial Hospital; in New York City, the People's Hospital; and in Baltimore, the Hebrew Hospital and Asylum.[8] (See Appendix, Table 1.)

After World War II, changing demographics in industrial cities were catalytic in mergers of Jewish hospitals in Philadelphia, Los Angeles, and the New York boroughs of Manhattan, the Bronx, and Brooklyn. The same changing demographics spurred the establishment of new Jewish hospitals: the Sinai hospitals of Miami, Minneapolis, and Detroit; Weiss Memorial in Chicago; and Long Island Jewish in New York's Nassau County. The Jewish hospitals underwent mergers of their identities and facilities. Some Jewish hospitals chose new identities, as did Brooklyn Maimonides Hospital, created in 1947 when Beth Moses and Israel Zion merged.[9] The Philadelphia Jewish hospitals and their nursing schools consolidated their strengths and responded to the shift in the Jewish population to suburbs by creating the newly named Albert Einstein Medical Center that operated three satellite divisions: Mount Sinai Hospital in the south, Northern Liberties to the north, and Jewish Hospital in the east. Jewish hospitals absorbed others entirely, as happened in the 1957 closure of Maimonides Hospital in San Francisco, its assets absorbed into Mount Zion Hospital. There were uneasy mergers, like that of the Jewish Hospital of St. Louis and the Washington University Medical School and Barnes Hospital in 1962, after a bitter fight during which Barnes Hospital resisted.[10] Mergers of Jewish hospitals, wishing to retain their identities produced hyphenated names: Cedars-Sinai in Los Angeles, formed from the merger of Cedars of Lebanon and Mount Sinai Hospitals; and Bronx-Lebanon in New York City, retaining the separate facilities of the former Bronx and Lebanon Hospitals less than a mile apart. Thus, the number of postwar voluntary nonprofit general hospitals under Jewish auspices fluctuated during the next cycle of mergers around Danzis's count.[11]

Another cycle of mergers was triggered in 1966 by factors that included the advent of Medicare, which required that hospitals abide by the provisions of the 1964 Civil Rights Act, and the inclusion of hospital employees under the provisions of the federal minimum-wage law. In July of that year, *Modern Hospital* identified nearly thirty-two mergers that had occurred within the previous decade.[12] A study revealed that these consolidations were attempting an economy of size and function, an approach praised by Dr. Anthony J. J. Rourke, who had engineered the merger that created Newark's United Hospitals Medical Center (later United Healthcare Systems, Inc.) in 1957: "No single step could do more for the advancement of hospital care, both as to the quality and cost than pooling our efforts into hospitals of optimum size."[13] The Hospital Review and Planning Council of Southern New York was limiting its recommendations for Hill-Burton modernization funding to mergers of small community hospitals that would create new hospitals of at least four hundred beds, a move that would broaden the scope of services and expand teaching programs with medical colleges. The hospitals that did not choose to merge were ripe for takeover by the for-profit hospital chains.[14] (See Appendix, Table 2.)

U.S. hospitals were on the brink of another cycle of mergers in the last decades of the twentieth century.[15] With the federal government pressing regional health-care decision makers to contain costs and prevent duplication of services, mergers might produce mega-hospitals capable of providing enough beds for an entire region, as smaller, less efficient hospitals were felled by economic strain.

The mega-hospital was not a new idea. A half century earlier, Dr. S. S. Goldwater had cautioned against such medical "super structures." He did not believe that a hospital of 1,500–2,000 beds in a single physically consolidated facility could sustain an economy of maintenance and medical efficiency or have the flexibility to respond to changes in medicine and technology. Consolidated management of hospitals within cities would work only if each hospital was granted a degree of local autonomy with respect to its internal affairs. Maintaining the individual identity of hospitals under consolidated management would promote local pride, encourage healthy rivalry among hospitals, develop a keen sense of responsibility to patients, and, especially, foster a warm personal devotion to all employees, without which the morale of an institution is speedily impaired.[16]

Goldwater also cautioned that mergers would be more difficult among hospitals that possessed distinct traditions, especially if they were denominational in origin. He advised that in such situations, a community would be wise to let the separate hospital institutions continue until they outgrew their defects and became more amenable to change. The 1982 consolidation of Brooklyn Jewish Hospital and Saint John's Episcopal Hospital to create the

Interfaith Medical Center demonstrated the problems that might develop
when two financially troubled hospitals merged prematurely. Brooklyn
Jewish Hospital had been founded by insurance broker Nathan Jonas with
the financial support of Abraham Abraham, founder of Brooklyn's Abraham
& Straus Department Store. Abraham wanted the hospital run as efficiently
as his store. In 1935, Abraham Lichtman had asked Joseph Baker, the president of Brooklyn Jewish, to address the Beth's board on how to operate the
hospital as a business. In 1979, Brooklyn Jewish Hospital filed for bankruptcy.[17] Grants and donations allowed its clinics to continue to provide care
to the indigent in the community. The Episcopal and the Jewish hospitals
consolidated their operations, but each medical staff continued to identify
with the former entity. By 1989, Interfaith Medical Center was running out
of money for basic equipment; the payroll checks bounced; and renovation
began at the Saint John's facility, while plans were made to close the Jewish
Hospital as a general hospital, sell its equipment, reduce its staff, and reopen
the building as a mental health center.[18]

The ecumenical merger that consolidated the most voluntary hospitals
into one medical care entity occurred in 1988 in Minneapolis, bringing
together the Episcopal, Swedish, Lutheran, Catholic, and Jewish hospitals.[19]
The consolidation had begun in 1970 when Saint Barnabas Hospital merged
with the Swedish Hospital to form the Metropolitan Medical Center (MMC).
In 1988, MMC, which had absorbed other voluntary hospitals, merged with
the Mount Sinai Medical Center to form the Metropolitan Mount Sinai
Medical Center (MSMC). The hospitals merged their staffs, while their auxiliaries and foundations continued to operate separately. But these hospitals
also had financial troubles that continued after the merger. Mount Sinai
Hospital was closed in 1991, laying off nearly 1,200 hospital employees.
What was most appalling to its doctors and staff was a "numbness and tolerance" for just another hospital closing.[20] The head of the MSMC sadly noted
that "a hospital could have a good facility, a positive location, a large medical staff, and a sizable patient volume and still lose money."[21]

Similar mergers of Jewish and non-Jewish hospitals were negotiated
between 1987 and 1991. Menorah Hospital in Kansas City reduced the
number of medical residency positions and entered into a contractual relationship with Kaiser Health Plan. In Milwaukee, the Sinai Hospital merged
with the Good Samaritan Medical Center to become Aurora Health Care, a
not-for-profit system. Mount Sinai in Hartford, Connecticut, was absorbed
into Saint Francis Hospital and Medical Center, the largest Catholic hospital in New England. Sinai Hospital in Detroit merged with Grace Hospital
and became a suburban outpatient center. Two Jewish hospitals merged

with university hospitals and medical schools in their cities: Mount Zion Hospital integrated with the University of California San Francisco Medical Center, giving it full responsibility for its governance and operation; and Montefiore Hospital in Pittsburgh was sold to the University of Pittsburgh and its medical college.[22]

The Cautionary Tale of Chicago's Michael Reese Hospital

The demise of Chicago's Michael Reese Hospital and Medical Center offered a cautionary tale to all Jewish hospitals looking warily to the future, including Newark Beth Israel. The legacy of Michael Reese, who had amassed a fortune in the California gold rush, was sufficient to create an endowment that enabled the construction of the first building in 1881 and a second larger building in 1907 to the west of Chicago's Jewish enclave, the Maxwell Street neighborhood. Junk Town, as it was called, resembled Newark's Prince Street, crowded with butcher shops and other stores whose signs were in Yiddish. Chicago's German Jewish businessmen pursued business opportunities and social acceptance, and, still unacceptable in many of the city's best clubs, had created the Standard Club, even as those in Newark had founded the Progress Club.

Michael Reese Hospital was surrounded by specialized hospitals such as the Sarah Morris Children's Hospital. In 1909, Sarah Morris's husband, Nelson, gave Michael Reese $250,000 to build the Nelson Morris Institute of Medical Research, recruiting researchers from the newly established Rockefeller Institute. The new institute continued to receive legacies exceeding $100,000 that enabled its staff to engage in advanced studies in the 1930s, providing a haven for Jewish physicians, including refugees from Nazi Germany. By 1946, Michael Reese had founded its own postgraduate school for training in the sciences. The postwar Jewish hospital absorbed the old office buildings and homes in the surrounding neighborhood, even taking over the Keeley Brewery. It was situated in a deteriorating neighborhood, increasingly like Newark's Central Ward, thrice used by generations of migrants: Germans, Russians, and African Americans. Like the Beth's, Michael Reese's medical staff and board questioned whether the hospital should relocate to an outlying suburb and consulted the American Society of Planning Officials to assess the best direction for the Jewish hospital. Their decision was to remain in place and "revitalize the neighborhood and Reese itself."[23]

The hospital began a steady program of land acquisition and demolition of the houses in the blighted streets around it, creating a forty-five-acre campus of new buildings while entering into agreements to build new public housing projects. The Illinois Blighted Areas Act of 1947 enabled the Chicago Land Clearance Commission to invoke the right of eminent domain and demolish housing declared to be slums. The land was then purchased by the hospital and private corporations. Together they financed a cluster of unadorned functional housing projects; the apartment houses were designed to match the new hospital buildings. By the mid-1960s, Michael Reese had grown to a 1,000 beds.

In 1981, Reese celebrated its centennial and began a new campaign for its second century. The hospital opened an outpatient clinic to care for a new generation of Russian-Jewish immigrants. Reflecting the national trend, the hospital began to suffer a low bed census and decided to reduce the number of beds. Medicare reimbursements became a staple of its income. In 1985, its board began to explore a merger with the University of Illinois Medical School in Chicago (UIC), a move opposed by some of the city's residents, who feared that the university hospital would close. During the negotiations many Reese physicians had been appointed to the UIC departments, and these physicians chose not to retain their appointments at Reese. Michael Reese Hospital, for the first time in its history, had too few physicians. In October 1990, Reese officials informed the Chicago Board of Health that the hospital had lost $17 million and could no longer continue to operate.

Michael Reese Hospital and its 240,000-member HMO was sold on October 1, 1990, to Humana Inc., a Louisville, Kentucky, for-profit chain of hospitals. Five months after the takeover, its new executive officer resigned. Three years later, the hospital was sold again. The buyer was Columbia/HCA, which had sought community support for the transaction by spreading rumors that the hospital's land was to be sold to real estate speculators for condominiums if Columbia's efforts to buy it failed.[24]

News of the sale sent shock waves rippling through the Jewish health-care community. The Jewish hospital's rich history, traditions, and legacies could not save it from perishing in the crucible of the late twentieth-century health-care economies. When Michael Reese Hospital lost its Jewish identity, other Jewish hospitals not already in the midst of mergers began to seriously ponder their own futures.

New Jersey Mergers and the Newark Beth Israel Medical Center

By the 1970s, the Beth Israel Healthcare Services Corporation (BIHSC) had entered into a number of affiliations, including that with the

Theresa Grotta Restorative Center in Redwood, to strengthen its economic position and to preserve its status as a voluntary nonprofit medical center. Other Beth affiliations were at the level of particular services. In 1973, for example, the Beth affiliated with Elizabeth General Hospital in the pediatrics service of both institutions and two years later in their ob/gyn departments.[25] Similar arrangements involved Saint James, Saint Michael's, and Rahway Hospitals. By 1986, the Newark Beth Israel Medical Center could claim two tiers of affiliations. The first involved close affiliations with East Orange Hospital, John F. Kennedy Memorial, Beth Israel Hospital of Passaic, and Irvington General Hospital; partial affiliations were made with Bayonne Hospital, West Hudson Hospital, and Montclair Community Hospital.

In 1989, the BIHSC was presented with its first opportunity to formally create a suburban presence: the Livingston Community Hospital, a ninety-four-bed facility, declared bankruptcy in 1988, and its board voted to sell the hospital to BIHSC. An agreement to set up a satellite program at Livingston Community Hospital became a prelude to taking over its buildings and land. However, at a subsequent bankruptcy auction, Saint Barnabas Medical Center in Livingston also bid for the hospital, proposing to use it for outpatient services, a nursing home, and a residential health-care facility that would be close to its own Livingston campus.

The New Jersey Board of Health chose the Saint Barnabas proposal.[26] Shortly afterward, the NBIMC's Certificate of Need (CON) application to acquire a magnetic resonance imaging unit was rejected. Morale at the Beth plummeted. In April 1990, NBIMC physicians, board members, and administrators attended a retreat to discuss how the hospital could best remain in the forefront in the wake of these setbacks.[27] The result was a resolve to form alliances with former competitors. In 1995, it was agreed that the NBIMC would form an alliance with Saint Michael's Hospital, which would increase the Beth's programs in heart surgery.[28] In addition, Beth physicians expressed a desire to form alliances with four New Jersey hospitals to reduce costs in biomedical engineering, mental health services, account collections, occupational health programs, and continuing medical education programs.

One alliance that did not endure was that with University of Medicine and Dentistry of New Jersey (UMDNJ). By the mid-1990s, "virtually every medical student from UMDNJ passed through Newark Beth Israel Medical Center at one time or another during his/her undergraduate medical years."[29] But the relationship of the medical school and the Jewish hospital began to unravel. By 1994, the two institutions were continuing an affiliation in only three medical specializations: cardiovascular surgery, oncology, and transplants.[30] There was some brief discussion of creating a new affiliation of the UMDNJ with the NBIMC thoracic surgery program, which would include the assignment of Beth surgeons to work at the medical school's cardiology clinic, a move that would "increase efficiency, decrease backlog, thereby increasing the caseload for the University Hospital cardiac program."[31]

In May 1995, to discuss the "deteriorating" relationship of the two institutions, a meeting brought together Dr. Stanley S. Bergen Jr., president of UMDNJ; Lieberman; Bornstein; Dr. D. Brief, director of the Beth's Department of Surgery; and Dr. M. Kirschner, director of the Beth's Department of Medicine. The issue of tertiary care quickly ignited rancorous exchanges. The NBIMC proposed to "develop new tertiary services at both institutions" and then "tithe these tertiary subspecialties to support new and needed academic programs," such as cardiothoracic surgery, transplantation surgery, and medical oncology. Others might include neurosurgery, orthopedics, urology, medical nephrology, and geriatrics. Lieberman noted that the alternative to cooperation was not bright: "If both our institutions proceed along independent lines, each institution will develop its own program, greatly increase costs, increase bad feelings between our institutions and set the stage for counterproductive animosities."

To UMDNJ, NBIMC represented a serious threat as a tertiary institution competing within the same geographical area; at the meeting, the Beth representatives learned that it was no longer considered a valuable affiliate and the current affiliation agreement with the medical school would be phased out. The UMDNJ decision provoked an angry response from them, couched in words that made it clear that they would not be bullied: "Over the past few years, the University Hospital and its administration have chosen to enter into the arena of expanded tertiary services. In effect we have supported the development of tertiary services at University Hospital. But we have not, and we will not destroy our existing tertiary program, which remains our lifeline of survival."

Over the summer months, discussions explored the possibility of the NBIMC joining the University Health Systems HMO begun by UMDNJ. In October, Bergen suggested that the NBIMC and his own institution "issue a joint press release concerning the fact that we are discussing possible joint ventures, or combining of the clinical and educational programs and components of the two medical centers to better serve the citizens of the Greater Newark area and in some selected programs statewide and regionally." But, distrust surfaced in a later paragraph: "We have increasingly found that many individuals and organizations are willing to talk and to accept the educational programs of the University without committing to any further joint efforts. Therefore, we must begin to narrow the field as to potential partners for the University and University Hospital." Lieberman demurred, calling such a joint statement "premature." Instead, he asked for "a short document outlining the areas and nature of potential collaboration" that he might use in exploring the BIHSC options with the entire board in the weeks ahead.[32]

BIHSC had entered into discussions for a possible ecumenical affiliation with the Cathedral Health Care system, composed of Saint James, Saint Michael's, and Columbus Hospitals. Discussion never progressed beyond the initial stages. By 1995, board president Lester Lieberman recognized that the Beth was in the midst of a crisis that it could not resolve by remaining an individual hospital. He pondered the old saying that "once you reach the summit of a mountain, there is no place to go but down." And he began to think that the institution he had built might have reached its crest and be declining in worth.[33]

The Options for the Future of Newark's Jewish Hospital

On November 20, 1995, Lieberman convened a special combined meeting of the NBIMC boards, the senior medical staff, and the BIHSC in the hospital's Max Danzis Auditorium to hear a report on the "strategic and business alternatives" available to the both boards. In painstaking detail, Lieberman and the BIHSC attorneys outlined the choices: to "manage the changing environment or simply react to the forces of change now pervading health care."[34]

To a shocked and silent audience, Lieberman presented the options for the future of their hospital: remain in its present individual configuration as a 580-bed medical center and hospital; attempt to create its own network system; merge with the small hospitals of Morristown, Overlook, and Mountainside (MOM) as a small system; create a limited partnership with Primary Health; become a member of the UMDNJ consortium of teaching hospitals; or transfer ownership of the NBIMC to the Saint Barnabas Corporation.

The points Lieberman made addressed the conditions many were facing. In the postwar period, he observed: "State and Federally regulated payment systems were favorable—even generous—to both the hospital and physicians. A 'cost plus,' fee-for-service commercial insurance system financially rewarded both physicians and the hospital and incented [*sic*] growth in patient volume and clinical programs." The Diagnosis Related Group (DRG) system that had initially worked so well to provide proactive fees was now overwhelmed by the expanding components of treatments and protocols, each with a separate fee. This system had changed as "business and government will no longer tolerate 'cost-plus' forms of payment to either hospitals or physicians and government and commercial payers." Now the payers wanted a "capitation" payment, with all "subsidy" components such as bad debts reduced by the receiving institution.

The government and insurance companies were instituting a new structure of global fees that bore a resemblance to the all-inclusive rate offered by hospitals nearly sixty years earlier. They proposed a return to a flat fee for a surgical procedure or a treatment that included all components, from bed to laboratory to diagnostic tests. The new system would not cover much of the costs, and not all patients would be able to pay the difference between the reimbursement and the charge. The shortfall in cash in-flow would bankrupt individual hospitals and entire networks of for-profit corporations who would realize no profit.

A second development was that in response to fee caps, hospitals had constructed "'vertical and horizontal systems' of in-patient, out-patient, nursing home, physician and other health-care services on a scale to achieve the cost effective management of covered lives," an expensive strategy that only large and wealthy institutions could employ. In the past few years, a number of national, for-profit HMOs were "deploying systems of capitated payment designed to shift financial risk away from the payer to the provider." This, Lieberman observed, placed at risk smaller, undercapitalized hospitals and their physicians.

Medicare payments to institutions were down. Medicaid reimbursements were also declining as enrollments increased and block grants to states were reduced, tightening eligibility requirements. The New Jersey Hospital Association projected a $150 million reduction in hospital income over a seven-year budget period. The commercial shifts to HMOs meant that when the projected enrollment reached 50 percent by the year 2000, the payments to NBIMC would have to be discounted at 25–30 percent below hospital charges. Moreover, there was a reduction in charity care and the income from government programs that subsidized it.

In addition to the problems that all voluntary hospitals were facing, there were problems specific to NBIMC. First, the medical education program showed a dramatic loss of revenue over expenses; with Medicare's medical education payments expected to fall, a $14 million subsidy would be reduced, making development of new residency program "financially difficult" at best. Most critical, the system of "franchise" protection provided by the issuance of CONs had been discontinued, which meant that other medical institutions were free to establish cardiac surgery units and transplants units to compete with the NBIMC program.

Lieberman concluded with his hope that the outcome of the meeting would call for a motion to initiate negotiations with Saint Barnabas Corporation. He proposed that the NBIMC be sold to its staunchest rival, but only under conditions that would preserve the hospital's existence, quality, and heritage. First, the Jewish hospital's original mission statement must be honored, including maintenance of its Jewish identity and the name "Newark Beth Israel Medical Center"; Stars of David would remain on the premises. Second, there must be protection for NBIMC physicians. Third, similar employment protection must be extended to all staff employees. Finally, there must be "maintenance of the high integrity of the Medical Center's specialized programs." This opaque language was a reference to coronary and pulmonary programs, among others, and reflected the apprehensions that once the medical center was sold, the buyer would strip it of its signature programs.

The men and women in the auditorium had listened silently, but now erupted in anguished outbursts. The immediate reaction to Lieberman's presentation was vocal and contentious. Dr. Murray Belsky, chair of the medical staff, expressed a strong concern about "being dominated by a larger hospital," and reported that four hospital CEOs had told him that "St Barnabas would eat us up" and take the programs the Beth had built into Livingston, where Saint Barnabas Medical Center was located. He also wanted reassurance that those involved in negotiations would recall the "mission of the Medical Center as one of dedication to the South Ward community and the community that makes up the Beth's primary service area." Others, such as board member David Rothschild, recognized that in addition to the "financial assurances," he and other board members were seeking "emotional assurances" because of the role that the Beth had played in their lives and in the community "over these many years."

Finally, board member George Grumbach formally moved to submit a letter of intent to Saint Barnabas Medical Center for a potential sale of NBIMC, with the proceeds paid to the Beth Healthcare Foundation or equivalent, per the legal doctrine of *cy pres*. In a second resolution the

officers of the corporation with the advice of counsel were authorized to
negotiate an agreement that would later be approved by the boards of
NBIMC and the BIHSC.

The hospital employees were all aware of the meeting, and Bornstein
recalled the palpable tension in the hallways outside the Danzis Auditorium.[35]
The motion carried, but not unanimously. Negotiations with Saint Barnabas
began. The news shook the Beth. The most vocal opposition came from the
physicians; nearly four hundred signed a petition to prevent the sale and one
group hired an attorney to try to stop it.[36] Many physicians and hospital staff
had an unvoiced reason for their opposition: the memory of a time long passed
when Saint Barnabas Hospital had refused privileges to Jewish physicians.
Cultural memories endure, and the stories related by previous generations of
Jewish doctors raised doubts and concerns. Dr. S. S. Goldwater had written in
1928 that institutions that are allowed the time to grow and expand can out-
grow their deficiencies. Could the doctors trust that the anti-Semitism practiced in the early part of the century had been outgrown?

One among the Many Mergers

By April 1996 an agreement was reached to sell the NBIMC to the
Saint Barnabas Health Care System for $125 million.[37] The terms of the
transaction offered the assurances that the historic mission of the Beth to
serve the needy would be continued, the "rights, privileges and independence" of the medical and dental staffs of NBIMC and its various departments and divisions were protected, and the Newark hospital campus would
continue as a teaching institution with the name "Newark Beth Israel
Medical Center." Most important, the NBIMC would continue its tertiary
programs, including cardiac surgery and heart and lung transplants. A new
NBIMC board would be comprised of 20 percent of the current board members, 20 percent of the medical staff, and the majority, 60 percent, nominated by Saint Barnabas.[38]

The Beth Healthcare Services Corporation Board would become the
new foundation, later named the New Jersey Healthcare Foundation, which
would with the proceeds from the sale offer assistance in addressing
Newark's health needs and those of the surrounding community.

Federal regulators on April 23, 1996, gave the approval for the Saint
Barnabas Health Care System to form a network of eight hospitals, including NBIMC and Saint Barnabas; six geriatric centers; five outpatient clinics;
and seventeen mental health clinics—a health-care system of 3,225 beds and

more than 20,000 employees, the largest in the state.[39] Ron Czajkowski, a spokesperson for the New Jersey Hospital Association, applauded the move, noting that the state is "'playing catch-up with the nation' in hospital consolidations . . . which should improve care by cutting duplicate services." Ronald J. Del Mauro, president and chief executive of the Saint Barnabas Health Care System, anticipated that "each year, it will handle some 166,000 hospital patients, 30,000 emergency rooms and 1 million outpatient visits, according to officials." The new venture would give New Jersey the nation's fifth-largest transplant center. Del Mauro promised New Jersey consumers of medical care greater access to services in three to six months.[40]

As expected, the UMDNJ severed the university's ties with the Saint Barnabas system, including the newly acquired NBIMC. However, in November 1996, the new giant merger of the New York Mount Sinai and NYU health-care systems created an affiliation with Saint Barnabas for medical residents from the Mount Sinai School of Medicine. Students from a traditional Jewish medical institution, wearing the blue logo of Mount Sinai on their white coats, would come from New York City to Newark to learn the practice of medicine in another Jewish hospital rich in the Jewish voluntary hospital tradition.[41]

The merger of the Beth with Saint Barnabas was one of many in 1996. In New Jersey alone, the Liberty Health System merged with the Columbia Health System; Morristown Memorial, Overlook, and Mountainside merged as Atlantic Health Systems; and the UMDNJ took over the Orange Memorial Medical Center. The states of Mississippi, New Mexico, and Nebraska each had one merger; there were two mergers in Montana, three in Minnesota, a merger of several small community hospitals in Nevada, and New Hampshire's regional medical center merged with a physician group practice of one thousand members. In Missouri, there were five mergers, including the Barnes Hospital and Jewish Hospital, Saint Louis, which had previously merged their ownership into the NJC Health system. New York City had nine mergers, including that of the hospitals and medical schools of Mount Sinai and New York University.[42]

The year 1996 was the culmination of nearly a decade of mergers and sales, more than exceeding the total number of mergers that had occurred in 1930 and 1966. Once again, U.S. hospitals were melted in the crucible of the health-care system, this time to produce the health-care configuration of the twenty-first century.

Epilogue

❧❦❧

A century after the birth of Beth Israel Hospital, Newark is once again a city of economic opportunity and a city of immigrants. While the tanneries and breweries are gone, banks, insurance companies, and small businesses flourish. Newcomers from Africa, China, Mexico, and El Salvador have replaced the Italians, Irish, Germans, and Eastern European Jews. African Americans whose parents or grandparents migrated to Newark from the South for jobs and to escape Jim Crow are now among Newark's older families.

Walking the streets and neighborhoods, one can still pass reminders of an earlier Newark. Old synagogue buildings such as the Anshe Russia Synagogue, Jewish cemeteries, and names on museums, concert halls, and buildings remind visitors that Jewish immigrants once came to Newark and flourished. The Star of David at Newark Beth Israel Medical Center is displayed at the front entrance of the hospital; the 1928 Spanish-style building at the top of the hill above Lake Weequahic is still faintly visible to those speeding by in cars and trains, a presence in the South Ward skyline and in the hearts of many Newarkers who were born there or who owe their lives to its medical staff.

Across the country there are similar Jewish hospital buildings, their bricks darkened with age. Of the thirty-six accredited Jewish hospitals identified by the Beth's Dr. Max Danzis in his 1940 *Medical Leaves* article, almost all are still components of the U.S. health-care system. As the historian Rosemary Stevens observed, "Voluntary hospitals have been successful organizations in the past hundred years because of their chameleon-like adjustments to changing conditions."[1] Some hospitals have evolved into powerful medical centers that bear names reflecting their Jewish ancestry, such as Cedars-Sinai Medical Center in Los Angeles and the Albert Einstein Medical Center in Philadelphia. Some are members of university medical systems, such as the Louis A. Weiss Memorial Hospital, a part of the University of Chicago Hospitals and Health System; and the Miriam Hospital in Providence, Rhode Island, a component of Tufts-Brown Lifespan. Some Jewish hospitals merged with other urban hospitals, as Jewish and Barnes Hospitals merged in St. Louis and then expanded into the BJC Health Care system, and Jewish Hospital in Louisville, which became the network called the Jewish Hospital Healthcare Service. Ecumenical mergers of voluntary hospitals founded under different religious auspices have become leading medical centers, such as the Beth Israel–Deaconess Hospital in Boston. The Mount Sinai New York Unity Health System in New York City is both an ecumenical merger and an amalgamation with a university medical system. Other hospitals, like the Milwaukee and Detroit Sinai Hospitals, and the Newark Beth Israel Medical Center, have been incorporated into health-care systems while retaining their individual names. (See Appendix, Table 2.)

Many of these contemporary incarnations of Jewish hospitals celebrate not only their religious heritage but also their medical heritage as voluntary hospitals. If the independent voluntary charitable hospitals have finally melted in the crucible of U.S. health care, their histories are reminders of a rich heritage. And they lasted far longer than was expected. Experts in health care were forecasting the voluntary hospital's demise even before World War II; while such predictions were premature, they were often grounded in sound analyses of the institutions' strengths and vulnerabilities.

Complex Arrays of Strengths and Weaknesses

Perhaps no American understood voluntary hospitals in the twentieth century better than Dr. S. S. Goldwater. A physician of German Jewish background and an eminent hospital administrator, Goldwater for nearly thirty years served as superintendent and director of New York's premier voluntary hospital, Mount Sinai (1903–1929). As commissioner of hospitals of Greater New York from 1930 to 1939, he witnessed the impact of the Depression on voluntary and public hospitals. From 1940 until his death in 1942, Goldwater was the president of the Associated Hospital Service, the New York Blue Cross Plan, just as prepayment insurance plans took hold in the United States. Through all the decades, he continued to serve on the editorial board of *Modern Hospital*, coauthoring articles on the hospitals of the

month and offering commentaries on the state of hospitals. On the eve
of World War II, in January 1940, he traveled to Chicago, the city he considered "the center of organized medical care for the entire country," to
address a meeting of the Chicago Hospital Council. His speech, published
in *Modern Hospital*, described the voluntary hospitals as complex arrays of
strengths and failings and the entire "tottering voluntary hospital system"
poised on the brink of failure.[2]

Chief among a voluntary hospital's assets, Goldwater observed, was its
flexibility in "patient load, its clinical intake" not available to most public
hospitals, and in economic allocation. Voluntary hospitals were not ham-
strung by the spending constraints imposed upon public institutions by non-
medical interests such as city councils and state legislatures. If voluntary
hospitals had these prerogatives, they also had the opportunity to convert
their flexibility of administration into an "experimental and normative function" that advanced therapy and care. As Goldwater observed, "Modern
medicine moves by leaps and bounds. The ideas of medical men are constantly changing"; these "novel ideas, little discoveries of [the medical
staff's] own, or adaptations of the progressive methods of others" could be
of great value, Goldwater believed. Voluntary hospitals' budgets were better positioned to take advantage of the medical staff's creativity than were
those of public hospitals, and voluntary hospitals could more easily try out
"new methods" and establish "new standards." Moreover, by so doing, voluntary hospitals could inspire "public hospital administrators to strive for
higher grades of service."

Voluntary hospitals of the kind Goldwater lauded had demonstrated
innovation inside and outside their walls. Inside, their laboratories and
research foundations permitted cutting-edge medical research, especially
clinical research, while never sacrificing state-of-the art care through the latest medical technology, which they could purchase without excessive red
tape. Their ability to quickly retrench and cope with the complexities of the
income streams offered by prepaid private insurance only enhanced their
ability to innovate medically. Outside the hospital, voluntary institutions led
the way in the development of outpatient services, ambulatory surgery, and
follow-up clinics.

The history of Newark Beth Israel Hospital and the other Jewish voluntary hospitals with which it has been compared in this narrative suggests
Goldwater's prescience. Newark's Jewish community created a voluntary
hospital that grew and survived the economic crisis of the 1930s. The community's philanthropy allowed the Beth to be flexible and experimental in

the way Goldwater described. In its laboratory and in its operating rooms, the Beth encouraged the "experimental" approach. It was that atmosphere that encouraged the research of Drs. William Antopol, Rita Finkler, Philip Levine, Aaron Parsonnet, Victor Parsonnet, and Seymour Ribot, and the surgical skills of Sam Diener, among so many others. The spirit of innovation created numerous medical journals at Jewish hospitals, including the *Journal of the Newark Beth Israel Hospital.*

Goldwater, the midwife of so many modern voluntary hospitals built in the 1920s, saw them as already outmoded by 1940. However, the managerial flexibility of voluntary hospitals thrust them into the vanguard of innovation. At such institutions, buildings and rooms could be redesigned and renovated to accommodate changes in anesthesia, occupational therapies, intake and admissions, and radiology. Hospital construction at the Beth and other voluntary institutions was planned in phases over lengthy periods, allowing them to develop adequate financing and revise their blueprints as needed to avoid erecting structures that were obsolete by the time the last construction worker departed.

The women of the voluntary hospital associations and auxiliaries were remarkable in pursuing entrepreneurial ideas. They were the force in founding Jewish hospitals and then a forceful presence in their survival. The auxiliaries of voluntary hospitals engaged in entrepreneurial experiments, such as tearooms and gift shops, which gently elicited contributions from patients and visitors, supplanting the charity boxes once adorning the counters of neighborhood stores. The auxiliaries donated state-of-the-art equipment to departments, bypassing the board and the budget process. The auxiliaries also were a source of unpaid labor, their members volunteering their time and then training themselves to perform duties in support of nurses and social workers. At times, the tasks they identified as worthy of their time evolved into jobs that became essential to the smooth operation of the hospital and, eventually, worthy of performance by full-time professionals. By the 1930s, prepaid health insurance plans were becoming an essential source of hospital revenue, and the voluntary hospitals led the way in making the administrative adjustments required to accommodate the redefinition of hospital–patient relations by Blue Cross and other insurance carriers.

If, by 1940, Newark Beth Israel Hospital had survived the Great Depression, it was because it demonstrated the strengths that Goldwater attributed to voluntary hospitals. Its evolution after World War II would follow Goldwater's prescient blueprint as well. But in the strengths of the voluntary hospitals lay their greatest weaknesses. According to Goldwater, it was their very institutional individuality that inhibited voluntary hospitals from joining forces with other private and public institutions for their own and the greater community's good. He contended that "in order to do a complete job for the medical profession and for the community," the voluntary hospitals must create relationships between public and private entities so that entire communities could be enveloped by organized care. It was the inability of the voluntary hospitals to heed Goldwater's warning at mid-century that ultimately fifty years later resulted in the mergers and sales compelled by the pressures of market forces.

Goldwater foresaw the possibility that the same private interests that founded voluntary hospitals—whether inspired by religion, ethnic identification, or some other motive—would curb charitable contributions and ruin these hospitals through "indifference and the lack of vigorous effort to support them." In such cases there might be no alternative to the "administration in dangerous doses of the sweet and tempting poison of government support." The siren call of public monies was dangerous, Goldwater believed, because such monies would be accompanied by mounds of regulations and piles of paperwork that would destroy the flexibility that was the voluntary hospital's greatest strength.

Goldwater had forecast that the diminished support from Jewish philanthropists and overburdened Jewish agencies would force voluntary hospitals to seek new sources for economic support, initially found in the third-party payment plans. By the 1960s, voluntary hospitals like Newark Beth Israel were ingesting ever larger doses of "the sweet and tempting poison of government support" in Medicare and Medicaid reimbursements and then a myriad of federal and state grants-in-aid for construction, renovation, training, and programs. The government aid was accompanied by increasing regulation to rationalize hospital growth through regionalization and impose cost reduction in the provision of medical services. The Certificate of Need (CON) requirement designed to avoid service duplication in geographically defined regions and the diagnosis-related groups (DRG) system to decrease the cost of medical care only increased the pressure on the Beth and other voluntary hospitals.

The Legacy of Jewish Voluntary Hospitals

As the independent Jewish voluntary hospital recedes into history, what remains to testify to the Jewish commitment to charity and healing that these institutions once embodied? What is their legacy apart from the hospital names and Stars of David hewn in their brick and mortar?

In 1966, two years before his retirement from public service, August F. Hoenack, the chief of the architectural, engineering, and equipment branch of the U.S. Public Health Service's Division of Hospital and Medical Facilities, the key government agency for the Hill-Burton Act program for hospital construction, paused to reflect on the impact of the hospital building program. He observed: "What really exists is the building, but a building does not exist until people use it. It then becomes a living entity. It becomes the focus of health activity in the community. It reflects our culture and becomes a symbol of our attitude."[3]

Increasingly, the entities that embodied the Jewish spirit of the old voluntary hospitals are the health-care foundations that the boards of Jewish hospitals founded with proceeds from sales and other financial settlements. Often the projects and services supported with health-care foundation grants were those once undertaken by voluntary hospitals or other community and educational institutions. The Beth's board, under the leadership of Lester Lieberman, founded the Healthcare Foundation of New Jersey (HFNJ) in the name of Newark's Jewish community with the proceeds of the 1996 sale. Its mission is to continue to act in the interests of Newarkers' health "through philanthropy."[4] Such a mission is consistent with the spirit that underlay the creation of Newark Beth Israel Hospital and many other Jewish voluntary hospitals as charitable institutions in the first place—the spirit of *tzedakah*, or justice.

In the early twentieth century, the Beth and other voluntary hospitals often held health fairs to which neighborhood families were encouraged to bring children for free examination and care. Publicly financed health care was also taken to children in the very schools that they attended. More recently, the public school has been neglected as a venue for health care, yet that is where ready access to children lies, especially poor children and the children of newly arrived immigrants. In 1998, the HFNJ decided to do what the Beth and the schools had traditionally done to ensure the health and well-being of Newark's children. The HFNJ began supporting comprehensive pediatric primary care services at nine Newark public schools, six on-school sites, and a mobile pediatric unit, staffed with a pediatrician, nurse practitioner, social worker, and dental hygienist, serving seven thousand children, as they progressed from elementary grades through high school.

The HFNJ also provided a grant to the Helen Keller World Wide Sight Vision Screening Services that in 1999, conducted on-site vision screening for every sixth grader in the Newark public schools, with eyeglass prescriptions filled on the spot. Nearly 20 percent of the screened students left the testing areas wearing eyeglasses. The HFNJ remains flexible and innovative and attuned to community needs, consistent with the earlier outreach efforts of the Maternity Auxiliary.

At the Beth, young ambitious students of science, such as the young Kenneth Tyson, could work in the very same pathology laboratory where clinical research projects of great importance were undertaken. A 2001 HFNJ grant introduced Newark students to the variety of occupational opportunities available in health care and to encourage through financial support those wishing to pursue careers as physicians, nurses, or other health-care professionals. With an annual grant of $489,000 the HFNJ's Service Scholarship program offered tuition assistance, paid internships, and bioethics seminars to ninety students from the Newark area pursuing careers in health care and attending one of eight local colleges or universities. In return, each awardee had to promise to work in the health-care field in Newark for at least one year after graduation. Thus, the foundation encouraged the young not only to work in health care, but also to serve their community.[5]

Education was always a priority at the Beth, although the medical staff suffered repeated disappointments in its desire for affiliation with a medical school. The HFNJ echoed that commitment with a grant awarded to recognize medical students and faculty members at area medical schools for their "commitment to compassion."[6] And in 2004, the concern with compassion in the medical community led the HFNJ to establish a $3.2 million center for humanism at the University of Medicine and Dentistry of New Jersey to train physicians to express compassion, the Jewish commitment to *tikkun olam*, healing the world, in their care of patients and to study the benefits of having physicians "treat the individual, not just the disease."[7]

The HFNJ embodies the Beth's spirit, even as the hospital building continues the daily work of offering cure and care. Its work is clear evidence that the culture which gave birth to the Beth's creed, drafted so long ago, is alive and well in Newark:

> Personal attention, notable for its warmth and sincerity, and inspired by a sympathetic recognition of the human element, is the powerful but gentle handmaiden of science employed by doctors, nurses, and attendants at Beth Israel Hospital. Patients are people—not cases— at this hospital. . . . The value of the human touch as a power for healing is never lost sight of at Beth Israel.[8]

ACKNOWLEDGMENTS

This history of Newark Beth Israel Hospital Medical Center was commissioned by the Jewish Historical Society of MetroWest (JHSMW) with funding from the Healthcare Foundation of New Jersey. The independence of the authors to pursue our scholarship in whatever direction it took us was contractually guaranteed, and neither the Jewish Historical Society nor the Healthcare Foundation exercised or sought to exercise any editorial control over this manuscript. Indeed, both organizations repeatedly made clear their commitment to a thorough, scholarly, and unbiased treatment of the subject.

We are grateful to many organizations and special individuals who graciously shared their time, expertise, and memories with us. We are deeply appreciative of the support given to us by Lester Z. Lieberman, whose leadership on the board of the Healthcare Foundation of New Jersey and membership on the JHSMW's Book Committee made his encouragement and support doubly valuable. His kindness, generosity of spirit, and respect for the academic enterprise contributed greatly to the completion of this volume. Truly, Lester Lieberman gave his heart for this history of the Beth.

We are most grateful to the Healthcare Foundation of New Jersey for its support and to its executive director, Ellen W. Kramer, Esq., for her kindness, cooperation, and patience as we completed our project. Thanks, too, to the Jewish Historical Society of MetroWest and to its past president, Warren Grover, who encouraged us to undertake the project, and more recently, Robert Max, who has been so cooperative in its completion. The JHSMW Publications Committee chaired by Alan Sagner offered advice on sources and intelligent, nonintrusive criticism. Our warmest thanks to all its members.

Specific individuals shared their knowledge of Newark Beth Israel Hospital (NBIH) and Newark's Jewish community with us, sometimes in formal interviews and often in informal discussion in person or on the telephone. These include Dr. Murray Belsky, the late Dr. Arthur Bernstein and his family, Lester Bornstein, Dr. Frederic Cohen, the late Dr. Samuel Diener Donna Dinetz, the late Harold Grotta, James Hopkins, Max Kleinman, the late Cecil Lichtman, Sima Jelleff, Leonard Lieberman, Lester Z. Lieberman, Dr. Alan Lippman, Alan Lowenstein, Dr. Victor Parsonnet, Dr. Seymour Ribot, Alan Sagner, Susan Schottenfeld, Bruce Shoulson, Dr. Edward Shapiro, Dr. Myron Jack Shapiro, Robert Skeist, Susan Spielman, Kenneth Tyson, and Leon Yanoff.

We greatly appreciate the support and help of Paul Mertz, the Executive Director of the Newark Beth Israel Medical Center, who enabled us to review the administrative minutes of the Board of Beth Israel Hospital, and shared with us his vision for the second century of the institution. He and Kenneth Tyson provided the opportunity for us to conduct interviews of hospital staff on site. Barnarbas Healthcare has since donated these papers to the JHSMW for their archive.

The archivists of the JHSMW, Jennifer McGillan, who succeeded Joseph Settanni, were unfailingly patient and efficient in responding to our inquiries and have worked with us as we pored through the collections. Archivist Lois R. Densky-Wolff offered valuable assistance in providing materials from the rich collections of the George F. Smith Library of the Health Sciences at the University of Medicine and Dentistry of New Jersey (UMDNJ).

Linda Forgosh, the JHSMW outreach coordinator, has been instrumental in obtaining donations of materials and unique documents. She was the curator of the JHSMW exhibit, "Born at the Beth: Newark's Jewish Hospital since 1901." She provided answers to key questions concerning the history of the hospital that greatly enriched this book. We appreciate her kindness and generosity.

A number of readers offered valuable editorial suggestions. Special thanks to Dr. Sarah Larson for her keen editorial eye and to M. Denise Miles and Shelby Shapiro for their careful reading of the entire manuscript Dr. Dale Smith, chair of the History of Medicine Department at the Uniformed University of the Health Sciences in Bethesda, Maryland, offered sound advice throughout the project. Dr. Gerald Grob, professor emeritus at Rutgers University and historian of medicine, offered the encouragement and insight that has been his trademark in assisting colleagues over the years. Dr. Howard Gillette Jr. of Rutgers University, Camden, offered us his great knowledge of New Jersey in conversation and his own fine volume on Camden. Janet Golden, a historian of medicine who teaches on the same faculty, offered useful suggestions and asked the right questions, as did historian of medicine Dr. Naomi Rogers of Yale University. Dr. Gail Wilensky of Project Hope offered a careful reading of our work and made certain that we did not err in our description of the complex relationship of the federal government to medical care in the period after 1960. The late James W. Mooney, a dear friend and American University colleague, was an astute student of U.S. institutions whose thoughtful insights were invaluable for the preparation of this manuscript. Our thanks to Dr. Melissa Kirkpatrick for the index. Also, special gratitude to Dr. Kay Mussell, the dean of the American University College of Arts and Sciences, for her constant friendship and support. The efforts of American University students who assisted in the newspaper research, especially Anne Marisic, Matt Clavin, and Michael Giese, are much appreciated.

Marlie Wasserman, our editor at Rutgers University Press, has been enthusiastic about this project from the beginning and we much appreciate her confidence, as well as Marilyn Campbell who guided us through the production process.

We would like to thank our friends and colleagues, especially the members of the Temple Micah Torah study group, who were most supportive of a husband and wife who embarked on that most perilous task of writing a book together. Ditto our dear friend of more than thirty years, Dr. Scott Parker. Drs. Fulvia Veronese, Bonnie Mathieson, Olivier Roumy, and Gail Wolfson were of great support as the work on the book progressed, and especially, at the moments, when it didn't.

Individually, we would like to reaffirm our love for each other and declare one final time that the other was correct in all things and oneself stubborn and just plain wrong in every instance. *Pacem.*

Our daughter, Julia Rose, graduated from law school (with high honors!) and grew into young adulthood during the preparation of this book. She managed to navigate through our editing and revision rants while retaining her love of history and remaining a loving daughter to her parents, Scylla and Charybdis. We love her and hope that our book offers her a reminder of the richness of the Jewish past and her parents' belief in that tradition, as well as anecdotes about her parents' collaboration with which to entertain friends and family for years to come.

APPENDIX

TABLE 1   *American Jewish Hospitals Identified by the American Jewish Yearbook and their Recognition by the American Medical Association and the American College of Surgeons, 1899–1940.*

American Jewish Yearbook	City, state	AMA *American Medical Directory* hospitals and sanitaria, 1906	AMA Council on Medical Education hospitals approved for internships, 1921	American College of Surgeons (ACS), first year accredited	American Hospital Association listed and ACS accredited, 1939	AMA Council on Medical Education Hospitals approved for internships, 1940
Leo N. Levi Memorial Hospital	Hot Springs, AR			1922	General	
Kuppenheimer Cottage of the Jewish Relief Society Hospital	Los Angeles, CA					
Mount Sinai Hospital	Los Angeles, CA					
Cedars of Lebanon Hospital (Kaspare Cohn Hospital)	Los Angeles, CA			1923	•	•
Mount Zion Hospital	San Francisco, CA		•	1921	•	•
Beth El Hospital	Colorado Springs, CO					
Beth Israel Hospital and Home	Denver, CO			1924	•	
National Jewish Hospital for Consumptives	Denver, CO	•		1928	•	Specialty fellowship
Jewish Consumptives Relief Solarium	Edgewater, CO	•				
Mount Sinai Hospital	Hartford, CT	•				
Roosevelt Memorial Hospital	Hartford, CT			1929	•	

	Location		Year		Specialty fellowship
Mount Sinai Dispensary	Wilmington, DE				
Albert Steiner Clinic for Cancer and Allied Diseases	Atlanta, GA		1929	•	•
Michael Reese Hospital	Chicago, IL		1919	•	•
Mount Sinai Hospital (Maimonides Kosher Hospital)	Chicago, IL	•	1922		
Lying-In Hospital	Chicago, IL		1939		
Willing Workers Shack of the Chicago Tuberculosis Sanitarium	Winfield, IL				
Jewish Hospital	Louisville, KY	•	1922	•	•
Touro Infirmary	New Orleans, LA	•	1919	•	•
Sinai Hospital	Baltimore, MD		1928	•	•
Frank Memorial Hospital	Baltimore, MD				
Hebrew Home Hospital and Asylum	Baltimore, MD	•	1919		
Hebrew Hospital and Maternity Building	Baltimore, MD				
Mount Pleasant Hospital	Baltimore, MD				
Leopold Morse Home for Infirm Hebrews and Orphans	Boston, MA				
Beth Israel Hospital	Boston, MA		1922	General	
Jewish Memorial Hospital	Boston, MA				
Frauen Verein Home for Convalescent Jewish Women					
New England Sinai Hospital		•	1919	•	•
Jewish Hospital of St. Louis	St. Louis, MO				•
Jewish Sanitorium	St. Louis, MO				

(Continued)

TABLE 1 (Continued)

American Jewish Yearbook	City, state	AMA American Medical Directory hospitals and sanitaria, 1906	AMA Council on Medical Education hospitals approved for internships, 1921	American College of Surgeons (ACS), first year accredited	American Hospital Association listed and ACS accredited, 1939	AMA Council on Medical Education Hospitals approved for internships, 1940
Miriam Rosa Bry Rehabilitation Hospital	MO					
Menorah Hospital (Formerly Jewish Memorial)	Kansas City, MO			1932	•	•
Isaac M. Wise Memorial Hospital	Omaha, NE	•		1923		
Newark Beth Israel Hospital	Newark, NJ	•	•	1919	•	•
Jewish Maternity Hospital	Newark, NJ				Merged	
Nathan and Miriam Barnart Memorial Hospital	Paterson, NJ	•	•	1922	•	•
Deborah Sanitarium and Hospital	Browns Mills, NJ				TB	
Theresa Grotta Convalescent Home	Caldwell, NJ				Convalescent	
Beth Israel Hospital	Passaic, NJ				General	
Jewish Seaside Home for Invalids	Atlantic City, NJ					
Beth Moses (Bokur Cholim Kosher Hospital)	Brooklyn, NY			1922	•	•

Hospital	Location	Year					
Beth-El Hospital (formerly Brownsville and East New York Hospital, briefly Menorah Hospital)	Brooklyn, NY	1922			•		•
Hebrew Maternity Hospital	Brooklyn, NY	1922	Maternity				
Jewish Hospital	Brooklyn, NY	1922	•	•	•	•	•
Jewish Home for Incurables	Brooklyn, NY						
Menorah Home and Hospital for the Aged	Brooklyn, NY						
United Israel Zion Hospital	Brooklyn, NY	1923	•				•
New Utrecht Hospital	Brooklyn, NY						
Williamsburg Maternity Hospital	Brooklyn, NY						
Beth David Hospital	New York, NY	1919	• •	•	•	•	•
Beth Israel Hospital	New York, NY						•
Beth Abraham Hospital	Bronx, NY	1923	•				•
Bronx Hospital and Dispensary	New York, NY						
Home and Hospital of the Daughters of Jacob	New York, NY						
Jewish Hospital for Deformities and Joint Diseases	New York, NY	1925	•	•	•		•
Jewish Memorial Hospital (formerly Philanthropin Hospital)	New York, NY	1923	General	•			•
Jewish Maternity Hospital	New York, NY	1922	Merged				
Lebanon Hospital	Bronx, NY	1919	General	•	•	•	
Montefiore Hospital	Bronx, NY	1922	Ob/gyn	•	•		
Bronx Jewish Maternity Hospital*	Bronx, NY						
Mount Sinai Hospital	New York, NY	1919	•	•	•	•	•
Mount Moriah Hospital	New York, NY	1922					
People's Hospital	New York, NY	1922**					

TABLE 1 (Continued)

American Jewish Yearbook	City, state	AMA American Medical Directory hospitals and sanitaria, 1906	AMA Council on Medical Education hospitals approved for internships, 1921	American College of Surgeons (ACS), first year accredited	American Hospital Association listed and ACS accredited, 1939	AMA Council on Medical Education Hospitals approved for internships, 1940
Sydenham Postgraduate College Hospital	New York, NY	•	•	1928	•	•
Zion Hospital	New York, NY					
Nathan Littauer Hospital	Gloversville, NY	•				
Maimonides Hospital	Liberty, NY			1922	General	
Workmen's Circle Sanitarium	Liberty, NY				TB	
Monticello Hospital	Monticello, NY					
Sternberger Hospital for Women and Children*	Greensboro, NC				General	
Jewish Hospital	Cincinnati, OH	•	•	1919	•	•
Mount Sinai Hospital	Cleveland, OH	•	•	1922	•	•
Jewish Hospital	Philadelphia, PA	•	•	1919	•	•
Mount Sinai Hospital	Philadelphia, PA		•	1922	•	•
Northern Liberty*	Philadelphia, PA					
Jewish Maternity Hospital	Philadelphia, PA		•			
Guggenheim Hospital for Private Patients	PA			1925	Merged	
Eagleville Sanitarium for Consumptives	Eagleville, PA				Chronic care	
Willow Crest for Convalescents	Willow Crest, PA					

Hospital	Location			
Montefiore Hospital	Pittsburgh, PA	•		•
Miriam Hospital	Providence, RI	•	1923	
Jewish Hospital	Norfolk, VA	•	1928	
Mount Sinai Hospital	Milwaukee, WI	•	1922	•

Sources: The American Jewish Yearbook was published by the American Jewish Committee. Volume 1 was published by Lord Baltimore Press, Baltimore, Maryland. Subsequent volumes were published by the Jewish Publication Society, Philadelphia, Pennsylvania. Volumes were published in conjunction with the Jewish calendar, so that Volume 1, 1899–1900, corresponded to 5660. C. Adler was the first editor, then by H. Szold; by 1908, the editing is attributed to the American Jewish Committee. Jewish hospitals appear in state-by-state lists of Jewish associations and institutions in volumes 1–25, and 32.

The names of the Jewish hospitals cited in the Yearbook were compared with the lists prepared by Daniel Ethan Bridge, "The Rise and Development of the Jewish Hospital in America 1950–1984" (Ordination thesis, Hebrew Union College, Jewish Institute of Religion, 1985).

American Medical Directory, Vol. 1 (Chicago: American Medical Association Press, 1906) presented a state-by-state list of medical colleges, hospitals and sanatoria, and licensed physicians.

Bulletin of the American College of Surgeons, Hospital Standardization Series, Vol. 4, no. 4, presented the report for 1919 of accredited hospitals of 100 or more beds (Chicago: American College of Surgeons, 1919).

Modern Hospital published the complete lists of hospitals that received American College of Surgeons accreditation in its November issues, 1920–1933.

"Hospitals Registered by the American Medical Association, including those identified as accredited by the American College of Surgeons," Journal of the American Medical Association 126 (March 30, 1940); "Approved Hospitals for Residency Training," Journal of the American Medical Association 126 (August 31,1940).

Notes:

*Did not appear in the American Jewish Yearbook.

**1922 was the only year that People's Hospital received ACS accreditation.

TABLE 2 *American Jewish Hospitals Identified by the American Jewish Yearbook, Status as of 1969 and 2005*

Hospital	City, state	Founded	AHA member, 1969	JCAHO approved hospitals or other functioning facility, 2005
Leo N. Levi Memorial Hospital	Hot Springs, AK	1914	•	Levi Hospital
Cedars-Sinai Medical Center	Los Angeles, CA	1961	•	Cedars-Sinai Medical Center
Cedars of Lebanon		1910	Merged	
Mount Sinai Hospital		1920	Merged	
Mount Zion Hospital	San Francisco, CA	1887	•	UCSF Healthcare System
Maimonides Hospital		1950	Merged	
Levine Hospital	Hayward, CA	1951		Now served by Kaiser Permanente Medical Center
National Jewish Hospital	Denver, CO	1899	•	National Jewish Medical and Research Center
General Maurice Rose Hospital and Medical Center	Denver, CO	1946	•	Rose Medical Center
Beth Israel Hospital and Home	Denver, CO		•	
Mount Sinai Hospital	Hartford, CT	1923	•	Saint Francis–Mount Sinai Campus for Rehabilitation
Hebrew Home for the Aged	Hartford, CT			Hebrew Healthcare Inc.
Mount Sinai Hospital of Greater Miami	Miami Beach, FL	1949	•	Aventura–Mount Sinai Medical Center
Albert Steiner Clinic for Cancer and Allied Diseases	Atlanta, GA		Merged with Grady Memorial 1947	
Michael Reese Hospital	Chicago, IL	1882	•	Doctors System

Hospital	City	Founded	Status	Current name / Notes
Mount Sinai Hospital	Chicago, IL	1918	•	Sinai Health System–Mount Sinai Hospital
Louis A. Weiss Memorial Hospital	Chicago, IL	1953	•	University of Chicago Hospital and Health System–Weiss Memorial Hospital
Willing Workers Shack of the Chicago Tuberculosis Sanitarium	Winfield, IL			Absorbed by Central DuPage Hospital
Jewish Hospital	Louisville, KY	1903	•	Jewish Hospital Healthcare Services Jewish Hospital
Touro Infirmary	New Orleans, LA	1862	•	Touro Infirmary
Sinai Hospital	Baltimore, MD	1868	•	LifeBridge Health–Sinai Hospital
Levindale Hebrew Home and Infirmary	Baltimore, MD		•	Merged with Sinai Hospital in 1998 Life-Bridge Health Levindale Hebrew Geriatric Center and Hospital
Beth Israel Hospital	Boston, MA	1915	•	Beth Israel Deaconess Hospital
Jewish Memorial Hospital	Boston, MA		•	Jewish Memorial Hospital and Rehabilitation Center
Sinai Hospital	Detroit, MI	1951	•	Detroit Medical Center System Sinai-Grace Hospital
Mount Sinai Hospital	Minneapolis, MN	1951	•	Closed 1991
Jewish Hospital Miriam Rosa Bry Rehabilitation	St. Louis, MO	1900	Merged 1951 •	BJC Health Care Barnes-Jewish Hospital
Jewish Sanatorium	St. Louis, MO	1912	Closed 1963	

(Continued)

TABLE 2 (*Continued*)

Hospital	City, state	Founded	AHA member, 1969	JCAHO approved hospitals or other functioning facility, 2005
Menorah Hospital	Kansas City, MO	1931	•	HCA-Midwest Menorah Medical Center Relocated to Overland Park
Newark Beth Israel Hospital and Medical Center	Newark, NJ	1902	•	Saint Barnabas Health Care System–Newark Beth Israel Medical Center
Nathan and Miriam Barnart Memorial Hospital	Paterson, NJ	1908	•	Barnert Hospital
Deborah Sanitarium and Hospital	Browns Mills, NJ	1923	•	Deborah Heart and Lung Center
Theresa Grotta Home	Caldwells, NJ	1916	•	Closed 1992
Beth Israel Hospital	Passaic, NJ	1926	•	Beth Israel Passaic Hospital Substance Abuse Treatment
Brookdale Hospital Medical Center (Beth El)	Brooklyn, NY	1963	•	Brookdale University Hospital and Medical Center teaching hospital
Metropolitan Jewish Geriatric Center (formerly Brooklyn Hebrew Home and Hospital for the Aged)	Brooklyn, NY	1932 1953	•	Metropolitan Jewish Geriatric Center
Jewish Hospital	Brooklyn, NY	1906	•	Extended care facility of the Interfaith Medical Center

Hospital	Location	Year	Status	Current name/Notes
Kingsbrook Jewish Medical Center	Brooklyn, NY	1968	•	Kingsbrook Jewish Medical Center
Jewish Home for the Incurables		1925	Merged	
Jewish Chronic Disease Hospital		1950		
Maimonides Hospital	Brooklyn, NY	1951	•	Mount Sinai NYU Health Care System Maimonides Medical Center
Beth Moses		1917	Merged	
United Israel Zion		1914	Merged	
Unity Hospital	Brooklyn, NY			Closed in 1978 as hospital, methadone maintenance drug program continued
Beth Abraham Hospital	New York, NY	1919		UJA Federation System facility
Beth David Hospital	New York, NY		Relocated and then closed 1966	
Beth Israel Hospital and Medical Center	New York, NY		•	Beth Israel Medical Center
Bronx-Lebanon Hospital	New York, NY	1962	•	Bronx-Lebanon Hospital Center 1969 teaching affiliation with Albert Einstein Medical College
Bronx Hospital and Dispensary		1909	Merged	
Lebanon Hospital		1890	Merged	
Bronx Jewish Maternity Hospital	New York, NY		•	Bronx-Lebanon Hospital Center component
Jewish Hospital for Deformities and Joint Diseases	New York, NY		•	Mount Sinai NYU Health System–Hospital for Joint Diseases
Montefiore Hospital	New York, NY		•	Montefiore Medical Center–Jack D. Weiler Hospital of Medical College
Albert Einstein Medical College of Medicine (merged)			•	
Mount Sinai Hospital	New York, NY	1852	•	Mount Sinai NYU Health System Mount Sinai Hospital

(Continued)

TABLE 2 *(Continued)*

Hospital	City, state	Founded	AHA member, 1969	JCAHO approved hospitals or other functioning facility, 2005
Sydenham Hospital	New York, NY			Sydenham Neighborhood Family Care Center
Long Island Jewish Hospital	Floral Park, NY	1954	•	North Shore–LI Jewish Health System
Nathan Littauer Hospital	Gloversville, NY		•	Nathan Littauer Hospital and Home
Maimonides Hospital	Liberty, NY			Maimonides Hospital
Monticello Hospital	Monticello, NY			Hospice
Sternberger Hospital for Women and Children	Greensboro, NC			Surplanted by Moses H. Cone Hospital and Health Center founded 1951
Jewish Hospital	Cincinnati, OH	1850	•	Heathcare Alliance of Greater Cincinnati
Mount Sinai Hospital of Cleveland	Cleveland, OH	1903	•	University Hospitals Health System–Mount Sinai East
Benjamin Rose Hospital	Cleveland Heights, OH	1953	Merged	Elder facility and hospice
Montefiore Hospital		1968	•	Short-term residential care
Kesher Home for the Aged		1882		
Albert Einstein Medical Center	Philadelphia, PA	1950	•	Albert Einstein Medical Center
Jewish			South division	
Mount Sinai			East division	
Liberty			North division	

Name	Location	Year	JCAHO	Current status
Eagleville Sanitarium for Consumptives	Eagleville, PA			Treatment facility for drug and alcohol addiction
Willow Crest for Convalescents	Willow Grove, PA			Restorative-care facility located on Albert Einstein Healthcare Network main campus
Montefiore Hospital	Pittsburgh, PA	1901	•	University of Pennsylvania Medical Center UPMC Montefiore
Miriam Hospital	Providence, RI	1925	•	Lifespan Miriam Hospital
Mount Sinai Hospital	Milwaukee, WI	1901	•	Aurora Health Care System Aurora Sinai Hospital

Sources: "American Hospital Association Members," *Hospitals* 43 (March 1969). The 2005 Joint Commission on Accreditation of Healthcare Organizations (JCAHO) data was obtained on-line from the Web page: http://www.jcaho.org. The status of facilities was identified through Web-based searches of the name listed in the *American Jewish Yearbook*, completed in 2006.
*Registered hospital of the American Hospital Association (AHA) (note that registration does not denote JCAHO accreditation)

NOTES

Abbreviations used in the notes

Administrative Committee Minutes	Minutes of the Administrative Committee of Newark Beth Israel Hospital, NBIH Papers at Jewish Historical Society of MetroWest (JHSMW)
Annual Meeting Minutes	Minutes of the Annual Meeting of the Newark Beth Israel Hospital, NBIH Papers at JHSMW
Annual Report	Annual Report of the Newark Beth Israel Hospital (various years), NBIH Papers at JHSMW
Board Minutes	Minutes of the Board of Directors of Newark Beth Israel Hospital, NBIH Papers at JHSMW
Board of Trustees Minutes	Minutes of the Board of Trustees of Newark Beth Israel Hospital, NBIH Papers at JHSMW
JHSMW	Jewish Historical Society MetroWest, Alex Aidekman Family Jewish Community Campus, Whippany, N.J.
Journal	Journal of Newark Beth Israel Hospital
Lazaron Papers	Rabbi Morris Lazaron Papers, American Jewish Archives, Cincinnati, Ohio
Maternity Auxiliary Minutes	Minutes of the Auxiliary of the Newark Maternity Department of the Beth Israel Hospital, 1930–1939, NBIH Papers at JHSMW
Medical Staff Minutes	Minutes of the Executive Committee of the Medical Staff, 1901–1918, Box Parsonnet Papers, JHSMW
	Newark Beth Israel Hospital Papers, JHSMW
News	*Newark Evening News*
Official Ledger	Official Ledger of the Medical Staff of the Newark Beth Israel Hospital, held by the Parsonnet family
UMDNJ Archives	University of Medicine and Dentistry of New Jersey Archives, Newark

249

Introduction

1. "Salutatory," *Modern Hospital* 1 (September 1913): 32.
2. Samuel S. Kottek, "The Hospital in Jewish History," *Review of Infectious Diseases* 3 (July/August 1981): 636–639.
3. The single most comprehensive volume on the evolution of the hospital in the United States is Charles E. Rosenberg, *The Care of Strangers: The Rise of America's Hospital System* (New York: Basic Books, 1987), 4. Also, for the gradual removal of the mentally ill from almshouses to state institutions, see Gerald N. Grob, *Mental Illness and American Society, 1875–1940* (Princeton: Princeton University Press, 1983), 76. For the twentieth century, see Rosemary Stevens, *American Hospitals in the Twentieth Century* (New York: Basic Books, 1989).
4. In addition to Rosenberg's *Care of Strangers*, two volumes that describe the hospital as a charitable institution that cared for the impoverished, but also often served as a venue for the dying who were bereft of families are Morris J. Vogel, *The Invention of the Modern Hospital: Boston, 1870–1930* (Chicago: University of Chicago Press, 1980); and David Rosner, *A Once Charitable Enterprise: Hospitals and Health Care in Brooklyn and New York, 1885–1915* (Princeton: Princeton University Press, 1982).
5. A brief discussion of this broader history of religious and ethnic hospitals can be found in Alan M. Kraut, *Silent Travelers: Germs, Genes, and the "Immigrant Menace"* (New York: Basic Books, 1994), 43–49, 197–210.
6. An overview of the Jewish hospital in the United States is Ethan Bridge, *The Rise and Development of the Jewish Hospital in America* (Rabbinical thesis, Hebrew Union College, 1985). There have been a number of individual hospital studies. Two notable published volumes are Dorothy Levenson, *Montefiore: The Hospital as Social Instrument, 1884–1984* (New York: Farrar, Straus and Giroux, 1984); and Arthur J. Linenthal, *First a Dream: The History of Boston's Jewish Hospitals, 1896 to 1928* (Boston: Beth Israel Hospital in association with the Francis A. Countway Library of Medicine, 1990).
7. Bridge, "Rise and Development," 18.
8. Jews' Hospital of the City of New York, *Act of Incorporation and By-Laws*, 1852.
9. Richard C. Cabot, *Social Service and the Art of Healing*, 2nd ed. (New York: Dodd, Mead, 1931), 4–5.
10. Linenthal, History of Boston's Jewish Hospitals, 20.
11. John T. Cunningham, *Newark*, rev. ed. (Newark: New Jersey Historical Society, 1988), 8–27.
12. William B. Helmreich, *The Enduring Community: The Jews of Newark and MetroWest* (New Brunswick, N.J.: Transaction, 1999), 8–9, 12–13.
13. Ibid., 14–16.
14. Ibid., 17.
15. Nathan Kussy, "Early History of the Jews of Newark," in *The Jewish Community Blue Book of Newark* (Newark: Jewish Community Blue Book, 1925), 30–31.
16. Helmreich, *The Enduring Community*, 20–22.
17. Benjamin Kluger, "Growing Up in Newark," *[Newark] Jewish News*, September 8, 1977.

18. August Hoenack, quoted in "Hill-Burton after 20 Years: The Men, the Money, the 360,000 Beds," *Modern Hospital* 107 (August 1966): 99.

CHAPTER 1   *"Trouble at the Betch Israel Hospital Association"*

1. "Seven Important Phases of Newark's Development Told," *Newark Evening News*, October 16, 1907 (hereinafter, *News*).
2. John T. Cunningham, *Newark*, rev. ed. (Newark: New Jersey Historical Society, 1988), 8–27. We are indebted to John T. Cunningham, Newark's foremost historian. The best overview of Newark's history is Cunningham, *Newark*. On the sorry state of public health in Newark at the turn of the century, see Stuart Galishoff, *Safeguarding the Public Health: Newark, 1895–1918* (Westport, Conn.: Greenwood Press, 1975). For the earlier era, see Galishoff, *Newark: The Nation's Unhealthiest City, 1832–1895* (New Brunswick, N.J.: Rutgers University Press, 1988).
3. Galishoff, *Newark: The Nation's Unhealthiest City*, passim.
4. "Prince Street Like a Small Section of Russia; the Hebrews There Retain Old Country Customs," *Newark Sunday News*, February 11, 1901.
5. "New Hospital Wing Nearly Completed," *News*, July 19, 1900. See a description of the tall oaks in "Work at City's Pioneer Hospital," *News*, March 3, 1901.
6. "Rapid Growth of a Hospital," *Newark Sunday News*, March 17, 1901.
7. "To Improve the German Hospital," *Newark Sunday News*, March 10, 1901.
8. "Scandal at a Hospital—Newark Grand Jury May Bring Indictment against Officials," *New York Times*, November 27, 1900. The report was rebutted the following day by the hospital superintendent, who stated that the scum was the grease from one patient and that the attendant had not had time to clean the bathtub ("Newark Hospital's Condition," *New York Times*, November 28, 1900).
9. "Turned from City Hospital—Severely Burned and Scantily Clad, Charles Loeffler and His Son Sent into the Street," *News*, December 24, 1900.
10. Cyrus Adler, ed., *The American Jewish Yearbook: 1899–1900* (Baltimore: Lord Baltimore Press, 1899). In the nineteenth and early twentieth centuries, Jews often preferred the designation "Hebrew" and named their institutions accordingly. They regarded the term "Jewish" as disparaging. Earlier German Jews had used the self-designation "Israelite" but largely abandoned it by the end of the century.
11. "Hebrew Orphan Asylum Dedicated," *News*, October 18, 1899
12. "At Odds over a Hospital," *News*, October 22, 1900.
13. Charles M. Robbins, "The Newark Beth Israel Hospital," *Medical Leaves* 5 (1943): 108.
14. "To Dedicate the New Dispensary," *News*, December 21, 1900.
15. "Daughters of Israel Meet," *News*, January 9, 1901.
16. "Prince Street Like a Small Section." See also Guenther B. Risse, "The Renaissance of Bloodletting: A Chapter in Modern Therapies," *Journal of the History of Medicine and Allied Sciences* 34 (January 1979): 3–22.
17. Nettie Katchen, "The First Ten Years," *Jewish News*, December 28, 1951.
18. "In Aid of a Hospital—Junior Daughters of Israel Managed a Highly Successful Ball at Columbia Hall Last Night," *News*, February 24, 1901.

19. "Daughters of Israel Have Disagreement," *News*, April 24, 1901.

20. "Objections to Choosing the Sabbath," *News*, May 2, 1901.

21. First entry of the Official Ledger of the Medical Staff of the Newark Beth Israel Hospital, July 18, 1901, 1 (hereinafter, Official Ledger). The ledger has been held by the Parsonnet family; Katherine Pawloski, grand-niece of Dr. Victor Parsonnet, transcribed the handwritten minutes.

22. "No Obstacle in Way of Hospital," *News*, March 19, 1902. The account of the pesthouse appeared in "Pest House Burned," *News*, March 10, 1901.

23. "An Act to regulate the erection of hospitals for sick and diseased persons," Assembly of the State of New Jersey, no. 102, February 10, 1902.

24. "No Obstacle in Way." It is interesting to note that a Catherine Guenther, RN, is listed in the Beth Israel 1926 annual report as superintendent of nurses for the Beth Israel Hospital.

25. "Hebrew Hospital Dedication Begun," *News*, September 1, 1902.

26. "Beth Israel Hospital Will Be Formally Opened on August 31, 1902," *News*, August 18, 1902. This front-page article includes a photograph of the "Pennington" Beth Israel Hospital.

27. Edward C. Atwater, "The Physicians of Rochester, N.Y., 1860–1910: A Study in Professional History, II," *Bulletin of the History of Medicine* 51 (1977): 96–97. Also, Atwater, "Women, Surgeons, and a Worthy Enterprise: The General Hospital Comes to Upper New York State," in *The American General Hospital*, ed. Diana Elizabeth Long and Janet Golden (Ithaca, N.Y.: Cornell University Press, 1989), 40–66.

28. Robyn Muncy, *Creating a Female Dominion in American Reform, 1890–1935* (New York: Oxford University Press, 1991), is the best work describing the trend toward women's shaping of social policy.

29. "Study Club Honors Woman Suffragist," *News*, March 2, 1900.

30. Several articles in Pamela Nadell and Jonathan D. Sarna, eds., *Women and American Judaism* (Hanover, N.H.: University Press of New England, 2001), suggest that Jewish women participated in the expression of religious ideals through social service. See Karla Goldman, "The Public Religious Lives of Cincinnati's Jewish Women," 107–127; William Toll, "From Domestic Judaism to Public Ritual: Women and Religious Identity in the American West," 128–148; and Felicia Herman, "From Priestess to Hostess: Sisterhoods of Personal Service in New York City, 1887–1936," 148–181.

31. Mary Lowe Dickinson, "Work That Women Can Find to Do," *Newark Sunday News*, April 26, 1901.

32. The following summer, the *New York Times* reported that the Board of Health of South Orange had appointed Elizabeth M. Devine to be a health inspector: "Her salary was fixed at the nominal sum of $1 per year. The Board of Health will communicate with a committee representing several women's clubs that favored the appointment of a woman health inspector and will pay the salary to the inspector" ("Woman Health Inspector in Orange, N.J.," *New York Times*, August 24, 1901).

33. "Women as Inspectors of City Tenements," *News*, November 9, 1900. Mrs. Von Wagner, the sanitary inspector for the Board of Health of Yonkers, New York, addressed the members of the Saint Barnabas Guild of Memorial Hospital in

Orange. In 1896, the Women's Civil League of Yonkers engaged her as an inspector for tenement houses and, by guaranteeing her salary and showing the officials of the city the practical results of a woman's work, secured her regular appointment in January 1900 after she passed the civil service examination. This was not a novelty; in 1888, Glasgow was the first city in the world to appoint women as sanitary commissioners. An overview of the Jewish hospital in the United States is Ethan Bridge, *The Rise and Development of the Jewish Hospital in America* (Rabbinical thesis, Hebrew Union College, 1985). See also Dorothy Levenson, *Montefiore: The Hospital as Social Instrument, 1884–1984* (New York: Farrar, Straus and Giroux, 1984); and Arthur J. Linenthal, *First a Dream: The History of Boston's Jewish Hospitals, 1896 to 1928* (Boston: Beth Israel Hospital in association with the Francis A. Countway Library of Medicine, 1990).

34. Alvin Rogal and Karen Wolk Feinstein, *Strength to Strength: A History of Montefiore Hospital and Jewish Health Care in Pittsburgh* (Pittsburgh: Jewish Healthcare Foundation, 1992), 19–22; "History of Mt. Sinai of Cleveland," *Cleveland Jewish News*, February 12, 1937; "Historical Perspective," Cedars-Sinai Medical Center, Los Angeles, www. csmc.edu/pdf/HistPersp703.pdf.

35. John Allen Hornsby, "Equipment of a Small Hospital: Making Over a Dwelling House" (Paper presented at the American Medical Association Meeting, Minneapolis, July 17–20, 1913), abstracts printed of the meeting were published in the October 1913 issue of *Modern Hospital.*

36. Alan M. Kraut, *Silent Travelers: Germs, Genes, and the "Immigrant Menace"* (New York: Basic Books, 1994), 203–206.

37. "How It All Began," Levi Hospital, www.levihospital.com.

38. Willie Maye Harman, "Four Women and a Sanatorium," reprinted from "The Buzzer," November 1943, papers of the Mountain Sanatorium, New Jersey. The article describes Mrs. E. A. Prieth and Miss Mary Wilson, the former dressed in black and the latter in a gray tailored suit and hat with a long blue ostrich plume, who cornered every assemblyman and were lauded in the *Morning Star*, April 15, 1907, under the headline "Two Frail Women Rout Five Hundred Wise Men by Hard Work." The Deborah Consumptive Association was founded the Deborah Sanitarium for Jewish patients in 1928.

39. Rosemary Stevens, *In Sickness and in Wealth: American Hospitals in the Twentieth Century* (New York: Basic Books, 1989), 21; David Rosner, *A Once Charitable Enterprise: Hospitals and Health Care in Brooklyn and New York, 1885–1915* (Princeton, NJ: Princeton University Press, 1982), 99.

40. Barbara Rogers and Stephen M. Dobbs, *The First Century: Mount Zion Hospital and Medical Center* (San Francisco: Mount Zion Hospital and Medical Center, 1987), 4–14.

41. Rogal and Feinstein, *Strength to Strength*, 19.

42. Sidney Bolkosky, *Harmony and Dissonance: Voices of Jewish Identity in Detroit, 1914–1967* (Detroit: Wayne State University Press, 1991), 412–441.

43. David A. Gee, *216 S.K.: A History of the Jewish Hospital of St. Louis* (St. Louis: Jewish Hospital of St. Louis, 1981), 13–15.

44. Richard C. Dujardin, "Miriam: 75 Years of Care," *Providence Journal*, September 27, 2001.

45. "History of Mt. Sinai of Cleveland," *Cleveland Jewish News*, February 12, 1937.
46. Tina Levitan, *Islands of Compassion: A History of the Jewish Hospitals of New York* (Manchester, N.H.: Olympic Marketing, 1998), 120–150.
47. "Hebrew Women Plan Nursery: Movement Started to Establish Creche to Aid Mothers Who Must Work," *News*, May 19, 1905.
48. The description of Feitzinger's daily cleaning was given to Nettie Katchen by Augusta Parsonnet; see Katchen, "The First Ten Years."
49. Official Ledger, December 10, 1904, 42.
50. Ibid., May 11, 1906, 52. Misses Katharine Sinis, Sadie Kaufer, and Bertha Hunkele posed for "Three Young Women Receive Their Diplomas as Trained Nurses," *News*, May 18, 1906.
51. Caroline Feitzinger, "Brief Historical Review," Annual Report of the Newark Beth Israel Hospital and Dispensary from January 1, 1901 to January 1, 1906, 8–9, NBIH Papers at JHSMW.
52. Dale C. Smith, "Appendicitis, Appendectomy, and the Surgeon," *Bulletin of the History of Medicine* 70 (fall 1996): 414–441.
53. Feitzinger, "Brief Historical Review." Subsequent histories of the hospital state that the number of beds in the first Newark Beth Israel Hospital was twenty-one, e.g., Katchen notes, 1937 booklet issued by the hospital public affairs section. However, Feitzinger does not cite the number of beds.
54. "Report of the Sewing Circle," Report of the Newark Beth Israel Hospital and Dispensary from January 1, 1901 to January 1, 1906, NBIH Papers at JHSMW, 37.
55. Ibid., 55.
56. Ibid., 36.
57. "Gechete Damen und Herren!" ibid., 41–44.
58. This concept is advanced most articulately in Linda Basch, Nina Glick Schiller, and Cristina Szanton Blanc, *Nations Unbound: Transnational Projects, Postcolonial Predicaments, and Deterritorialized Nation-States* (Amsterdam, Netherlands: Gordon and Breach, 1994).
59. "Prince Street Like a Small Section of Russia; The Hebrews There Retain Old Country Customs," *Newark Sunday News*, second section, February 11, 1901. See also Guenther B. Risse, "The Renaissance of Bloodletting: A Chapter in Modern Therapies," *Journal of the History of Medicine and Allied Sciences* 34 (January 1979): 3–22.
60. See *News*, May 15, 16, 17, 20, 1903.
61. "The Spirit of the Passover," *News*, April 3, 1904.
62. "Aid for Russian Jews Nearing $12,000 Mark," *News*, November 23, 1905.
63. "Beth Israel's Year of Work," *News*, January 24, 1905.
64. Louis Frank was both partner and brother-in-law, having married Louis Bamberger's sister. Upon Frank's death, Felix Fuld, already a partner, also became a brother-in-law when he married Frank's widow.
65. "Contribute to Hospital Fund," *News*, May 22, 1905.
66. "Plan Accepted for New Beth Israel Hospital—Beth Israel Managers to Put Up $80,000 Building at High and Kinney Streets," *News*, January 31, 1906. The article includes a sketch of the hospital building.

67. "Lay Hospital's Corner-Stone—Thousands of Spectators Witness Ceremony at Beth Israel's New Building," *News*, October 29, 1906. The building committee consisted of William Rich, Dr. Armin Fischer, Nathan Salzman, Adolph Hollander, Henry Gross, Max Krasner, Joseph Mann, Joseph Steiner, Dr. Victor Parsonnet, and Dr. Max Danzis; Katchen, "The First Ten Years."
68. "Beth Israel Hospital Board Again at Odds—President Okin Tenders Resignation—Takes Exception to Action of Woman Member," *News*, October 7, 1907.
69. "Hospital Row at Acute Point—Okin's Resignation Accepted, but He Declares Action of Board Irregular," *News*, October 9, 1907.
70. "Want Okin to Continue Head—Movement to Have Former President of Beth Israel Hospital Reorganize Association," *News*, October 14, 1907.
71. Report of the Newark Beth Israel Hospital and Dispensary, 1909, 57.
72. "Hebrews Open New Hospital," *News*, January 30, 1908.
73. "Fort's Tribute to the Hebrew," *News*, January 31, 1908.
74. "Parade Closes Hospital Fete," *News*, February 3, 1908.
75. "Fort's Tribute to the Hebrew." Rabbi Silberfeld made his remarks at the January 29, 1908, dedication ceremonies held at the hospital. See also "Programme of the Dedication of the Newark Beth Israel Hospital," NBIH Papers at JHSMW.

CHAPTER 2 *The Formative Years*

1. "Two Bonfires Cause Deaths—Anne Krotowitz and Alice Nash Fatally Burned in Similar Accidents—Both Suffered Great Agony," *News*, August 3, 1903.
2. "Seven Important Phases of Newark's Development Told," *News*, October 16, 1907.
3. "Fifteen Girls Die in High Street Factory Fire—Have to Leap for Their Lives," *News*, November 26, 1910. The *News* printed extra editions during the day, each edition reporting the names of more dead and injured.
4. Ibid.
5. "Miss Haag, Heroine of Fire, Succumbs, Making Twenty-fourth Death," *News*, November 29, 1910. Haag persuaded many women to follow her and survive instead of leaping to their deaths.
6. "Five Hospitals to Get Estate—Residuary Estate of Joseph Nichols Was Left to 'The Newark Hospital,'" *News*, February 4, 1909. The will specified a Newark hospital that was created under a special act of the state legislature in 1857 and no longer existed when the estate was probated. The *News* article stated, "The report makes application of the rarely used legal doctrine *cy pres*, which means, the power of a court of equity to substitute for a particular charity that has failed another of the same kind as nearly may be." The special master appointed for the case designated five Newark charitable hospital institutions.
7. "Three Sisters Perish in Fire," *News*, November 28, 1910.
8. "Hospital Work for Year Told," *News*, January 28, 1909.
9. Official Ledger of the Medical Staff, minutes of the first meeting, July 18, 1901. The ledger listed the following physicians as attending the meeting: from the Hebrew Hospital and Dispensary Association, Emanuel Schwartz, S. Greenbaum,

Armin Fischer, Alex Fischer, M. Seidman, Theodore Teimer, B. H. Greenfield, E. D. Newman; from the Daughters of Israel Hospital Association, Maurice Asher, G. A. Rogers, Clarence Rostow, Victor Parsonnett [*sic*], M. Danzis.

10. Official Ledger, March 10, 1902, 22.

11. Minutes of the Executive Committee of the Medical Staff, October 8, 1902, in Minutes of the Executive Committee of the Medical Staff, 1901–1918, Box 1, Parsonnet Papers, at JHSMW (hereinafter, Medical Staff Minutes).

12. Ibid., May 19, 1904.

13. Ibid., July 18, 1907, 55.

14. William G. Rothstein, *American Medical Schools and the Practice of Medicine: A History* (New York: Oxford University Press, 1987), 134.

15. Official Ledger, August 12, 1908, listed the examining physicians and their specialties: Dr. Solomon Greenbaum, eye, ear, nose, and throat; Dr. Armin Fischer, chemistry; Dr. Max Feldman, children; Dr. Bernard H. Greenfield, physiology; Dr. Maurice Asher, material medicine; Dr. Emanuel Schwartz, medicine; Dr. Max Danzis, surgery; Dr. Victor Parsonett [*sic*], gynecology; Dr. George A. Rogers, obstetrics.

16. Medical Staff Minutes, August 15, 1911.

17. Kenneth M. Ludmerer, *Time to Heal: American Medical Education from the Turn of the Century to the Era of Managed Care* (New York: Oxford University Press, 1999), 96.

18. "A Martyr to Science," *Newark Sunday News*, September 1, 1901. The Newark German Hospital was renamed four times: in 1918, it was renamed Newark Memorial Hospital, then Lutheran Hospital, in 1952, renamed in honor of their most famous graduate nurse as Clara Maas Memorial Hospital, and finally Clara Maas Medical Center.

19. Stuart Galishoff, *Safeguarding the Public Health: Newark, 1895–1918* (Westport, Conn.: Greenwood Press, 1975).

20. "Three Doctors on the Carpet—Health Board Exonerates Clark and Sharply Criticizes Danzis and Seidman," *News*, February 8, 1905.

21. Dr. Eugene Parsonnet, recorded interviews transcribed by his son, Dr. Victor Parsonnet, sec. 1.2, Parsonnet Papers at JHSMW.

22. "Ejected from Hospital Ball—Socialists Who Went As Advertisements for Another Ball Complain," *New York Times*, December 15, 1907.

23. "Court Upholds Surgeon's Act—Patient's Consent to Emergency Change of Operation Not Necessary," *News*, July 15, 1912.

24. Dr. Eugene Parsonnet recorded interviews transcribed by his son, Dr. Victor Parsonnet, sec. 19.5, 90.1, Paronnet Papers at JHSMW.

25. Ibid., secs. 19.5, 2.6, 90.1.

26. Medical Staff Minutes, 1902.

27. Ibid., June 18, 1912, 105.

28. Ibid., July 25, 1911.

29. Annual Report, 1911.

30. Ibid.

31. Medical Staff Minutes, September 19, 1911.

32. "Miss Schmoker Gets Back Former Position—Board Appoints Her to City Hospital—Leaves Beth Israel—Superintendent Also Retires," *News*, April 22, 1908.

33. "Beth Israel Hospital Superintendent Quits," *News*, December 10, 1908.

34. "Again Tries to Take Her Own Life—Miss Rosa Rosensohn, a Nurse, Blames Misfortunes on Dr. Saul Rubinow," *News*, October 31, 1908.

35. Official Ledger, November 3, 1912, 107.

36. Medical Staff Minutes in 1911 also refer to Fischer but do not cite her official position.

37. Medical Staff Minutes, August 1, 1911.

38. Ibid., November 21, 1913.

39. Ibid.

40. Ibid.

41. Ibid., March 30, 1916.

42. Ibid., April 19, 1916. In June 2001, James Hopkins, telephone interview by Deborah A. Kraut, said he was told that the incident had occurred in the kitchen of the hospital in Weequahic.

43. "Hospital News," *Journal of the Newark Beth Israel Hospital* 1, 1 (January 1950): 94. Notes state that Dr. Danzis visited Israel and met Paula Ben Gurion. The *[Newark] Jewish News* expands upon the anecdote.

44. A. B. Tipping, "The Intern Question—Where Lies the Trouble?" *Modern Hospital* 6, 4 (April 1916): 257–260.

45. Medical Staff Minutes, September 19 and October 28, 1911.

46. Ibid., May 27, 1911.

47. Ibid., September 16, 1913, 113.

48. "In Ill Health Girl Ends All—Father, Returning from Synagogue Finds Her Lifeless on Bed in Her Room," *News*, October 2, 1905.

49. Among males, despair was often traceable to the shame of unemployment. Jacob Rausch, only fourteen years old, swallowed carbolic acid after losing his errand-boy job ("Boy Ends Life with Carbolic—Only Reason Known for His Act Is That He Lost His Job," *News*, February 4, 1904).

50. "Hold Physician in Fatal Case," *News*, November 8, 1912. Physicians were indicted for deaths attributed to complications after performing illegal operations, i.e., abortions.

51. Dr. Eugene Parsonnet interview, sec. 19.4.

52. Annual Report, 1909.

53. Annual Report, 1911, 19–23.

54. "Girl Dead, Hold Doctor in Case—Manslaughter Charge against Dr. Shapiro Involves Alleged Illegal Practice—Court Refuses Him Bail," *News*, February 12, 1913.

55. It is not known whether McKenzie was related to the nurse-supervisor McKenzie who had resigned after being accused of making anti-Semitic comments. As county medical examiner, he would visit the Beth Israel Hospital twice more in 1913 in order to assess two suicides: a young woman who had jumped from a second-story window of the hospital ("Leap from Beth Israel Window Ends in Death," *News*, May 15, 1913) and a young woman who had tied a bed sheet around her neck ("Invalid Strangles Herself to Death—An Attendant Nearby," *News*, November 3, 1913).

56. "Dr. N. J. Shapiro Is Found Guilty," *News*, January 30, 1914; "Dr. Shapiro Given Long Prison Term," *News*, February 3, 1914.

57. Was Shapiro a Beth Israel Hospital staff member? Although his name does not appear in the Official Ledger or the Medical Staff Minutes, it is possible that he had just been hired when he was involved in the scandal.

58. Medical Staff Minutes, March 26, 1916.

59. On midwives, see Judith Walzer Leavitt, *Brought to Bed: Child-Bearing in America, 1750–1950* (New York: Oxford University Press, 1986); Richard W. Wertz and Dorothy C. Wertz, *Lying-In* (New York: Free Press, 1977); Virginia A. Metaxas Quiroga, *Poor Mothers and Babies: A Social History of Childbirth and Child Care Institutions in Nineteenth-Century New York* (New York: Garland, 1990); and Charlotte G. Borst, *Catching Babies: The Professionalization of Childbirth, 1870–1920* (Cambridge, Mass.: Harvard University Press, 1996).

60. City of Newark Annual Reports, 1914, Board of Health, 704–732, Newark Public Library, Newark, N.J.

61. "Midwives Listen to Hygiene Talk, Board of Health Officials Also Instruct Them Regarding Provisions of Statutes," *News*, June 25, 1915.

62. The Jewish Maternity Hospital was not affiliated with the Newark Beth Israel Hospital and the medical staffs did not have joint appointments from 1912 to 1930. In 1930, the Jewish Maternity Hospital was amalgamated into the Newark Beth Israel Hospital.

63. Editorial, *Modern Hospital* 2 (September 1914).

64. Annual Report, 1915–1916, 9, 8.

65. Ibid., 9, 7–17.

66. Ibid., "Special Appeal," 8–10.

67. "Report of Nathaniel G. Price, M.D., Secretary Medical Staff," Annual Report, 1920, 25–26.

68. Abraham Flexner, *Medical Education in the United States and Canada: A Report to the Carnegie Foundation for the Advancement of Teaching*, Bulletin 4 (1910; rpt. New York: Carnegie Foundation, 1972), 275.

69. Ibid., 111.

70. Ibid., 112. For added insight on Flexner's views, see Thomas Neville Bonner, *Iconoclast: Abraham Flexner and a Life in Learning* (Baltimore: Johns Hopkins University Press, 2002).

71. "Otho Fisher Ball, M.D., June 20, 1875–July 19, 1953," *Modern Hospital* 81 (August 1953): 47–51.

72. Otho Ball, editorial, *Modern Hospital* 1 (September 13, 1913): 32.

73. Ibid.

74. "Outlines Duty of Board of Health," *News*, February 17, 1915. Mayor Raymond, while advocating qualifications for a new director of the Board of Health, was also answering for his failure to meet a campaign promise. He was unable to get a woman appointed to the Board of Health as promised, and blamed the aldermen. The mayor eventually made good on his promise, appointing Elizabeth Aitken as supervisor of the Division of Child Hygiene. Aitken held the RN degree and passed the civil service examination ("Strict Curb on Midwives in Force," *News*, June 17, 1915).

75. "Pneumonia Grows in Fatal Effects," *News*, November 12, 1915.

76. "Is Newark Penny-Wise and Pound-Foolish?" *Survey* 36 (May 13, 1916): 173–174.

77. "All Unite to Check Infant Paralysis—Health Department, Rockefeller Institute, and Private Doctors Organize Campaign," *New York Times*, June 30, 1916.

78. Naomi Rogers, *Dirt and Disease: Polio before FDR* (New Brunswick, N.J.: Rutgers University Press, 1992), 41.

79. "Cause of Disease Unknown, *American* Editor Says, Therefore We Can't Control It," *New York Times*, July 9, 1916.

80. "Government Aid in Paralysis Fights 133 New Cases," *New York Times*, July 7, 1916.

81. Medical Staff Minutes, March 26, 1916.

82. John R. Paul, *A History of Poliomyelitis* (New Haven: Yale University Press, 1971), 149–151.

83. "Government Aid in Paralysis Fights 133 New Cases," *New York Times*, July 7, 1916.

84. Ibid.

85. Ibid.

86. Charles V. Craster, "Poliomyelitis, Some Features in City Prevalence," *Journal of the American Medical Association* 68 (May 26, 1917): 1535–1539.

87. Ibid. The necropsies were performed by Dr. Harrison Stanford Martland.

88. Medical Staff Minutes, October 3, 1916, 131.

89. "Newark Sniffles, Then Ah-Kerchoos—Health Officials Do Not Admit There's Epidemic, but Say Grip Habit Is General," *News*, December 28, 1915.

90. "Looks for Lull in Grip Epidemic, Dr. Park Believes a Few Days of Clear Weather Will Stop Its Spread," *New York Times*, January 7, 1916.

91. "Physicians See Change in Grippe," *News*, January 16, 1902.

92. "Cause of Disease Unknown, *American* Editor Says."

93. The report is cited by Henderson J. Donald, "Dependents and Delinquents," *Journal of Negro History* 6 (October 4, 1921): 458–470, quote on 459.

94. Medical Staff Minutes, February 23, 1917.

95. Richard E. Schmidt, "Hospitals for Communicable Diseases," *Modern Hospital*, 10 (March 1918).

96. On the impact of influenza on the military during World War I, see Carol R. Byerly, *Fever of War: The Influenza Epidemic in the U.S. Army during World War I* (New York: New York University Press, 2005).

97. Two books on the influenza epidemic in the United States are: Alfred W. Crosby, *America's Forgotten Pandemic: The Influenza of 1918* (New York: Cambridge University Press, 1989) and John M. Barry, *The Great Influenza: The Epic Story of the Deadliest Plague in History* (New York: Viking, 2004).

98. "Influenza Chief Cause of Death in Home Camps," *New York Times*, January 26, 1919.

99. "Two Soldiers from Newark among Pneumonia Victims at Camp Dix," *News*, September 23, 1918.

100. Crosby, America's Forgotten Pandemic, 47.

101. Ibid.

102. "Scenes at City Hall and Military Park as Fourth Liberty Loan Campaign Opens," *News*, September 28, 1918.

103. "Influenza Total Is 1,024, but Only Two More Die," *News*, October 2, 1918. The article reported that three anti-influenza serums were being tested. The serum was prepared by subjecting the germs to heat and then suspending them in a salt solution.
104. "State-Wide Closing to Curb Influenza," *News*, October 7, 1918.
105. "City's Grip Total Near 11,000 Cases, Craster Thinks 20,000 Ill Here," *News*, October 17, 1918.
106. "Rigid Quarantine in Newark Is Ordered, Plan Emergency Hospitals Here," *News*, October 10, 1918.
107. Ibid.
108. Medical Staff Minutes; the last entry is dated November 6, 1917.
109. George M. Price, "Influenza, Destroyer and Teacher—A General Confession by the Public Health Authorities of a Continent," *Survey* 41 (December 21, 1918): 367–369.
110. "Dr. Polevski Rites Held," *New York Times*, July 30, 1936.
111. Dr. Eugene Parsonnet interview as transcribed by his son, Dr. Victor Parsonnet, sec 22.1, Parsonnet Papers at JHSMW.
112. Nathanial G. Price, "Dr. Victor Parsonnet, in Memoriam," Annual Report of the Newark Beth Israel Hospital, 1921.

CHAPTER 3   *From Little House on the Hill to Modern Institution*

1. "Hospital Drive Slogan Revived," *Newark Star-Eagle*, February 4, 1928. (The same full-page advertisement appeared in *Der Tog*, the Yiddish-language newspaper published in New York City.) The Ladies Auxiliary conducted a door-to-door campaign wearing hearts to signify Miss Beth.
2. Nancy Tomes, *The Gospel of Germs: Men, Women, and the Microbe in American Life* (Cambridge, Mass.: Harvard University Press, 1998), 62–67, 150–154. Also, Suellen Hoy, *Chasing Dirt: The American Pursuit of Cleanliness* (New York: Oxford University Press, 1995); Charles Goodrum and Helen Dalrymple, *Advertising in America: The First 200 Years* (New York: Harry Abrams, 1990), 249–255.
3. Harvey Green, Fit for America: Health, Fitness, Sport, and American Society (New York: Pantheon Books, 1986). Also, Clifford Putney, Muscular Christianity: Manhood and Sports in Protestant America, 1880–1920 (Cambridge, Mass.: Harvard University Press, 2001).
4. Edward Alaworth Ross, The Old World in the New: The Significance of Past and Present Immigration to the American People (New York: Century, 1914), 282.
5. Annual Report, 1921.
6. "Society Proceedings," *Modern Hospital* 7 (November 1919): 472.
7. Ibid., 472–473.
8. M. R. Kneifl, "The Catholic Hospital Association," in *American and Canadian Hospitals: A Reference Book* (Chicago: Physicians' Record Company, 1937), 36–40.
9. E. E. Hanson, "American Protestant Hospital Association," in ibid., 41–42.
10. "Society Proceedings," *Journal of the American Medical Association* (March 14, 1914): 876.

11. Malcolm T. MacEachern, "The American College of Surgeons," in *American and Canadian Hospitals*, 49.

12. "More Than 1,000 Hospitals of Fifty or More Beds Meet Minimum Standard of A.C.S.," *Modern Hospital* 19 (November 1922): 424–425.

13. "Hospitals Approved for Internships," *Bulletin of the American College of Surgeons* 4 (1921):27–32.

14. "Attacks Jewish Hospitals—Dr. Danzer Says Politics Dominates Smaller Institutions," *New York Times*, October 5, 1925.

15. Arthur J. Linenthal, *First a Dream: The History of Boston's Jewish Hospitals, 1896 to 1928* (Boston: Beth Israel Hospital in association with the Francis A. Countway Library of Medicine, 1990), 145, 171.

16. "Women Praised at Dedication of Ward for Kiddies," *[Newark] Jewish Chronicle*, November 25, 1921.

17. "Beth Israel Board Asks More Nurses—Miss Rafter, New Chief of Nurses Ready to Enroll New Students," *Jewish Chronicle*, December 16, 1921. The article notes that the position was left vacant by Sarah Van Gilder [*sic*] after more than ten years service.

18. This ACS requirement and those that follow in the text were published in the November 1922 issue of *Modern Hospital* accompanying the list of the ACS-accredited hospitals. *Modern Hospital* had extracted the information from the report of the 1922 American College of Surgeons on Hospital Standardization.

19. Linenthal, *First a Dream*, 145.

20. The other Newark hospitals that were accredited in 1922 were Newark City Hospital, Saint James Hospital, and Newark Memorial Hospital (formerly German Hospital). Newark Presbyterian Hospital received an asterisk next to its name, indicating that although it met the spirit of the ACS criteria, it had not developed the criteria sufficient to deserve full accreditation.

21. *Modern Hospital* 19 (October 1922): 327.

22. "Start Construction of Y.M.-Y.W.H.A. Building," *Jewish Chronicle*, June 16, 1922.

23. Ibid., January 26, 1923.

24. "Grad at 80, Reviews 56 Years in Career as Major Architect," *Jewish News*, March 29, 1963.

25. Frank Grad, A.I.A., to the Ways and Means Committee, September 28, 1923; "City Plans Hospital with 1,000 Beds," *Newark Star Eagle*, April 4, 1935.

26. "Plans for New Building Outlined at Dinner of Beth Israel Hospital Staff," *Jewish Chronicle*, May 4, 1923.

27. On the great migration, see Nicholas Lemann, *The Promised Land: The Great Black Migration and How It Changed America* (New York: Knopf, 1991), and James R. Grossman, *Land of Hope: Chicago, Black Southerners, and the Great Migration* (Chicago: University of Chicago Press, 1989).

28. Henderson H. Donald, "The Effects of the Migration upon the Migrants Themselves," *Journal of Negro History* 6 (October 21, 1921): 449. "The Negro Migration of 1916–1918," *Journal of Negro History*, October 1921, cites F. D. Tyson, *Negro Migration in 1916–1917*, report of the U.S. Department of Labor, 121; H. B. Pendleton, *Survey* 37 (February 17, 1917): 569.

29. "Dice Game Dispute Causes Race Riot—Through Streets of Hill Section Negroes and Whites Battle with All Sorts of Weapons," *News*, September 4, 1917.
30. Ibid.
31. Frank J. Prial, "Weequahic Wondering," *Newark Sunday News*, June 18, 1961.
32. "May Move Beth Israel Hospital." *Jewish Chronicle*, February 15, 1924.
33. "Give Many Motives for Helping Beth Israel," *Jewish Chronicle*, May 30, 1924. The streets named were not wholly accurate, as the northern boundary beyond Irving would be Lehigh Avenue.
34. "City Leaders Hail Plans for Fuld Memorial; Nation's Jewry Mourns Late Philanthropist, Acclaim Civic and Charitable Deeds," *Jewish Chronicle*, January 25, 1929.
35. Daniel Spear, "Newark Will Respond to Appeal, Predicts Hollander as Beth Israel Campaign Nears," *Jewish Chronicle*, April 11, 1924. A. Hollander and Sons was a fur dyer and dresser company located in Newark, NJ.
36. "The Story of Dynamic Michael A. Stavitsky," *Jewish Chronicle*, June 20, 1941.
37. Ibid.; "Launching the Campaign for the New Beth Israel Hospital—$1,500,000 Mark Ignored as Drive Enthusiasm Rises," *Jewish Chronicle*, June 6, 1924.
38. Anton Kaufman, "We Scan the History of the *Chronicle*," *Jewish Chronicle*, May 29, 1931. No copy of the first issue of the newspaper has been found.
39. "Morris Rachlin, Master Builder," *Jewish Chronicle*, September 23, 1927.
40. "Campaign for $1,500,000 for Beth Israel Hospital to Begin in May," *Jewish Chronicle*, March 14, 1924.
41. Rachlin's obituary notes that he had arranged for the purchase of the new hospital site; see "Dr. Israel J. Rachlin, Physician since 1903," *New York Times*, December 6, 1949.
42. "Beth Israel Completes Hospital Site Purchase—Silencing Rumors That Original Site Has Been Abandoned," *Jewish Chronicle*, March 7, 1925; Annual Report, 1926, 2.
43. "Agreement Filed for Beth Israel," *Jewish Chronicle*, September 19, 1926.
44. Board Minutes, April 25, 1949. On the inside cover of the Beth Israel Nurses Training School Catalogue is an aerial view of the hospital that clearly shows the corner plot behind the main tower that had not been sold in 1925. The lot was still vacant in the early 1960s.
45. Cartoon, *Jewish Chronicle*, August 20, 1926. "Break Ground for Beth Israel Hospital," *New York Times*, August 19, 1926. Straightforward accounts were published in the *New York Times* and *Modern Hospital*.
46. "Construction on Bergen Street Block Is Started," *Jewish Chronicle*, January 8, 1926.
47. "Personal Service Is a Paramount Matter in the Weequahic Section," *Jewish Chronicle*, April 24, 1925.
48. Paul Keller, "The Beth Israel of the Present and the Future, Outline of the Medical Staff Organization Including a List of the Complete Personnel of the Local Hospital," *Jewish Chronicle*, December 11, 1925.
49. Ibid.
50. Annual Report, 1926, 25.
51. Ibid.

52. "Local Medicos, Dentists to Match Science on the Basketball Court," *Jewish Chronicle*, November 26, 1926.
53. "Launching the Campaign," *Jewish Chronicle*, June 6, 1924.
54. "Agreement Filed for Beth Israel," *Jewish Chronicle*, September 17, 1926.
55. "Trio Who Will Head Beth Israel Hospital Drive," *News*, January 13, 1928. (The *Jewish Chronicle* issues for September 1927 through April 1928 are not held at the JHSMW and have not been found in other libraries or archives.)
56. "Women Outline Hospital Drive—Mrs. Augusta Parsonnett [*sic*] Named Chairman of Division for Campaign," *Newark Star-Eagle*, January 25, 1928.
57. "Hospital Gifts Will Be Marked," *Newark Star-Eagle*, January 21, 1928.
58. "Gives Last $5 to Beth Israel," *Newark Star-Eagle*, February 13, 1928.
59. "25,000 Throng to Beth Israel," *Newark Star-Eagle*, February 13, 1928. Keller reduced the visiting hours for touring the hospital when the crowds of families with children began to affect the hospital staff's ability to ready the wards for patients ("Inspection Time Cut at Hospital," *Newark Star-Eagle*, February 14, 1928).
60. "WOR in Program for Beth Israel—Bamberger Station Will Broadcast Dedication Exercises Sunday," *Newark Star-Eagle*, February 17, 1928.
61. A two-minute silent film exists of this dedication ceremony. Mr. Thomas Coulihan, the Beth Israel Hospital Medical Center medical photographer, retained the film, which he states was made by members of the Rachlin family. The film was donated to the JHSMW.
62. "$200,000 Given to Beth Israel—Mayor Delivering Address at Beth Israel Hospital Opening," *Newark Star-Eagle*, February 21, 1928.
63. "Great House Replaces Little House on the Hill," *News*, February 19, 1928.
64. "Patients Being Quickly Moved," *Newark Star-Eagle*, February 21, 1928.
65. Jules E. Tepper, "Back through the Years, a History of the Home for the Aged," *Jewish News* special supplement, March 1962. The founders included Rachel Parsonnet (Victor Parsonnet's mother), Ida Ascher, Anna Berman, Bessie Cohn, Frieda Elias, Mollie Hoffman, Zlota Kleinman, Frieda Lesser, Annie Nelson, Sarah Rader, Esther Sabo, Yetta Scher, Rose Simon, and Esther Yadkowsky.
66. Tepper, "Back through the Years." Also, Rachel Parsonnet was an active member of the Daughters of Israel.
67. *The Beth*, 1974, Opening of the New Pavilion, NBIH Papers at JHSMW.

CHAPTER 4 *A Modern Hospital Surviving Depression and War*

1. "25,000 Throng to Beth Israel," *Newark Star-Eagle*, February 13, 1928.
2. C. Stanley Taylor, "Modern Trends in Hospital Construction," *Modern Hospital* 30 (March 1928): 59.
3. Frank Grad and S. S. Goldwater, "Newark Beth Israel Hospital Has Unique Features," *Modern Hospital* 30 (April 1928): 67–75; quote on 67. The detailed description that follows in the text is drawn from this article.
4. Tonsillectomies and adenoidectomies were common surgeries performed on children.
5. Grad and Goldwater, "Newark Beth Israel Hospital," 67, 71.
6. Ibid.

7. Dr. Paul Keller to Board of Directors, Monthly Report, in Board Minutes, June 4, 1928. Keller explained that when the walls were washed the paint peeled off the walls, leaving blotchy surfaces.

8. Administrative Committee Minutes of Newark Beth Israel Hospital, April 9, 1929, NBIH Papers at JHSMW (hereinafter, Administrative Committee Minutes).

9. Administrative Committee Minutes, October 25, 1928. Included in the minutes are the letters to Frank Liveright from Abbott, Merkt, and Company, March 16, 1929, and to Mr. Bazemore, Chief Engineer, October 8, 1929.

10. Dr. Paul Keller to Board of Directors, Monthly Report, in Board Minutes, June 4, 1928.

11. Reports of the Administrative Committee, in Board Minutes, March 12 and 28, and April 9, 1928.

12. Administrative Committee Minutes, October 2, 1929.

13. Sarah Gordon, ed., *All Our Lives: A Centennial History of Michael Reese Hospital and Medical Center, 1881–1981* (Chicago: Michael Reese Hospital and Medical Center, 1981), 104.

14. Chairman of Training School Committee to Chairman, Administrative Committee, in Board Minutes, March 20, 1928.

15. Administrative Committee Minutes, May 10, 1928.

16. Board Minutes, October 21, 1929.

17. "City Leaders Hail Plans for Fuld Memorial," *[Newark] Jewish Chronicle*, January 25, 1929.

18. "Felix Fuld Dies, a Philanthropist," *New York Times*, January 21, 1929.

19. This description was distilled from the following: William E. Leuchtenberg, *The Perils of Prosperity: 1914–1932*, 2nd ed. (Chicago: University of Chicago Press, 1993); Studs Terkel, *Hard Times: An Oral History of the Great Depression* (New York: Avon, 1971); and Albert U. Romsaco, *The Poverty of Abundance: Hoover, the Nation, and the Great Depression* (New York: Oxford University Press, 1965).

20. John T. Cunningham, *Newark*, rev. ed. (Newark: New Jersey Historical Society, 1988), 280–281.

21. Benjamin Kluger, "Growing Up in Newark," *[Newark]Jewish News*, September 8, 1977.

22. "American Hospital Standards," supplement to *Science* 74 (October 23, 1931): 10.

23. "Help the Hospitals," *Survey* 67 (November 15, 1931): 202.

24. "Woman to 'Ride' Hospital Bus, Four Newarkers Qualify to Enter," *Jewish Chronicle*, January 10, 1930.

25. "City Plans Hospital with 1,000 Beds—Main Structure Would Rise Eighteen Stories," *Newark Star-Eagle*, April 6, 1935.

26. Board Minutes, November 13, 1933. Subsequently, Frank Van Dyk, Executive Secretary of the Hospital Council of Essex County, to Board Member, November 22, 1933. Board president Lichtman also wrote to Franklin, offering a hundred beds for ward service to meet the needs of the city.

27. Mary Ross, "Crisis in the Hospitals," *Survey* 22 (July 1933): 364.

28. Rosemary Stevens, *In Sickness and in Wealth: American Hospitals in the Twentieth Century* (New York: Basic Books, 1989), 142.

29. "Bronx Hospital May Be Forced to Close," *Jewish Chronicle*, January 29, 1932.

30. Executive Directors' Report to the Board of the Beth Israel Hospital, Board Minutes, October 8, 1929.

31. Board Minutes, January 13, 1930.

32. Minnie Edelschick, "Analysis of the Monthly Report for January 1939," in Board Minutes. The report analyzes admissions to the hospital and clinic by diagnosis, as well as by referrals from social service agencies.

33. Ibid.

34. Bessie Glassman, "The Effects of the Depression on the Department of Social Work, Jewish Hospital, St. Louis Missouri," *Transactions of the American Hospital Association* 35 (1933): 496–504.

35. "Rate Information for Physicians," Newark Beth Israel Hospital, effective May 15, 1937, pamphlet, NBIH Papers at JHSMW. The earlier iterations of the rate information have not been found. This rates pamphlet is quoted for its completeness.

36. Compensation Bureau of the Newark Beth Israel Hospital, Annual Report, 1931.

37. Dr. Lee K. Frankel, Introduction, Annual Report, 1930, n.p.

38. "Federation Plans Survey of Hospitals in Newark," *News*, December 19, 1928. Felix Fuld offered to defray the cost of a complete survey of Newark hospitals, which would be prepared for the Welfare Federation.

39. Joseph P. Peters, "Necessity Is Often the Mother of Mergers," *Modern Hospital* 107 (July 1966): 90.

40. "News," *Bulletin of the American Hospital Association* (February 1930).

41. Mrs. Abraham Schindel, "Maternity Hospital's Service Needed, Reply of President to Survey of City's Institutions," *Jewish Chronicle*, January 24, 1930. Dr. James C. Doane's report is quoted.

42. "New Hospital Unit to Hold Ceremony," *New York Times*, June 6, 1937. The merger of the Women's and Children's Hospital into Saint Barnabas Hospital was completed January 1, 1932, in conjunction with the construction of a six-story red brick addition ("News of the Month," *Modern Hospital* 38 [February 1932]).

43. Ibid.

44. Ibid.

45. Board Minutes, November 22, 1927.

46. The Special Committee Report recommendations are listed in Administrative Committee Minutes, September 16, 1931.

47. Ladies Guild summary report to the Beth Israel Board for 1931, Board Minutes, January 18, 1932.

48. The minutes of the Auxiliary of the Newark Maternity Department of the Beth Israel Hospital, March 27, 1931, JHSMW (hereinafter, Maternity Auxiliary Minutes). The minutes, handwritten, span the years 1930 to 1939. On January 1, 1940, the Maternity Auxiliary merged with the Ladies Guild to become the Ladies Auxiliary.

49. Maternity Auxiliary Minutes, October 15 and March 27, 1931.

50. Seventh Annual Report of the Maternity Auxiliary, January 30, 1939, JHSMW.

51. Maternity Auxiliary Minutes, June 1, 1931.

52. "Our Voluntary Hospitals," editorial, *Bulletin of the American Hospital Association* 6, 7 (July 1932).
53. B. C. MacLean, MD, "Depression Developments in Relation to Hospital Economics," *Bulletin of the American College of Surgeons* 16 (December 1932): 38–41.
54. Administrative Committee Minutes, September 10, 1931.
55. Plan to reduce the operating expenditures for Newark Beth Hospital, Plan No. 1, in Administrative Committee Minutes, March 13, 1933.
56. President Frank I. Liveright to all Board and Members of the Senior Staff, "a crisis in the life of Newark Beth Israel is imminent," May 4, 1932, in Board Minutes, May 11, 1932.
57. Administrative Committee Minutes, September 10, 1931; the lunch meeting was held at the Bamberger Department Store restaurant.
58. Minutes of the Joint Meeting of Board of Directors and Senior Medical Staff, April 13, 1933, NBIH Papers at JHSMW.
59. Minutes of the Board of Directors Meeting, January 30, 1933.
60. The Louis Schlesinger Real Estate company submitted a list of properties owned by the hospital to the board in a letter dated April 13, 1931, that includes a diagram of their locations. The properties identified were: 647–651, hospital, occupied by the Daughters of Israel; 646 High Street, nurses home, old three-story brick mansion, abandoned; 643–645 High Street, two-story frame, abandoned; 643–645 High Street, two-story brick; 133–135 West Kinney, two-story frame, abandoned; 137 West Kinney, three-story frame; 139–141 West Kinney, three-story stucco.
61. Board Minutes, December 14, 1931.
62. "Charles Sumner Ward—a tribute from the Ward, Well and Dreshman Company, lauding his accomplishment in designing the short-term money-raising campaigns of pledges to raise money for hospitals and his work in directing the national Red Cross campaigns," *Modern Hospital* 33 (September 1929): 139. Ward died two months before the stock-market crash.
63. Minutes of the Annual Meeting of the Newark Beth Israel Hospital, January 30, 1933, JHSMW.
64. Cecil Lichtman, interview by authors, at his home in New Jersey, September 26, 1999.
65. "Proposed Plan with Recommendations to Further Reduce the Operating Expenditures," Newark Beth Israel Hospital, presented at a Joint Meeting of the Board of Directors and Senior Medical Staff, April 13, 1933.
66. Minutes of Special Board Meeting, May 8, 1933.
67. Administrative Committee Minutes, August 14, 1933.
68. Board Minutes, June 14, 1933.
69. Abraham Lichtman, "17th Annual Report on Beth Israel Hospital," *Jewish News* February 1, 8, 1952.
70. Board Minutes, June 14, 1933.
71. "Mob of 1,000 Raids Jersey Nazi Rally," *New York Times*, May 22, 1934. For further information, see Warren Grover, *Nazis in Newark* (New Brunswick, N.J.: Transaction, 2003).
72. Minutes of Emergency Board Meeting, with Board Minutes, July 20, 1934. Everyone in the room knew that Leber literally held Hollander's letter in his hand, but before he could speak, Liveright said: "Any talk; any discussion, regarding

reorganization, or Mr. Hollander's report is out of order. We are not concerned with Mr. Hollander's report of reorganization at the present time. He went abroad."

73. Ibid.
74. Ibid.
75. Ibid.
76. Board Minutes, August 24, 1934.
77. Board Minutes, January 31, 1935.
78. President's Annual Report, Board Minutes, January 27, 1935.
79. Administrative Committee Minutes, December 12, 1928; Board Minutes, September 23, 1935.
80. Annual Meeting Minutes, January 27, 1936.
81. Lichtman, "17th Annual Report on Beth Israel Hospital."
82. Joseph Baker, speech, appended to Board Minutes, February 6, 1935.
83. Stevens, *In Sickness and in Wealth*, 39.
84. Baker speech appended to Board Minutes, February 6, 1935.
85. "New Pathologist for Beth Israel," *Jewish Chronicle*, August 30, 1935. Dr. Antopol had interned in Beth El Hospital in Brooklyn, then won a fellowship in pathology at the New York Mount Sinai Hospital, went on to study at the Institute of General and Experimental Pathology in Vienna, and returned to the United States to become assistant pathologist at Mount Sinai.
86. Schwarz to Lichtman, January 20, 1936, NBIH Papers at JHSMW.
87. "Newark Health Post Given Dr. Keller," *Newark Star-Eagle*, April 2, 1935.
88. The Baylor University prepayment plan for teachers required that if 75 percent of those eligible, agreed to pay fifty cents each month to the plan, the hospital would regard their monthly payments as prepayment for their hospital care when needed. The hospital collected the funds, underwrote the risk, guaranteed the benefits, and controlled the medical resources.
89. American Hospital Association, *The Individual Hospital* (Chicago: American Hospital Association, September 1945), 52. The characteristics were emphasis on public welfare, limitation to hospital charges, enlistment of professional and public interests, free choice of physicians at hospital, nonprofit organization, economic soundness, and cooperative and dignified promotion.
90. "100 Hospitals Open a 3-Cent-a-Day Plan," *New York Times*, May 8, 1935. The first groups of employees to subscribe to the plan were from: the Central Park Zoo, a local high school, and two companies. Jewish hospitals in New York City that were members of the plan included: Beth David, Beth El, Beth Israel, Jewish, Israel-Zion, Mount Sinai, and Montefiore. The Newark Beth Israel Hospital was a member of the plan.
91. Seventh Annual Report of the Maternity Auxiliary, January 30, 1939.
92. Beth Israel Hospital Board Resolution on the death of Dorothy Silverman Lichtman, Board Minutes, March 27, 1939.
93. "A. Schindel, Head of Newark Store," *New York Times*, December 22, 1939. Schindel, after twenty-nine years of service at Bambergers and seven years at Kresge's, had become the store manager of the Hearns Department Store. He had been at the store continuously through the Christmas Holidays, and was stricken with a heart attack at the store and died shortly after being admitted to the Newark

Beth Israel Hospital. At Kresge's, Schindel had opened an art gallery; in addition, he had established a junior aviation group for 1,500 Newark boys, and served as an advisor on the construction of the Newark Museum.

94. Winford H. Smith, "Role of Civilian Hospital in the Program of Preparedness," *Hospitals* (October 1940): 23–28.

95. "Lichtman Predicts New Era in Hospitalization," *Jewish Chronicle*, February 2, 1940; "Organize U.S. Hospital for 'Emergency,'" *Newark Star-Ledger*, May 25, 1940.

96. Board Minutes, November 25, 1940.

97. "Dr. Parsonnet off to Serve," *Jewish Chronicle*, August 23, 1940.

98. Board Minutes, May 26, 1941.

99. Annual Meeting Minutes, January 27, 1941.

100. "Thousands Stricken by Flu," *Newark Star-Ledger*, January 13, 1941; "1,000 under Quarantine at Dix," *Newark Star-Ledger*, January 17, 1941; "Chlorine Fells Many in Jersey," *New York Times*, August 8, 1941.

101. Board Minutes, December 22, 1941; "Airport Closing to Start Drive for Federal Funds," *Newark Star-Ledger*, May 30, 1940. Newark Mayor Meyer Ellenstein negotiated a temporary closure in order to have the U.S. government buy, lease, or subsidize the airport facility.

102. Board Minutes, January 25, 1943.

103. Board Minutes, May 22, 1944; "Public to Get Penicillin through 1,000 Hospitals," *New York Times*, May 5, 1944. In Newark, the Beth, as well as Newark Memorial, Newark City, Saint Barnabas, Saint Michael's, and Saint James, were designated as depots.

104. Board Minutes, September 27, 1943. The federal government paid the hospital for the training of each nurse, and awarded each student a monthly stipend.

105. Annual Meeting Minutes, January 26, 1942; Report of the Inspection of the Hospital made Thursday December 4, 1941, by the House Committee.

106. Board Minutes, January 25, 1943.

107. Board Minutes, December 27, 1943.

108. Board Minutes, January 24, 1944.

109. "Dr. Keller, Expert on Hospital Plan—Medical Director of Associated Service Here, a Pioneer in the Field, Dies at 52," obituary, *New York Times*, December 23, 1943.

110. Board Minutes, March 27, 1944.

111. Minutes of Dinner Meeting of Board of Directors, December 18, 1944. The meeting began with Dr. Danzis reminiscing over the "old days," followed by Dr. Robbins, who spoke of the Beth Israel of the future. Then those assembled literally burned the mortgage papers, after which the ashes were placed "in their last resting place"—most likely an ashtray.

112. Board Minutes, November 27, 1944.

113. Board Minutes, December 26, 1945.

114. American Hospital Association Report, *The Individual Hospital* (Chicago: American Hospital Association, 1945), 7–11. Subsequent quotes and details in the text are drawn from this report.

115. Ibid.

CHAPTER 5   *Medicine at the Beth, 1928–1947*

1. "Poison Gas Kills 100 in Cleveland Clinic; Explosions Spread Fumes, Fire Following; Patients, Nurses, Doctors Die in Flight," *New York Times*, May 16, 1929, 1.
2. Administrative Committee Minutes, June 4, 1929.
3. N. P. Colwell, secretary, to Dr. Paul Keller, in Board Minutes, May 18, 1929.
4. F. H. Arestad, "Report of Inspection of Newark Beth Israel Hospital," May 6, 1929, in Administrative Committee Minutes, 1.
5. The high percentage of autopsies is not explained as Jewish halachic law forbids such actions.
6. Michael M. Davis, "Middle Class Hospitals and Clinics," *Survey* 63 (January 1930): 423.
7. Dr. Arthur Bernstein, interview by the authors, Maplewood, NJ, May 7, 2000.
8. Dental Executive Committee Minutes, September 11, 1929, NBIH Papers at JHSMW
9. Administrative Committee Minutes, April 2, 1929, NBIH Papers at JHSMW.
10. Ibid., November 10, 1930, and House Committee Minutes, December 10, 1931, NBIH Papers at JHSMW.
11. Committee for the Study of Nursing Education (Josephine Goldmark, Secretary), *Nursing and Nursing Education in the United States* (New York: Macmillan, 1923), 26. Also see Philip A. Kalisch and Beatrice J. Kalisch, *American Nursing: A History*, 4th ed. (Philadelphia: Lippincott Williams and Wilkins, 2004), 226–228.
12. "Gives Last $5 to Beth Israel," *Newark Star-Eagle*, February 13, 1928.
13. "Report of the Director of the Nurses Training School to the Beth Israel Hospital Board," in Board Minutes, January 28, 1929.
14. Ibid.
15. Nurses Training School Committee Minutes, May 8, 1929, NBIH Papers at JHSMW.
16. Administrative Committee Minutes, January 28, 1930.
17. Ibid., September 8, 1930. The chain of command was Dr. Keller, the Nurses Training School director; Miss Marx, assistant director; and a new position of night nurse supervisor.
18. Outpatient Committee Minutes, March 30, 1929, NBIH Papers at JHSMW.
19. Annual Report, 1930.
20. "$3,000 Radium Found in Ashes after 4-Day Hunt in Newark," *New York Times*, October 6, 1930.
21. Dr. Lee K. Frankel, Introduction, *Annual Report, 1930*.
22. "Report of the Superintendent, presented at the Annual Meeting of the Board of Beth Israel Hospital," January 18, 1932.
23. "Dental Clinic of Beth Israel to Open Monday," *News*, February 24, 1928.
24. "Report of the Superintendent," January 18, 1932.
25. "Bamberger Gives $5,000,000 for Study—He and Sister, Mrs. Felix Fuld, Set Up Foundation in Newark to Aid Advanced Learning," *New York Times*, June 12, 1930.

26. "Latest Gift of $5,000,000 for Institute of Advanced Study Brings Bamberger, Fuld Philanthropies to Ten Millions," *Jewish Chronicle*, June 13, 1930.
27. "Flexner Gives Views on New Institute Here," *Jewish Chronicle*, July 18, 1930.
28. "Dr. Flexner to Speak Here Monday: Louis Bamberger to Act as Chairman," *Jewish Chronicle*, December 18, 1931.
29. "Name Einstein to Faculty of New Institute," *Jewish Chronicle*, October 14, 1932. The news story appeared next to the headline, "Dr. Meyer C. Ellenstein Elected to City Commission; First Jew to Hold High Office Here." Ellenstein would be appointed mayor by the city commissioners shortly afterward.
30. Outpatient Committee Minutes, May 5, 1931.
31. Samuel I. Kessler, Joel L. Schlesinger, and Sidney C. Keller, "Report of Special Committee on Personnel and Salaries, May 1932," Administrative Committee Minutes, May 11, 1932.
32. Administration and Medical Executive Committee Minutes, May 24, 1932.
33. Annual Meeting Minutes, January 16, 1934.
34. Dr. Eugene Parsonnet, recorded interviews transcribed by his son, Dr. Victor Parsonnet, secs. 7.6, 8.1, and 8.2, Parsonnet Papers at JHSMW.
35. Administrative Committee Minutes, January 23, 1935, May 25, 1936.
36. Paula Marx, "Report to the Board of Directors," Board Minutes, January 21, 1936.
37. "President's Annual Report," Board Minutes, January 27, 1936.
38. Rita Finkler, typewritten manuscript, Rita Finkler papers, University of Medicine and Dentistry of New Jersey Archives, Newark, 71 (hereinafter UMDNJ Archives).
39. Ibid., 141.
40. Leonard S. Morvay, "Relation of Dental Service to Medical Hospital Service," *Journal of the American Dental Association* 23 (June 1936): 960–972.
41. "Dr. Philip Levine New Bacteriologist Aid at Beth Israel," *Jewish Chronicle*, October 18, 1935; Board Minutes, December 28, 1936.
42. Maxwell M. Wintrobe, *Blood, Pure and Eloquent: A Story of Discovery, of People, and Ideas* (New York: McGraw-Hill, 1980), 695–703. Also, Douglass Starr, *Blood: An Epic History of Medicine and Commerce* (New York: Knopf, 1998), 209–210.
43. "President's Annual Report," Board Minutes, January 25, 1937.
44. *Medical Leaves* Inc. published five annual volumes, ceasing publication in 1943. All proceeds were contributed to the Histadruth, the Israel Labor Federation, which was dedicated to building a Jewish homeland on the basis of social justice and productive labor.
45. Goldenberg and Wolff quoted in Barry A. Lazarus, "The Practice of Medicine and Prejudice in a New England Town: The Founding of Mount Sinai Hospital, Hartford Connecticut," *Journal of American Ethnic History* 10 (spring 1991): 21, 35.
46. Leon Sokoloff, "The Rise and Decline of the Jewish Quota in Medical School Admissions," *Bulletin of the New York Academy of Medicine* 68 (November 1992): 498. See also Edward C. Halperin, "The Jewish Problem in U.S. Medical Education, 1920–1955," *Journal of the History of Medicine* 56 (April 2001): 140–167.
47. Kenneth M. Ludmerer, Time to Heal: American Medical Education from the Turn of the Century to the Era of Managed Care (New York: Oxford University Press, 1999), 64.

48. Sokoloff, "Rise and Decline," 500–501. Sokoloff derives much of this information from a report compiled by an investigating committee of the New York City Council in 1946.

49. C. Bachmeyer to Rabbi Morris S. Lazaron, February 24, 1934, and Arthur C. Curtis, MD, to Rabbi Morris S. Lazaron, February 20, 1934, in *Jews in Medicine Survey of Medical Schools, 1930–1934*, collection 71, file 37/16, Rabbi Morris Lazaron Papers, American Jewish Archives, Cincinnati, Ohio (hereinafter Lazaron Papers). Also, Sokoloff, "Rise and Decline," 500–501.

50. Dr. Arthur Bernstein interviews, January 21 and July 28, 1994, quoted at length in William B. Helmreich, *The Enduring Community: The Jews of Newark and MetroWest* (New Brunswick, N.J.: Transaction, 1999), 92.

51. Ludmerer, *Time to Heal*, 64.

52. Ibid.

53. Max Danzis, MD, "The Jew in Medicine," *American Hebrew and Jewish Tribune*, March 23, 1934, photocopy in Lazaron Papers.

54. Morris S. Lazaron, "The Jewish Student in Medicine," Lazaron Papers.

55. Burton D. Meyers to Rabbi Morris S. Lazaron, October 30, 1934, in *Jews in Medicine Survey*.

56. C. C. Bass, MD, to Rabbi Morris S. Lazaron, March 8, 1934, and Meyers to Lazaron, October 30, 1934, ibid.

57. Leon Sokoloff, "The Question of Antisemitism in American Medical Faculties, 1900–1945," *Patterns of Prejudice* 31 (1997): 47, 45.

58. Ibid., 53.

59. Gert H. Brieger, "Classics and Character: Medicine and Gentility," *Bulletin of the History of Medicine* 65 (spring 1991): 88–109.

60. Dan Oren, *Joining the Club: A History of Jews at Yale* (New Haven: Yale University Press, 1986), 136.

61. Dr. Arthur Bernstein, interview for the Jewish Historical Society, October 27, 1994, JHSMW.

62. Dr. Bernstein was joined by Dr. H. H. Kessler, who became chief of orthopedic services.

63. Aaron E. Parsonnet, MD, FACP, and Albert S. Hyman, AB, MD, FACP, coauthored two books: *Applied Electrocardiography: An Introduction to Electrocardiography for Physicians and Students* (New York: Macmillan, 1929) and *The Failing Heart of Middle Life: The Myocardosis Syndrome, Coronary Thrombosis and Angina Pectoris* (Philadelphia: F. A. Davis, 1932), with a section on the medico-legal aspects of sudden death from heart disease. Three Parsonnet brothers—Victor, Thomas, and Aaron—would die of sudden massive myocardial infarctions.

64. Dr. Arthur Bernstein, interview with the authors, Maplewood, NJ, September 12, 1999.

65. Max Danzis, MD, "The New Jersey State Committee for Refugee Physicians," *Medical Leaves* 5 (1943): 116.

66. Board Minutes, March 27, 1939.

67. Board Minutes, April 28, 1940.

68. Ibid.

69. Board Minutes, June 23, 1941.

70. Board Minutes, October 26, 1942.
71. Dr. Arthur Bernstein, interviews with the authors, Maplewood, NJ, September 12, 1999, and August 4, 1994.
72. Board Minutes, January 23, 1943.
73. Dr. Eugene Parsonnet interview by son, Dr. Victor Parsonnet, sec. 11.4, Parsonnet Papers at JHSMW.
74. Dr. Samuel Diener, interview by author, Newark, NJ, July 17, 2000.
75. Newark Beth Israel *Bulletin* 2 (May 1943), NBIH Papers, JHSMW.
76. Board Minutes, January 24, 1944.
77. Bernice Anderson to Adele Zeiman, April 6, 1943, in Board Minutes, April 6, 1943.
78. "Cancer Clinics Approved," *New York Times*, January 4, 1943.
79. The information on the origin of residency programs is derived from Rosemary Stevens, *American Medicine and the Public Interest: A History of Specialization*, rev. ed. (Berkeley: University of California Press, 1998), 120–121, 156–157.
80. Max Danzis, "Jewish Hospitals and Facilities for Graduate Training," *Medical Leaves* 3 (1940): 65–74.
81. Ibid.
82. Ibid.
83. Dr. Eugene Parsonnet interview by his son, Dr. Victor Parsonnet, secs. 27.1–27.2, Parsonnet Papers at JHSMW.
84. Board Minutes, February 23, 1946.
85. Vannevar Bush, *Science, the Endless Frontier: a Report to the President* (Washington, D.C.: United States Government Printing Office, 1945). Also, Roosevelt to Bush, November 17, 1944, vii–viii.
86. Roosevelt to Bush, November 17, 1944, 47–48.
87. Dr. Eugene Parsonnet interview by son, Dr. Victor Parsonnet, sec. 11.4, Parsonnet Papers at JHSMW.
88. "Henry H. Kessler, Newark Orthopedist," obituary, *New York Times*, January 19, 1978.

CHAPTER 6   *The Modern Institution at Midcentury*

1. Rosemary Stevens, *In Sickness and in Wealth: Twentieth Century American Hospitals* (New York, Basic Books, 1989), 1, 14.
2. Ibid., 228.
3. "City Census Lists 420,000 Persons, Loss of 22,000," *Newark Star-Ledger*, May 1, 1940.
4. John T. Cunningham, *Newark*, rev. ed. (Newark: New Jersey Historical Society, 1988), 99.
5. Bartholomew Report quoted in ibid.
6. Charles V. Craster, "Slum Clearance," *American Journal of Public Health* 39 (September 1944): 936.
7. Ibid., 937.
8. "Orthodox Congregations Complete Merger Details," *News*, December 14, 1935.
9. In April 1928, the Administrative Committee approved for patients' rooms the purchase of fans that were permanently attached and had lock switches; the

portable fans initially supplied were "leaving" with discharged patients (Administrative Committee Minutes, April 25, 1928).

10. Donna Marie Rey, interview by Deborah Kraut, Newark Beth Israel Medical Center, Newark, NJ, June 20, 2001. Rey won a scholarship from Beth Israel Hospital for a two-year associate degree in nursing when the diploma school merged with Essex County College.

11. Dr. Fred Cohen, interview by Alan Kraut, Newark Beth Israel Medical Center, Newark, NJ, July 26, 2001.

12. "Boy's Faithful Dog Keeps Vigil at Hospital," *News*, April 16, 1951.

13. "Pike Dedication November 30," *Newark Star-Ledger*, November 21, 1951.

14. "Turnpike Route Is Set Here—Plans Call for 4.25 Miles across the Meadowlands," *Newark Star-Ledger*, May 7, 1950.

15. Steve Anderson, "The Roads of Metro New York 1996–2000," *www.nycroads.com*. Anderson refers to "New Roads with New Numbers Will Parallel Old U.S. Routes," *New York Times*, September 19, 1958. Interstate 280 was originally known as the Essex Freeway and began in the east at the Stickel Memorial Bridge, spanning the Passaic River that opened in 1948. The same year that I-78 was authorized, the proposal was to connect the New Jersey Turnpike with I-80, extending from the older suburbs of the Oranges west to still-rural Morris County. A freeway, I-75, was also proposed to connect I-78 with the proposed I-280, directly through Newark, extending north between Hillside and Belmont Avenues, then Prince, Boston, and Wilsey Streets. The interchange would extensively widen the exit at Fabyan Place, swallowing more streets from Meeker to Hawthorne Avenue in Weequahic ("To Link Freeways," *Newark Sunday News*, January 26, 1964).

16. "Freeway Network," *Newark Star-Ledger*, July 9, 1961, includes a good map of the roads that had been built by 1961 (Garden State Parkway and New Jersey Turnpike) and the freeways under construction, including I-78, I-280, I-287, that would connect them with I-80.

17. "Challenged Map," *Newark Star-Ledger*, May 25, 1961, presents a good diagram of the three paths of I-78. The Weequahic Plan would follow the path of the old Route 22 through Weequahic Park, but go through Hillside; the Mayor Carlin plan would bisect Hillside slightly north; and the state plan, which with slight variations ultimately prevailed, would run through Weequahic. This account draws on the *Newark Star-Ledger*'s coverage of the fight over I-78 from 1961 through 1964.

18. Frank Prial, "Weequahic: Troubled Eden," *Newark Sunday News*, June 25, 1961.

19. "Highway Path," *Newark Sunday News*, June 4, 1961. A diagram of the thirteen structures that were affected by the I-78 construction from Clinton Avenue to Chancellor Avenue included Torah Chaim Jewish Center, Bet Yeled School, Bragaw Avenue School, Bethlehem Evangelical and Reformed Church, Chevra Radfee Sholem, Congregation Tefereth Zion, Hawthorne Avenue School, South Ward Boys Club, Congregation Kehilah Israel, Congregation Talmud Torah, Mount Calvary Baptist Church, Peshine Avenue School, and Saint Charles Church and Parochial School.

20. The four stores were Argyle Men's Shop, Gertrude's, Sybil's, and Murray Lavigne Children's Shoes, *Jewish News*, February 19, 1965.

21. Dr. Eugene Parsonnet, recorded interviews transcribed by his son, Dr. Victor Parsonnet, sec. 29.4, Parsonnet Papers at JHSMW.

22. "Dr. Parsonnet Named as Chairman of United Jewish Appeal Campaign," *[Newark] Jewish News*, October 16, 1959. Dr. Parsonnet also became head of the new suburban YM-YWHA Jewish Community Center of Essex County (ibid., May 20, 1960). He was succeeded by Alan Sagner.

23. "Jewish Center Need Stressed," *News*, January 23, 1951. Also, "Center to Get New Quarters," *Jewish News*, November 2, 1951. The High Street Newark Center was sold to the King William Grand Lodge, AF&AM, Inc., in 1954.

24. Minutes of the Board of Trustees, Jewish Community Council, October 20, 1953, JHSMW. The Newark Y straddled two buildings during the 1950s, moving into a new center in 1959 that closed ten years later.

25. "B'nai Abraham Will Dedicate Facilities at Suburban House," *Jewish News*, June 5, 1958; Jose Ann Steinbock, "Congregation Oheb Shalom Moves—Goes to South Orange after 99 Years in Newark," *Jewish News*, July 11, 1958. The ceremonies at the High Street building included closing the doors with the same key that had been used to open them in 1911.

26. William B. Helmreich, *The Enduring Community: The Jews of Newark and MetroWest* (New Brunswick, N.J.: Transaction, 1999), 212–213.

27. "Will Close Children's Home; Has Been in Use since 1898," *Jewish News*, June 30, 1955.

28. The Theresa Grotta Center was established on March 21, 1916, through the Aid Society and named in honor of Grotta on the occasion of her eightieth birthday. The society sponsored walks in the forest and fresh air and supplied milk and eggs for needy patients, then rented a house in Verona in 1923, and later acquired a cottage in Caldwell that was expanded to a forty-two-bed facility, which became a rehabilitation center in 1942. By the mid-1950s, suburbs had replaced the forest. The Grotta rehabilitation center became a drug center, then a group home, and by the late 1980s was abandoned. By 1994 when the vacant building was purchased for $320,000, the facility was in the middle of an affluent residential community; efforts to convert it into a bed and breakfast were being fought by its neighbors in 1999 (Rebecca Goldsmith, "W. Caldwell Balks at Bed and Breakfast Proposal," *Newark Star-Ledger*, February 21, 1999).

29. "Letters on Newark and the Suburbs," *Jewish News*, September 26, 1958. The *Jewish News* began publication in 1950.

30. Board Minutes, October 24, 1949.

31. Administrative Committee Minutes, October 24, 1949.

32. Ibid., May 23, 1949.

33. Ibid., June 25, 1951.

34. Ibid., September 24 and October 22, 1951.

35. "Council Makes Grant of $100,000 to Newark Beth Israel Hospital for 1951— Added Funds to Be Contingent on Total Sum Raised by UJA," *Jewish News*, February 23, 1951.

36. Board Minutes, February 26, 1951.

37. Board Minutes, June 25, 1951.

38. "Positions on Issues between Council and Beth Israel Hospital Are Presented," *Jewish News*, December 4, 1953. Statements by Simond T. Shifman and Louis Stern, the president of the Jewish Community Council, were published in their entirety. Shifman was succeeded by Norman Karpf in January 1955.

39. Administrative Committee Minutes, February 24, 1953, NBIH Papers at JHSMW.

40. Minutes of the Board of Trustees, Jewish Community Council, April 20, 1954. The move toward reconciliation was developed on the morning of the UJA special-gifts dinner, March 25, 1954.

41. "Speech as Delivered by Leo Yanoff at Annual Meeting of the Jewish Community Council, December 17, 1959 at The Goldman, West Orange," JHSMW.

42. Stevens, *In Sickness and in Wealth: American Hospitals in the Twentieth Century*, 218.

43. Dorsey Woodson, "Colorado's Fighting General: Maurice Rose," *Empire Magazine (Denver Post)*, November 27, 1960. The opening date was given by Ms. Touchon, director of the Rose Medical Center volunteers.

44. "A History of Minneapolis: Religion, Social Services, and Medicine," Minneapolis Public Library, *www.mplib.org/history*. See also Pamela Hill Lampert, "Heritage Lives On after the Doors Close," *Minnesota Medicine* 74 (December 1991): 17–22.

45. "About Us," Weiss Memorial Hospital, *www.weisshospital.org*.

46. For the survey, see Tina Levitan, *Islands of Compassion: A History of the Jewish Hospitals of New York* (Manchester, N.H.: Olympic Marketing, 1998), 272; Eugene D. Rosenfeld, MD, and Louis Allen Abramson, "The Tenth Plan Passed All Tests," *Modern Hospital* 82 (May 1954): 70–72; the hospital was the May 1954 modern hospital of the month.

47. Material on the Hill-Burton Act is from Rosemary Stevens, *American Medicine and the Public Interest: A History of Specialization*, rev. ed. (Berkeley: University of California Press, 1998), 216–224. Also, Paul Starr, *The Social Transformation of American Medicine* (New York: Basic Books, 1982), 348–351.

48. See *www.nursing.upenn.edu/history/collections/aemc.htm*. In 1952 three Jewish hospitals merged in Philadelphia: Jewish Hospital became the eastern division, Mount Sinai the southern division, and Northern Liberties the northern division of the Albert Einstein Medical Center. Two hospital nursing schools also merged.

49. "Contributes $1 Million Dollars to Baltimore Medical Center," *Jewish News*, July 20, 1951. The Mount Pleasant building of the center opened in 1953 and the complete hospital in October 1959.

50. Malcolm M. Manber, "Hospitals Prepare for More Patients," *News*, November 13, 1964. Bernard Weinraub, "51 Patients Are Moved in Jersey as Old Hospital Gets New Home," *New York Times*, November 30, 1964; and "Century of Service Ends for Newark's St. Barnabas," *News*, November 30, 1964.

51. Donald M. Rosenberger, "How Mergers Begin and How They Work," *Modern Hospital* 107 (July 1966): 85.

52. Ibid., 89.

53. "Will Dedicate New Hospital Laboratory Building May 5," *Jewish News*, April 26, 1957.

54. "Event Honors Dr. Goldman," *Jewish News*, November 25, 1955.

55. Alan Sagner, interview by Alan Kraut, Morristown, NJ, July 18, 2000.

56. Board of Trustees Minutes, December 26, 1956.

57. Board of Trustees Minutes, January 28, 1957.

58. Board of Trustees Minutes, September 20, 1965. The concept of a master plan was presented by Isadore and Zachary Rosenfeld in "The Best Answer to Growing Pains Is a Master Plan," *Modern Hospital* 104 (March 1965), 112–115. See also "Architects Rendering of the Proposed New Addition to Newark Beth Israel Hospital," *News*, December 3, 1965.

59. "Five Newark Hospitals Join Forces to Raise $25 Million for Modernization and Expansion," *News*, August 25, 1961. Also, "Hospitals Obsolete, Crowded," *News*, April 25, 1961.

60. "Proposed New Building Program," approved by the Board of Trustees, October 26, 1965, NBIH Papers at JHSMW.

61. Alan Sagner, interview by Alan Kraut, Morristown, NJ, March 5, 2005.

62. James Hopkins, telephone interview with Deborah Kraut, June 2001.

63. Martin Cherkasky, MD, "Why We Signed a Union Agreement," *Modern Hospital* 93 (July 1959): 69–70. The hospital workers were covered by the Fair Labor Standards Act effective January 1966, as the hospitals began to prepare for Medicare (*Modern Hospital* 105 [September 1965]).

64. "Union Report Shows 750,000 Hospital Workers Are Outside Minimum Wage Law," *Modern Hospital* 98 (April 1962): 21.

65. "Beth Israel Has Crisis," *News*, November 16, 1950. The Beth could not match the new Veterans Hospital, which offered to nurses an entry-level salary of $3,400 with a maximum of 6,400.

66. "Sees Nurses Return," *News*, November 17, 1950.

67. Board Minutes, February 25, 1945.

68. Board Minutes, May 27, 1946.

69. "Value Clinical Cases," *News*, November 5, 1952.

70. Board Minutes, October 23, 1950. George Furst, the chair of the Nursing Committee, recommended that consideration be given to discontinuing the School of Nursing, as it was costing at least $3,000 to train each nurse and most were leaving the hospital upon graduation.

71. Barbara L. Brush, "The Exchange Visitor Program, 1945–1990," *Nursing History Review* 1 (1993): 171–180.

72. Board Minutes, October 25, 1954.

73. Nurses, interviews by Deborah Kraut, NBIMC, June 2001.

74. Ibid. The anecdote of being introduced to Ms. Champagne was told by several interviewees to Deborah Kraut.

75. Board of Trustees Minutes, June 27, 1966. The building was opened in June 1966, but dedication ceremony scheduled during the period that the United Nations was in session.

76. "A.N.A. Takes Play away from N.L.N.—Says All Nursing Personnel Should Be Trained outside Hospitals," *Modern Hospital* 106 (January 1966): 32.

77. Cherkasky, "Why We Signed a Union Agreement."

78. Sanford Gottlieb, "How Unions Are Doing in Hospital Campaigns," *Modern Hospital* 94 (March 1960): 109–111, 151.

79. Ibid.
80. Duane R. Carson, "Labor Union: Color It White, Black, or Red," *Modern Hospital* 105 (August 1965): 107–111, 182.
81. Martin Luther King Jr. communication to Moe Foner, given by Foner to the authors; and quoted in Leon Fink and Brian Greenberg, *Upheaval in the Quiet Zone: A History of Hospital Workers' Union, Local 1199* (Urbana: University of Illinois Press, 1989), 103.
82. "STAT—Hospital Union Wins Elections at Six New Jersey Medical Facilities," *Modern Hospital* 103 (November 1964): 21.
83. "New Jersey Hospitals Facing Massive Drive by Drug and Hospital Union," *Modern Hospital* 103 (October 1964): 20D.
84. "About People—Administrators," *Modern Hospital* 92 (May 1959): 80.
85. "New Beth Israel (Newsletter) Reports Activities at Hospital," *Jewish News*, March 17, 1961.
86. Edelschick, the director of the Social Services Department, retired in 1962 in name only; she continued to serve as a paid consultant to the new director and the new assistant director who replaced her. Schwarz, the director of the Outpatient Department that had averaged thirty thousand patients per year for thirty years, retired in September 1963; the thirty clinics began to decrease their services. Eight more long-time employees retired by 1966, including Sadie Paul, chief housekeeper, who received a gold watch from the board of trustees. In January 1967, Sophia L. Morris, MA, the director of Dietary Services since the opening of the hospital in 1928, retired.
87. Administrative Committee Minutes, September 22, 1964, NBIH Papers at JHSMW.
88. "STAT—Hospital Union Wins Elections," November 1964.
89. Administrative Committee Minutes, September 28, 1964. Also Malcolm Manber, "Hospitals Are Urged to Delay Unionizing," *News*, September 24, 1964.
90. Minutes of the Board of Trustees, September 18, 1964.
91. Ibid.
92. Board Minutes, March 28, 1949.
93. Robert Cunningham III and Robert M. Cunningham, Jr., *The Blues: A History of the Blue Cross and Blue Shield System* (DeKalb: University of Northern Illinois Press, 1997), 97.
94. Ibid.
95. Stevens, *In Sickness and in Wealth: American Hospitals in the Twentieth Century*, 262.
96. Administrative Committee Minutes, September 24, 1956.
97. "No Medicare Boycott for Beth," *Jewish News*, March 2, 1962.
98. "Doctors, Hospital Men Fear New Over-65 Care Will Strain Facilities," *Wall Street Journal*, August 20, 1965; "Many MDs Doubt Plan to Prevent Overuse of Hospitals Will Work," ibid., October 28, 1965.
99. Harry Becker, "Medicare: What It Means, What It Covers, How It Works," *Modern Hospital* 105 (August 1965): 27–42.
100. Medicaid was the related federal program funded with block grants to the states. Some expected it to dwarf the program for the aged, as it was predicted that

nearly 35 million Americans would be covered by the Title 19 programs (Frank J. Prial, "And Now 'Medicaid,' Sweeping Health Plans Open to All Age Groups May Dwarf Medicare," *Wall Street Journal*, September 2, 1966).

101. Stevens, *In Sickness and in Wealth, American Hospitals in the Twentieth Century*, 274–275.

102. History of Social Security Act during the Johnson Administration, 1963–1968, Social Security Online, www.ssa.gov/history/ssa.htm.

103. J. A. Rosenkrantz, "The Impact of Medicare," *Journal of Newark Beth Israel Hospital* 18 (July 1967): 157 (hereinafter, *Journal*).

104. Ibid., 152.

105. Ibid., 151–157.

106. Stanley S. Bergen, Jr., "A Medical School and Its Community: The Newark Experience," in *From Riot to Recovery: Newark after Ten Years*, ed. Stanley B. Winters (Washington, DC: University Press of America, 1979), 317.

107. "Author Awaits Ironic Ending," *News*, June 21, 1967.

108. Stanley B. Winters, "Medical Politics and Ghetto Resistance in the New Newark," in *From Riot to Recovery: Newark after Ten Years*, 45–52. See also these 1967 *News* articles: James Cusick, "Relocation Is Stressed," June 14; and Bob Shabazian, "Med School Protest," January 11; "Med School Value Told," January 12; "Medical Site Is Really Ailing," May 11; "Plan Board Postpones Interrupted Med School, " May 24; "Med School Pact Voted by Council," May 25; "Med School Foes May Block Funds," June 18.

109. "Negro for Top Court," "Protests Resume at Blight Hearing," and "Johnson Waiting," *News*, June 13, 1967.

110. "Interrupted Med School Hearing," *News*, May 24, 1967; and "Joachim Prinz Leaving Temple," *News*, May 17, 1967.

111. William Gordon, "A Neighborhood of Fear," *News*, January 26, 1967; and Douglas Eldridge, "Protest Resumes at Meat Market," *News*, April 9, 1967.

112. J. A. Rosenkrantz, MD, "Hospital Administration and the Emergency Service," *Journal* 14, 4 (October 1963): 245–251. The emergency room was essentially unchanged four years later. The October 1963 issue of the *Journal* was devoted to the review of the hospital's emergency room, noting an increase of 367 percent in the number of cases and admissions from 1947 to 1962, with little change in the physical configuration of the room from the original 1928 design. Articles addressed the medical conditions presented by those admitted for emergency treatment: acute appendicitis, cardiac arrest, gastrointestinal bleeding, anaphylactic reactions, fractures, accidental poisoning, and penetrating chest wounds caused by knives and bullets. Nearly half of the incoming to the emergency room presented non-urgent medical issues, indicating that the neighborhood regarded the Beth Israel emergency room as a de facto community health center.

113. James Cusick, "Trouble Centered on Man Few Knew," *News*, July 13, 1967.

114. "Snipers Fire on Newark Hospital," *Hospitals, JAHA* 31 (August 1, 1967): 19.

115. Edward Higgins, "Hospitals Swamped," *News*, July 14, 1967. Also, "Beth Israel Treated Many Victims of Riot," *Jewish News*, July 21, 1967.

116. John D. Kirwan, "One Man's Newark," *National Review*, August 8, 1967, 847. Kirwan provides an eyewitness account of the city during the four days of riots.

117. Charles Q. Finley, "Brothers Honor King in Newark," *Newark Star-Ledger*, April 8, 1968.
118. "Thousands Set to Walk," *Newark Star-Ledger*, April 5, 1968.
119. "Speech by Mrs. Samuel Einhorn to the Annual Women's Auxiliary Luncheon, June 10, 1968," NBIH Papers at JHSMW.
120. Ibid.
121. Alan Sagner, telephone interview with Alan Kraut, March 30, 2005.

CHAPTER 7   *Medical Research at Midcentury*

1. Autobiography of Dr. Rita Finkler, unpublished manuscript, UMDNJ, 85.
2. Kenneth Tyson, interview with Alan Kraut, NBIMC, June 5, 2001.
3. For the American Hospital Association creed, see " 'My Pledge and Creed' Wins Universal Approval at Buffalo Conference," *Modern Hospital* 23 (November 1924): 460–461. The Creed of the Newark Beth Israel Hospital first appears in the 1928 Beth Israel records and minutes, as well as on commemorative memorabilia; its author remains unknown.
4. Dr. Samuel Diener, interview with Alan Kraut, Short Hills, NJ, July 19, 2000.
5. Fiftieth Anniversary Celebration Committee Minutes, July 17, 1950, NBIH Papers at JHSMW.
6. For the establishment of the residencies, Board Minutes, November 27, 1944; for the discussion of salaries for residents also receiving an allowance under the Veterans Readjustment Act, "G.I. Bill," Board Minutes, April 25, 1949.
7. Administrative Committee Minutes, March 27, 1950, NBIH Papers at JHSMW. Also "Radioisotope Center's Opening to Be Held Tuesday Evening," *Jewish News*, February 25, 1951.
8. Administrative Committee Minutes, September 26, 1949.
9. Board Minutes, April 25, 1949.
10. Board Minutes, March 28, 1949. The scientific journal was estimated to cost $3,000 per year, the cost to be offset by ads and subscriptions
11. Catalogue of holdings, National Library of Medicine, Bethesda, Maryland. The catalogue is by no means exhaustive or complete.
12. Editorial, *Journal* 14 (1964), 1: 85.
13. A history of the hospital would appear only twice, both in reprints of speeches. The first, written by Dr. Danzis and excerpted from Dr. Robbins's article, was reprinted in the January 1952 *Journal*. The second was a speech that Dr. Eugene Parsonnet gave to the medical staff and was printed in the 1973 issue of the *Journal*.
14. Dr. Arthur Bernstein, interview with the authors, Maplewood, NJ, May 2000. Dr. Bernstein also recounted this story in an interview recorded in 1993, UMDNJ Archives. The obituaries of Beth physicians were intensely personal, such as the one for Dr. Julius Newman: "He was a fun-loving man who enjoyed life. He would always produce a story to fit the occasion be it in the doctor's room, at the lunch table, or at a dinner party. His descriptive stories of old Beth Israel incidents, his army life and the one that got away were gems. His loss leaves a void among us."

15. Dr. B. H. Greenfield was listed among those at the July 18, 1901, meeting that is the first entry of the Official Ledger. He practiced in Newark for forty years; his name appears in the Medical Staff Minutes. He retired to Miami Beach, where he died in 1962. "Dr. B. H. Greenfield, a Hospital Founder," obituary, *New York Times*, July 3, 1962.

16. Dr. Danzis was scheduled to speak on the history of medicine at the opening ceremony of the radioisotope center, but told others that when "the strong hand of the grippe 'gripped him'" he took to his bed and gave his speech to Dr. Harold Goldberg, the chief of staff, to read.

17. Seven of the films addressed cancer, with titles such as *The Traitor Within, Time Is Life*, and *Challenge: Science against Cancer.* Consistent with the socially conservative 1950s, the first afternoon was reserved for women only to watch the films *Having a Baby* and *Breast-Self-Examination.* The evening programs offered formal lectures delivered by professors from New York University (NYU) School of Medicine, Temple University School of Medicine, and Jefferson Medical College. The Thursday-evening program chaired by hospital superintendent I. E. Behrman featured greetings by board president Abraham Lichtman; Mayor Ralph Villani; Dr. Harold Goldberg, the president of the medical staff; J. Harold Johnston, the executive director of the New Jersey Hospital Association; and Alan Lowenstein, chair of the Jewish Community Council of Essex County. Dr. Danzis delivered a history of the hospital. The Friday program was chaired by Fannie Katz, RN, the newest director of the Nursing School; its evening speaker was Professor Estelle Osborne, assistant professor of nursing education at NYU (Program of Events, Dinner-Dance of the Fiftieth Anniversary of the Beth Israel Hospital, Newark Beth Israel Papers). The program for the dance listed the trustees, senior medical staff, emeritus medical chiefs, and officers of the Ladies Volunteer League, including the past presidents of the auxiliary and the guild, as well as a reprint of the 1928 Creed of Beth Israel.

18. In 1953, Newark also mourned the death of Dr. Charles Craster, who had served as its public health officer for thirty-eight years, and the hospital world mourned the death of Otho Ball, the founder and publisher of *Modern Hospital.*

19. "Honor Memory of Dr. Danzis at Dinner Tendered to Family," *[Newark] Jewish News*, February 5, 1955. Dr. Hossein Eslami, who enjoyed a long and fruitful career at the hospital, was the first recipient of the award

20. Dr. Finkler was the eldest member of the Essex County physicians branch of the United Jewish Appeal. Her oft-told stories of swallowing half the Red Sea while skin-diving in the Middle East were favorites of her Beth colleagues. See "Dr. Finkler Constantly Active with Endocrinology, Hobbies," *Jewish News*, February 24, 1956; www.umdnj.edu/libweb/speccoll/Finkler.html.

21. "New Hope in Blood Ailment Is Found in Study at Beth Israel," *Jewish News*, April 11, 1952. The hospital would open the first hemophilia center in the world in 1953.

22. "New Method Seen Aiding Hemophilia," *New York Times*, April 11, 1952.

23. "This Issue: An Innovation," *Journal* 3 (October 1952): 304.

24. Administrative Committee Minutes, September 22, 1958.

25. For a history of renal dialysis, see J. Stewart Cameron, *A History of the Treatment of Renal Failure by Dialysis* (New York: Oxford University Press, 2002).

26. Dr. Seymour Ribot, interview by Alan Kraut, at NBIMC, July 17, 2000.

27. See *Journal* 14 (April 1963): 95–117: Milton Shoskes, Louis J. Kampel, Jerold Moss, Bertram Levinstone, and Seymour Ribot, "The Use of Artificial Renal Dialysis Techniques for the Removal of Bilirubin in the Dog"; Maxwell Klausner, Seymour Ribot, and Gabriel Yelin, "The Role of the Artificial Kidney in the Treatment of the Anuric Phase of Acute Glomerulomnephritis"; Victor Parsonnet, Jacob Rabinowitz, and Seymour Ribot, "Superior Mesenteric Vein to Inferior Vena Cava Shunt: An Effective Method for Decompression of the Portal Venous System."

28. Annual Report, 1962, NBIH Papers at JHSMW.

29. Elie Faust, "Beth Israel Marks Advances in Heart, Cancer Research," *Jewish News*, August 11, 1961.

30. Editorial, *Journal* 14 (January 1963): 85

31. Phyllis J. Epstein, "Use Very Latest Techniques in Delicate Heart Operations," *Newark Jewish News*, June 10, 1955.

32. W. Bruce Fye, *American Cardiology: The History of a Specialty and Its College* (Baltimore: Johns Hopkins University Press, 1966), 216.

33. Dr. Eugene Parsonnet interviews, transcribed by his son, Dr. Victor Parsonnet, section. 32.3, Parsonnet Papers at JHSMW.

34. Faust, "Beth Israel Marks Advances," *Jewish News*, August 11, 1961.

35. John Y. Templeton III and John H. Gibbon, "Evaluation of Current Cardiac Surgical Procedures," *Journal* 9, 2 (April 1958): 87–96.

36. "Beth Israel Hospital Given New Hypothermia Machine," *Newark Jewish News*, July 15, 1961.

37. Annual Report, 1962.

38. Fye, *American Cardiology*, 272.

39. George H. Myers and Victor Parsonnet, "Biomedical Engineering: Current Applications at the Newark Beth Israel Hospital," *Journal* 15 (April 1964): 71–87.

40. Kirk Jeffrey and Victor Parsonnet, "From Bench to Bedside: Cardiac Pacing, 1960–1985: A Quarter Century of Medical and Industrial Innovation," 1978–1991," *Circulation* 97 (May 19, 1998): 1978–1991.

41. Ibid.

42. "Adult Cardiovascular Training Programs," *American Journal of Cardiology* 34 (1974): 449–456, as cited in Fye, *American Cardiology*, Table A9: "Cardiology Training Programs and Cardiology Fellows" (1941–1995), 346.

43. *Jewish News*, March 26, 1973.

44. In 1979, Drs. Parsonnet, Seymour Furman, Dryden Moore, and Warren Harthorne founded the North American Society of Pacing and Electrophysiology (NASPE).

45. J. A. Rosenkrantz, "Hospital Administration and Medical Staff Responsibilities," *Journal* 11 (January 1960): 5.

46. Ibid.

47. Administrative Committee Minutes, June 22 1964.

48. Editorial, *Journal* 1 (January 1950): 90.

49. "Might Be Medical School Base," *News*, July 23, 1950. The hopes were dashed again in 1954, when Jersey City won the competition for a medical school.

50. "Two Hospitals Study Plan for Big Center," *News*, May 19, 1950. See also, "New Hospital Need Is Told," *Newark Sunday News*, January 15, 1950.

51. "Two Medical Schools Are Accredited in 1962," *Modern Hospital* 99 (December 1962): 155.
52. "Mt. Sinai to Open Medical School," *New York Times*, July 8, 1963, 31. Eamanuel Perlmutter, "Medical School May Join City U.," *New York Times*, June 20, 1967, 1. See also M. A. Farber, "Medical School Joined to City U.," *New York Times*, August 3, 1967, 35.
53. "Medical Education in the Community Hospital," editorial, *Journal* 14 (April 1963): 166.
54. William G. Rothstein, *American Medical Schools and the Practice of Medicine: A History* (New York: Oxford University Press, 1987), 318.
55. Board Minutes, December 27, 1965.
56. "Medical College Moves from Jersey City Medical Center after City Cuts Bed Supply," *Modern Hospital* 106 (February 1966): 196.
57. The description of the national trend has been excerpted from Rosemary Stevens, *American Medicine and the Public Interest: A History of Specialization*, rev. ed. (Berkeley: University of California Press, 1998), 300–301.
58. Ibid.
59. Ibid., 381–382.
60. "The Resident-Intern Problem," *Journal* 5, 136.
61. Newark Beth Israel brochure, box 2–8, NBIH Papers at JHSMW.
62. " 'Beth' Names Dr. Applebaum Medical Education Director," *Jewish News*, October 6, 1961.
63. "Beth Israel Again Assigned Requested Quota of Interns," *Jewish News*, March 15, 1963.
64. "New Beth Israel 'Newsletter' Reports Activities in the Hospital," *Jewish News*, March 17, 1961.
65. "Newark Beth Israel Hospital a Story of Many Miracles," *Jewish News*, December 13, 1963.
66. Annual Report, 1966, 47–48.
67. Annual Report, 1967, 76.
68. Ibid., 75.
69. Dr. Seymour Ribot, interview by Alan Kraut, at NBIMC, July 17, 2000.
70. Annual Report, 1967, Parsonnet Papers, JHSMW.
71. Ibid., 95–99. The Personnel Department reported that eighteen employees in the hospital who were eligible for retirement, but had chosen to remain working through 1967. Among the staff who chose to remain rather than retire in 1967 were four stalwarts of the Beth: Elsie Berger, Gertrude Williams, Lois Kearney, and Gussie Cohen. Elsie Berger supervised eleven employees who inspected and sewed made thousands of repairs to the dietary, maintenance, volunteer, operating room, nursing, and technician garments, and to the white jackets of the interns, residents, and physicians. Every cloth article used in the hospital with the exception of the bed linen was sewn in the linen room, and that included including the draperies and sheet panels separating the beds, the plastic covers for the equipment, and the gauze and flannel bandages and the belly binders for the nurseries were also made on the cutting tables in these rooms. The sewing room also noted ruefully that they would sometimes make some tailoring alterations to the physicians' and interns' jackets—whether taking

in or letting out. Gertrude Williams supervised the sixteen women and three orderlies of the Central Supply Department who wrapped and sterilized trays for all medical supplies, using only a handwritten inventory system. Lois Kearny, the chief telephone operator, managed to maintain a telephone system that was inadequate for calls at peak hours, and remained hopeful that the new doctors might let her know when they left the hospital. Gussie Cohen was no longer sitting in the center of the lobby, but from her information desk on the first floor, still managed to receive everyone who came into the hospital, while updating the patient statistics, including births, discharges, and expirations.

72. The American Hospital Association still listed thirteen diploma nursing schools at Jewish Hospitals: Michael Reese Hospital and Medical Center, Mount Sinai Medical Center (Chicago), Touro Infirmary, Sinai Hospital (Baltimore), Jewish Hospital (Missouri), Newark Beth Israel Hospital, Beth Israel Medical Center (New York City), Jewish Hospital of Brooklyn, Mount Sinai Hospital (New York City), Jewish Hospital of Cincinnati, Mount Sinai Hospital (Cleveland), Albert Einstein Medical Center, Montefiore Hospital (Pittsburgh), Mount Sinai Hospital (Milwaukee). The JAHA list, *Hospitals* 43 (August 1, 1969): 446–450.

73. "Competition or Collaboration between NBIMC and UMDNJ," a report of a May 19, 1995, meeting accompanying Lester M. Bornstein to Stanley S. Bergen Jr., June 27, 1995, in personal correspondence of Lester Bornstein.

74. "Five Hospitals Affiliate with Brown University," *Modern Hospital* 43 (July 1, 1969): 127.

75. "Consolidation Announced by Two New York Hospitals," *JAHA* 43 (July 1969): 118.

76. *The Voice*, special issue 5 (1974): 3. NBIH Papers at JHSMW.

77. Ibid., 4.

78. Annual Report, 1975, 68–69, 20.

79. Board of Trustees Minutes, April 6, 1976.

80. John H. Kneels, "The Hospital," *Scientific American* 229 (September 1973): 130.

81. Ibid., 132.

82. "Answer to Soaring Hospital Costs," *Business Week* (July 7, 1975): 62–63.

83. "Special Announcement from the Publisher, Daniel McKelley," *Modern Hospital* 115 (February 1974): 5.

CHAPTER 8   *Redefining the Beth's Community*

1. Fred J. Cook, "Newark's Mayor Gibson—A Divided and Devastated City," *New York Times Magazine*, July 25, 1971.

2. Robert W. Maitlin, "State Promises to Clean Up Debris along Route 78," *Newark Star-Ledger*, October 2, 1968.

3. Cook, "Newark's Mayor Gibson."

4. "Hospital Reports Two More Assaults," *News*, January 3, 1968.

5. Cook, "Newark's Mayor Gibson."

6. Lester Bornstein had won the Bronze Star Medal for bravery in combat against the Nazis at the Battle of the Bulge. His hands shaking, he had unintentionally disabled two bazooka shells before he managed to load a third, his last one, and helped knock out a German tank headed directly for his position.

7. Richard L. Johnson, "Urban Hospitals Face Three Choices: Move, Grow, or Change," *Modern Hospital* 108 (November 1967): 93–97.
8. "End of Hospital Shortage: Why the Turn Around," *U.S. News and World Report*, September 6, 1971, 72–74.
9. Kenneth Tyson, interview by Alan Kraut, at NBIMC, June 5, 2001.
10. June H. Malone, "A Housing Program for the Housekeeping Department," *Modern Hospital* 75 (1951): 126–130.
11. Board Minutes, February 24, 1969 NBIH Papers at JHSMW.
12. Lawrenz, Madden, and Associates, Inc., "Report of Consultation to the Nursing Department of Beth Israel Medical Center, Newark, New Jersey, January 1989," 2, Board Minutes, NBIH Papers at JHSMW.
13. "Bornstein Reports to Board of Trustees," *Jewish News*, September 27, 1971.
14. J. Buford, J. Waller, and C. Wilson, "Improving the Quality of Life through the Organization of Municipal Health Services," in *From Riot to Recovery: Newark after Ten Years*, ed. Stanley B. Winters (Washington, D.C.: University Press of America, 1979), 367–368.
15. Report of the Community Health and Planning Committee, appended to Board of Trustees Minutes, March 23, 1970.
16. Fox Butterfield, "New Complex Highlights the 2 Worlds of Newark," *New York Times*, August 15, 1971.
17. Board Minutes, September 6, 1968.
18. Ibid.
19. Board of Trustees Minutes, April 7, 1969.
20. Board Minutes, April 17, 1969.
21. For a discussion of CONS see Rosemary Stevens, *In Sickness and in Wealth: American Hospitals in the Twentieth Century* (New York: Basic Books, 1989), 307.
22. See www.shpda.state.al.us/History.html#2.
23. Memo from M. Bernadrik [Grant Development, board member] to Lester Bornstein, November 10, 1975.
24. Board of Trustees Minutes, September 17, 1975.
25. Ibid., January 28, 1974.
26. In 1970, the loan was extended to 255 months and increased by $1 million (Board of Directors Executive Committee Minutes, December 15, 1970). For the 1974 agreement, see Secretary's Certificate of the Newark Israel Board of Trustees, August 1974, NBIH Papers at JHSMW.
27. Board of Trustees Minutes, December 23, 1974.
28. "Economizers," *Building Design and Construction*, December 1974, included in Board of Trustees Minutes, September 17, 1975.
29. Board of Trustees Minutes, September 23, 1974.
30. *The Voice* 5, special issue (1974): 1, NBIH Papers at JHSMW.
31. Richard J. H. Johnston, "Byrne and Gibson Lead the Dedication of Newark Beth Israel's New Pavilion," *New York Times*, November 11, 1974.
32. Board of Trustees Minutes, December 13, 1971.
33. Victor Parsonnet to Lester Z. Lieberman, July 13, 1976, memo attached to Board of Trustees Minutes of that date.
34. Board of Trustees Minutes, April 21, 1975.

35. Ibid., September 8, 1975.
36. Lester Bornstein, interview with Alan Kraut, West Orange, NJ, June 29, 2000.
37. Ibid.
38. Board of Trustees Minutes, December 11, 1978.
39. "The Promise Has Never Been Broken," Newark Beth Israel Medical Center Office of Development, publicity brochure, circa 1982, JHSMW. The brochure presents an excellent aerial from the southwest looking north for a view of the Pavilion and tower buildings, as well as buildings later replaced by the parking garage, and the ambulatory center with the pedestrian bridge over Osborne Terrace.
40. Lieberman, interview, July 18, 2000.
41. Bruce Shoulson, telephone interview with Alan Kraut, October 29, 2004.
42. Board of Trustees of Beth Healthcare Service Corporation Minutes, May 24, 1993.
43. Lieberman, interview, July 18, 2000.
44. Newark Beth Israel Medical Center House Staff Manual, prepared by Julia Dector, M.D., Director, Medical Education, and Dorothy E. Dennison, Director, Public Relations, circa 1980, 4, NBIH Papers at JHSMW.
45. Leda A. Judd, "Federal Involvement in Health Care after 1945," *Current History*, May/June 1977, 201–206.
46. Stevens, *In Sickness and in Wealth*, 323–327; "Between You and Your Doctor," *Wall Street Journal*, February 6, 1984.
47. Victor Parsonnet to Lester Bornstein, September 4, 1979 and Bornstein to Parsonnet, October 12, 1979, Bornstein personal correspondence.
48. Geraldine Dallek, "Hospital Care for Profit," *Society*, July/August 1986, 55.
49. Carolyn Phillips, "Harsh Medicine: Medicare's New Limits on Hospital Payments Force Wide Cost Cuts," *Wall Street Journal*, May 2, 1984.
50. "Grotta Center Affiliates with Beth Israel," *Newark Sunday News*, March 24, 1968.
51. Board of Trustees Minutes, January 22, 1973.
52. Doctors on Duty, Immediate Medical Care, "Client Employee Marketing," 1987. By 1987, shortly after the program was organized, the client list included such prominent companies as Hermans Sporting Goods, Holiday Inn, Lord and Taylor, and the Irvington Township Police.
53. Jennifer Bingham Hull, "Medical Turmoil: Four Hospital Chains, Facing Lower Profits, Adopt New Strategies," *Wall Street Journal*, October 10, 1985.
54. "Hospitals a Sick Industry," *U.S. News and World Report*, March 18, 1985.
55. Michael Waldholz, "Most Hospitals Quickly Learn to Be Profitable," *Wall Street Journal*, August 28, 1985.
56. American Hospital Association, "Guidelines for Managing Hospital Closures," *Report of the Ad Hoc Committee on Hospital Closures* (Chicago: American Hospital Association, 1990), 1.
57. Dr. Lee K. Frankel, Introduction, Annual Report, 1930, NBIH Papers at JHSMW.

CHAPTER 9 *The Changing Shape of Health Care*

1. David McKelly, "Special Announcement," *Modern Hospital* 115 (February 1974): 2.

2. Bradford H. Gray and Walter J. McNerney, "Special Report: For-Profit Enterprise in Health Care, the Institute of Medicine Study," *New England Journal of Medicine* 314 (June 5, 1986): 1528.
3. "Business Bulletin," *Wall Street Journal*, September 20, 1984, 1.
4. Rosemary Stevens, "Past Is Prologue," *Society*, July/August 1986, 32–39.
5. Christina Kent, ed., "Perspectives," *Medicine and Health*, September 14, 1992, 1–4.
6. Joseph P. Peters, "Necessity Is Often the Mother of Mergers," *Modern Hospital* 107 (July 1966): 90.
7. "Communal Organizations for the Promotion of Health, 1929–1930," *American Jewish Yearbook* (Philadelphia: American Jewish Committee, 1930), 175.
8. Max Danzis, "Jewish Hospitals and Facilities for Graduate Training," *Medical Leaves* 3 (1940): 65–74.
9. "Small Hospitals Should Merge, Consultant Urges," in "News Digest," *Modern Hospital* 98 (April 1962): 21. See the reference to the Rourke study in Donald M. Rosenberger, "How Mergers Begin and How They Work," *Modern Hospital* 107 (July 1966): 89. Also, Joseph P. Peters, "Necessity Is Often the Mother of Mergers," *Modern Hospital* 107 (July 1966): 90.
10. The board chair of Barnes Hospital responded to the Jewish Hospital offer of affiliation by declaring: "I don't want anyone else sleeping with my mistress" (David Gee, *A History of the Jewish Hospital of St. Louis* [St. Louis: Jewish Hospital, 1981], 101).
11. Danzis, "Jewish Hospitals and Facilities."
12. Mark S. Blumberg, "Changing Times Spur Hospital Mergers," *Modern Hospital* 107 (July 1966): 83–84.
13. In discussion of United Hospitals of Newark, Alexander Milch, "Full Medical Center Is Goal," *News,* April 24, 1961.
14. Peters, "Necessity Is Often the Mother of Mergers," 91.
15. Stevens, "Past Is Prologue," 37.
16. S. S. Goldwater, "The Drift toward Hospital Amalgamation," *Modern Hospital* 30 (January 1928): 52.
17. Board of Trustees Minutes, February 6, 1935.
18. "Interfaith Medical Center: A History of Triumph," www.Interfaithmedical.com/main/history.html.
19. Pamela Hill Lampert, "Heritage Lives on after the Doors Close," *Minnesota Medicine* 74 (December 1991): 17–22.
20. Quoting Marvin Segal, MD, vice president for medical affairs at [Minneapolis] Mount Sinai, ibid., 18.
21. Ibid., 19.
22. Mary Wagner, "Jewish Hospitals Yesterday and Today," *Modern Healthcare*, February 1991, 38.
23. Sarah Gordon, ed., *All Our Lives: A Centennial History of Michael Reese Hospital and Medical Center, 1881–1981* (Chicago: Michael Reese Hospital and Medical Center, 1981), 128.
24. The decline of Michael Reese continued through the 1990s, as it was warned in 1996 that there were serious violations of Medicare rules that threatened its

reimbursements. In 1998, a group of physicians sought to stop the hospital's decline by joining a management group. However, the takeover was a fiscal failure. By 2003, the hospital was in receivership.

25. Board of Trustees Minutes, June 2, 1975.
26. Ibid., September 19 and November 28, 1988; March 27, July 24, September 25, and November 27, 1989.
27. Ibid., May 21, 1990.
28. Ibid., September 18, 1995.
29. "Competition or Collaboration between NBIMC and UMDNJ," 12, a summary of the May 19, 1995, meeting between representatives of the two institutions, accompanying Lester M. Bornstein to Stanley S. Bergen Jr., June 27, 1995; private correspondence of Lester M. Bornstein, JHSMW (hereinafter, Bornstein correspondence).
30. Ray V. Lourenco to Lester M. Bornstein, January 19, 1994, Bornstein correspondence.
31. Ibid.; Bornstein to Lourenco, April 25, 1994, Bornstein correspondence.
32. Bergen Jr. to Lieberman, October 26, 1995; fax from Lieberman to Bergen Jr., October 30, 1995, Bornstein correspondence.
33. Lester Lieberman, interview with Alan Kraut, Morristown, NJ, July 18, 2000.
34. Minutes of a special combined meeting of the Boards of Trustees of Newark Beth Israel Medical Center and Beth Health Care Services Corporation, November 20, 1995. NBIH Papers at JHSMW
35. Lester Lieberman, interview with Alan Kraut, Morristown, NJ, June 29, 2000.
36. Lieberman, interview, July 18, 2000.
37. Agreement among the Saint Barnabas Corporation, Saint Barnabas Medical Center, Beth Health Services Corporation, and Newark Beth Israel Medical Center, April 1, 1996. Copy of the full agreement provided to the authors by Newark Beth Israel Corporation counsel Bruce D. Shoulson.
38. Minutes of combined Annual Meeting of the Board of Trustees of Newark Beth Israel Medical Center and Beth Health Care Services Corporation, April 12, 1996, 2–3. NBIH Papers at JHSMW.
39. Naz Namazi, "Saint Barnabas: NJ's Largest," Medical Data International: Managed Care IQ Resource System Daily "News Perspectives," September 26, 1996, 1.
40. David Schwab, "8 Hospitals Joining Forces to Cut Costs, FTC Approval Creates Largest System in State," *Newark Star-Ledger*, April 24, 1996.
41. Gale Scott, "Rebuffed Hospital Links with Mt. Sinai," *Newark Star-Ledger*, November 6, 1996.
42. "1996 Hospital Mergers, Acquisition, and Joint Ventures," *Modern Healthcare* (December 1996), 41.

Epilogue

1. Rosemary Stevens, *In Sickness and in Wealth: American Hospitals in the Twentieth Century* (New York: Basic Books, 1989), 360.
2. S. S. Goldwater, "Do American Cities Need Both Voluntary and Tax-Supported Hospitals?" *Modern Hospital* 14 (February 1940): 13–19.

3. August Hoenack, quoted in "Hill-Burton after 20 Years: The Men, the Money, the 360,000 Beds," *Modern Hospital* 107 (August 1966): 99.

4. "Our Mission," *Healthcare Foundation of New Jersey 2001 Annual Report* (Livingston, N.J: Healthcare Foundation of New Jersey, 2002), 1.

5. Ibid., 9.

6. Ibid., 11.

7. Sharon Waters, "Medical School Looks to Training Compassion," *[East Brunswick, N.J.] Home News Tribune*, March 30, 2004.

8. Creed of the Newark Beth Israel Hospital, circa 1928, author unknown.

A NOTE ON SOURCES

The history of Newark Beth Israel Hospital (NBIH) and Medical Center (NBIMC) is grounded in an ensemble of sources, official and personal. The Jewish Historical Society of MetroWest (JHSMW) is the repository for many of these sources and continues to acquire donations from the Beth Israel Hospital community.

In 2005, the JHSMW acquired the official minutes of the NBIH Board of Directors and its committees from the office of Paul Mertz, the executive director of the NBIMC, now part of the Barnabas Healthcare Network. The minutes provide a continuous summary of the decision-making process at the Beth from 1928 to 1989. Arthur Lindeman, the secretary of the Beth Israel board, hired two stenographers skilled in dictation to prepare transcriptions of the meetings held from 1928 to 1939. Lindeman's penchant for accuracy ensured that the minutes retained the voices of the board members during the period when the hospital nearly closed during the Great Depression. After Lindeman's death in 1939, the minutes, due to the scarcity of paper during wartime, became shorter summaries. The brevity continued with some notable exceptions during the next decades; when a specific issue generated discussion, the minutes offered fuller descriptions and quotations. The board of directors met monthly, then quarterly, and the numerous committees (such as the Nurse Training School Committee) met more frequently, often monthly. During the first decades, all committees reported to the Administrative Committee, which then produced summaries for the board meetings. The minutes also include the annual reports of the executive director. The Planning and Housing Committee, engaged in the issues of maintenance in the first decades, became the paramount committee from the 1960s onward when the ten phases of

construction were initiated. In the last decade of its existence as an independent voluntary hospital, the Beth Healthcare Corporation succeeded the
hospital's board of directors, and each of its entities, including the NBIMC,
presented reports to the corporation. Interspersed sporadically are the internal annual reports of the hospital departments, which provide an invaluable
summary of the hospital's accomplishments, especially valuable during the
turbulent years of the sixties and early seventies.

Minutes were also maintained by affiliate organizations of the Beth
Israel Hospital. In 1930, the Newark Jewish Maternity Hospital was amalgamated into the Beth Israel Hospital, and its all-women board of directors
became the Maternity Auxiliary of the hospital. The handwritten minutes of
the Maternity Auxiliary from 1930 to 1939 offer a vivid contrast to the board
minutes and mark the origin of the "Babies Alumni" born at the Beth society
and the gift shop and tearoom.

During its formative period from 1901 to 1919, the hospital medical
staff maintained minutes of its formal and informal meetings. A set of
handwritten notes exists that summarize the medical staff meetings, often
held in the home of Dr. Victor Parsonnet. A formal Ledger of the Newark
Beth Israel Hospital Medical Staff was also maintained from 1901 to
1917. The ledger provides a history of the Newark Jewish Dispensary,
which functioned until 1908. The ledger has been in the possession of
Dr. Victor Parsonnet and will be donated to the Jewish Historical Society of
MetroWest.

The JHSMW is the repository for the collection of the hospital's
annual reports and of personal accounts such as Nettie Katchen's typewritten description of her activities in the first decade of the hospital.
Dr. Eugene Parsonnet's reminiscences, dictated and transcribed by his son,
Victor, were made available for this book. The document is an invaluable
account of a Jewish physician's life in the twentieth century. The archives
of the University Medical and Dental School of New Jersey (UMDNJ) are
the repository for Dr. Rita Finkler's papers, including a three-hundred-page
typewritten autobiography. Finkler describes her research performed at the
hospital in the 1930s. Her papers provide a unique perspective, that of a
female Jewish physician engaged in research on fertility and birth control in
the early twentieth century. Dr. Victor Parsonnet graciously provided materials from his personal collection. Lester Bornstein also lent his materials
for review during the preparation of this book.

The JHSMW also is the repository for the papers of the Jewish
Community Council, which offer insight into the Jewish community's

perspective on Newark Beth Israel Hospital and the many other issues confronting the Jewish community.

The NBIMC published its own medical journal, *Journal of the Newark Beth Israel Hospital*, from 1951 until 1968, renamed the *Journal of Newark Beth Israel Hospital Medical Center* in 1968 and ceasing publication in 1978. The National Library of Medicine, located on the campus of the National Institutes of Health, maintains the journal volumes. Dr. Alan J. Lippman, a Beth physician and former editor of the journal, prepared an insightful summary of the trends in research.

The journal *Modern Hospital* (renamed *Modern Healthcare* in 1974) was founded by Otho Ball and first published in 1913. Ball's monthly publication was intended for the hospital administrators who hoped to create modern, well-managed institutions offering state-of-the-art medical care and run with businesslike efficiency. The journal features included a hospital of the month from 1922 to the post–World War II period, which inspired new building and renovation. The Beth Israel Hospital was the April 1928 designee, and an extensive article provides the vision of the architect and of Dr. S. S. Goldwater, an editor of the journal. Journal articles addressed the rise of unions and the importance of ancillary departments such as dietary, housekeeping, and record keeping, as well as mergers and the impact of federal legislation, such as the Hill-Burton Act and Medicare. The journal extolled the virtues of the voluntary Jewish hospitals, and many of the commissioned articles were written by the managers of these hospitals. Equally important was Ball's decision to include the annual American College of Surgeons complete list of accredited hospitals through 1933.

Local newspapers were an important source for comprehending the hospital's public face and for the context of the larger Newark community. The *Newark Evening News*, published between 1881 and 1968 and known as the *News*, offered ongoing coverage of the hospital and the larger Jewish community. The *Newark Star Eagle* often took a somewhat sensationalist approach to events, and after 1968, the *Newark Star-Ledger* became Newark's leading newspaper. For news of Newark Beth Israel Hospital from the perspective of the Jewish community, no newspaper exceeded the weekly *Jewish Chronicle* in coverage and depth. Under the inspired editorship of the tireless Anton Kaufman, the *Chronicle* began publication in 1921 and ceased publication in 1943 when he died. The JHSMW holds issues of the *Chronicle* from 1922 onward, but the issues from September 1927 through April 1928 cannot be located. The weekly *Jewish News* began publication in 1947 and is an important source of information about the postwar Jewish community of Essex County. It is valuable for understanding the impact of suburbanization on the Newark Jewish community.

We relied on a variety of secondary sources on the history of Newark. The most thorough is John T. Cunningham's *Newark*, first published by the New Jersey Historical Society in 1966; a revised and expanded edition appeared in 1988 and a third edition in 2002. A history of the Jewish community, William Helmreich's *The Enduring Community: The Jews of Newark and MetroWest* (1999), provided a broad history of Newark's Jewish life that contextualized the history of the NBIMC. A history of health conditions in Newark in the early twentieth century is Stuart Galishoff's *Safeguarding the Public Health: Newark, 1895–1918* (1975). A useful anthology documenting the rebuilding of Newark after the turmoil of the late 1960s is Stanley B. Winters's edited volume *From Riot to Recovery: Newark after Ten Years* (1979). Tremendous insight and a comprehensive perspective of the Newark African American experience was provided by historian Clement Price, Rutgers distinguished-service professor and founder of the Institute on Ethnicity, Culture, and the Modern Experience.

There is no single volume that documents the history of the Jewish hospital in the United States. Daniel Ethan Bridge's 1985 ordination thesis, "The Rise and Development of the Jewish Hospital in America, 1850–1984," written at Hebrew Union College under the direction of the late Dr. Jacob Rader Marcus, was useful in identifying hospitals in New York City. Tina Levitan's volume, *Islands of Compassion: A History of the Jewish Hospitals of New York* (1964) offers an overview of New York's Jewish hospitals. In addition, there have been a number of hospital histories that record in considerable detail the history of particular hospitals. Examples include physician Arthur J. Linenthal's *First a Dream: The History of Boston's Jewish Hospitals, 1896–1928* (1990); David A. Gee's *216 S.K.: A History of the Jewish Hospital of St. Louis* (1981); Arthur H. Aufses Jr. and Barbara J. Niss's *This House of Noble Deeds: The Mount Sinai Hospital, 1852–2002* (2002); Dorothy Levinson's *Montefiore: The Hospital as Social Instrument* (1984); *All Our Lives: A Centennial History of Michael Reese Hospital and Medical Center, 1881–1981,* edited by Sarah Gordon (1981), and Barbara Rogers and Stephen M. Dobbs's *The First Century: Mount Zion Hospital and Medical Center* (1987).

The articles published in *Modern Hospital* written by administrators of Jewish hospitals and the descriptions of their modern buildings are an excellent source of their histories. Several editions of the *American Jewish Yearbook* directories have lists by state of Jewish organizations from which one can cull the Jewish hospitals, although these listings are by no means complete. The 1899–1900 volume (Hebrew Year 5660) is a good source for identifying the initiatives that produced the second wave of Jewish hospitals. Occasional articles on Jewish hospitals appear in *Medical Leaves*, the journal published by progressive-minded Jewish physicians in the 1930s and 1940s. Hospitals and medical centers maintain digital Web pages, and these may include a subpage on the history of the institution; these may provide photographs and brief time lines of Jewish hospitals, although some caution needs to be applied to verify dates and captions with other sources.

The *Journal of the American Hospital Association* and the American College of Surgeons each prepared separate lists of hospitals, by state, annually, through World War II. Since 1954, the Joint Commission on Accredited Hospitals and Healthcare Organizations, which succeeded both, has published an annual list. These lists are the most complete and consistent source for identifying Jewish hospitals, especially for tracking the mergers and amalgamations that occurred during the 1930s and early 1950s. The credit for pursuing these lists belongs to the Beth's Dr. Max Danzis, who published a study of medical residencies in Jewish hospitals in *Medical Leaves* based on the ACS and AHA lists of 1939–1940 and who showed us this path.

Newarkers are imbued with a duty to chronicle their histories; many physicians and board members shared their memories with us. We are indebted to Lester Bornstein, Harold Grotta, Cecil Lichtman, Lester Lieberman, Alan Sagner, Bruce Shoulson, and Kenneth Tyson; and Drs. Arthur Cohen, Sam Diener, Seymour Ribot, Robert Skeist, and Jules Titlebaum. In 2001, during the centennial celebration of the hospital, many longtime hospital-staff members provided oral histories.

Those who offered contributions include Alma Beatty, Ethel Belcher, Mathilda Cohen, Estelle Crenshaw, Cynthia Fairley, Carmen Flores, Betty Harris, Rosemary Jaico, Peri Kamalaker, Susan Katz, Blanche Kornegay, Catherine Lubliner, Virginia Palencia, Solane Paul, Opal Rose, Cordelia Small, Cecilia Vasquez, and Yvonne Weatherington.

Our special thanks to Donna Dinetz and Patricia Skerko for their vivid memories of the Weequahic neighborhood of the 1950s and 1960s. And we are most grateful to James Hopkins for recounting the "frying-pan fight," first thought to be the Dietary Department's apocryphal anecdote, but to our delight, an incident well documented in the medical minutes written more than eighty years earlier.

INDEX

abortions, 47–49
Abrams, Dr. Abram, 165
accreditation, 63–66, 153; and medical
  advances, 164
Addams, Jane, 22
Addonizio, Hugh, 133, 157
affiliations: between hospitals and
  medical schools, 179–180, 223; with
  other hospitals, 217
African Americans: migration to
  northern cities, 68–69; and urban
  conflict, 69–70
Albert Einstein Medical Center, 141,
  180, 212, 225
American Association of Hospital
  Social Workers, 110
American College of Surgeons (ACS),
  6, 63–64, 67, 84, 107, 164
American Hospital Association (AHA),
  5–6, 62, 67, 90, 99, 103, 148, 153;
  and accreditation standards, 211; and
  Ad Hoc Committee on Hospital
  Closures, 206; and report *The
  Individual Hospital*, 103–104
American Jewish Yearbook, 6, 211
American Medical Association (AMA),
  53, 62, 153, 172; and accreditation of
  postgraduate medical training, 46,
107, 212; and *American Medical
  Directory*, 63; and Council on
  Medical Education, 6, 39, 62, 67, 172,
  174, 212; and *Journal*, 53
American Nurses Association, 147
American Society of Clinical
  Pathologists, 111
annual reports: 1906, 27–28;
  1915–1916, 51
anti-Semitism, 5, 94–95, 116–117,
  119–120, 158, 222
Antopol, Dr. William, 115, 116, 121,
  139, 227
Applebaum, Irving L., 115, 175
architecture and design, 67, 79–81, 104,
  108; of 1906 Beth Israel building,
  30–31, 67–68, 72
Arestad, Dr. Fritjof H., 106, 107
Aschheim, Dr. Selmar, 114
Asher, Dr. Maurice, 43
Association of American Medical
  Colleges, 117
Association of Hospital
  Superintendents, *see* American
  Hospital Association
Atomic Energy Commission, 170
Augenblick, Dr. Meyer "Gil," 59, 95,
  144

About the Authors

Alan M. Kraut is a professor of history at American University in Washington, D.C. His research interests combine immigration and ethnic history with the history of medicine and public health in the United States. He is the author or editor of seven books and many articles. *Silent Travelers: Germs, Genes, and the "Immigrant Menace"* (1994) won the Theodore Saloutos Prize from the Immigration and Ethnic History Society. *Goldberger's War: The Life and Work of a Public Health Crusader* (2004) received the Henry Adams Prize from the Society for History in the Federal Government, the Arthur J. Viseltear Prize from the American Association for Public Health, and the Watson Davis and Helen Miles Davis Prize from the History of Science Society.

Deborah A. Kraut is an analyst at the National Institutes of Health, U.S. Department of Health and Human Services. She coauthored *Pregnancy Bedrest: A Guidebook for the Pregnant Woman and Her Family* (1990) and authored *Supportive Services for Disadvantaged Workers and Trainees* (1973). In 1991, she was awarded a civilian citation for her work at the Bethesda Naval Hospital during the Gulf War.